Taking Care of Aging Family Members

A Practical Guide

REVISED AND EXPANDED

WENDY LUSTBADER
NANCY R. HOOYMAN

THE FREE PRESS

New York   London   Toronto   Sydney   Tokyo   Singapore

THE FREE PRESS
A Division of Simon & Schuster Inc.
1230 Avenue of the Americas
New York, NY 10020

Manufactured in the United States of America

10 9 8

Library of Congress Cataloging-in-Publication Data

Lustbader, Wendy.
 Taking care of aging family members: a practical guide / Wendy
Lustbader, Nancy R. Hooyman.—Rev. and expanded.
   p. cm.
 Prev. ed. cataloged under: Hooyman, Nancy R. Taking care of your
aging family members.
 Includes bibliographical references and index.
 ISBN 0–02–919517–9.—ISBN 0–02–919518–7 (pbk.)
 1. Aged—Care—United States. 2. Aged—United States—Family
relationships. 3. Life skills—Study and teaching—United States.
I. Hooyman, Nancy R. II. Hooyman,
Nancy R. Taking care of your
aging family members. III. Title.
HV1461.H655 1994   93–24322
649.8—dc20   CIP

ISBN 0–02–919518–7

In memory of my father-in-law
ISRAEL GROSSKOPF
—W. L.

In memory of my parents,
DORIS STRATTON RUNKLE
HUGH RUNKLE
—N. R. H.

Contents

Preface

Most books about aging are targeted either to professionals or to families, artificially separating these audiences. This book attempts to reflect the partnership between professionals and families that is a vital part of successful care arrangements. Theory and practice are blended, with the goal of suggesting solutions to care dilemmas that are clinically sound and applicable to everyday life. Included in the text are practical tools, such as a medical bill accounting sheet, a guide for delegating tasks among family members, a phone search guide for community resources, and a checklist for comparing retirement homes. These are designed to be duplicated and used by professionals, students, and family members.

This revised and expanded edition has been updated to keep pace with developments in the field of aging. Subheadings have been added to ensure easy access to information. Suggested resources at the end of each chapter direct readers to relevant articles, books, and organizations. New sections have been added on self-neglect, men as caregivers, spirituality, and crossing cultural boundaries.

Acknowledgments

This book grew out of our friendships and working relationships with many older people and their families. The questions and concerns they raised made the need for such a book clear to us. It was their voices which motivated us when other professional and caregiving demands made the task arduous.

For help with the section on spirituality, special thanks to the members of New Visions for Aging: Mary Liz Chaffee, Bonnie Genevay, Nancy Holloran, Marty Richards, and Denise Klein. This group has been a support on every level: personal, professional, and spiritual.

For offering their insights for the section on ethnicity, many thanks to Pauline Agbayani-Siewert, Mary Chavez, Alicia Mei, Bettye Mitchell, Melissa Talamantes, Susan Tomita, Laura Trejo, and Mary Watson. Any misunderstandings or errors remaining in this section are my responsibility.

Many thanks to our editor at Free Press, Susan Arellano, and her assistant, Allesandra Stapleford, for their enthusiasm toward this project and their understanding the value of addressing professionals and family members in a single book.

Special thanks to my mother-in-law, Evelyn Grosskopf, for her patience, encouragement, and good humor as I rushed around the house in the last months of preparing the manuscript.

To my husband, Barry Grosskopf, I owe every appreciation. His belief in my work supplied much of the stamina for getting this second edition accomplished.

—W. L.

Special appreciation to my boys—Kevin and Christopher—who want copies of the book so that they can use it "when Mom gets old," and to my husband, Gene, who is struggling with his own long-distance parent care issues.

To the dean's office staff—Carole Crawford, Lorna Chong, Ingeborg

Dolan, Sarah Resah, Christa Wells, Olivia Zapata—for their ongoing caring support along with their assistance with production details.

N.R.H.

Introduction

M ost people face a continual tug-of-war between their desire to
take good care of their aging relatives and other pressures impinging on their lives. Finding time for caregiving in the midst of other
obligations is not easy. The societal emphasis on making money and
enhancing individual goals has made caregiving an interference, rather
than part of the natural rhythm of living and dying. The opportunities
for personal discovery and satisfaction inherent in caregiving are not
widely acknowledged, detached as they are from economic gain or social achievement.

Rather than have their lives disrupted by care demands, families
often grasp at the first solution which occurs to them: "If only we could
find someone to live with Mom, she'd have help whenever she needed
it." The idea of obtaining help in exchange for room and board seems attractive, especially when compared to the cost of hiring hourly help.
When families attempt to find live-in helpers, however, they quickly realize that few people are willing to accept such positions without a high
salary. When they try on their own to hire hourly help, without resorting to agencies' expensive rates, they often discover that a great deal of
effort must be exerted to make sure helpers show up and do their work
reliably. Many families learn that managing services furnished by
others can be almost as difficult as providing services themselves.

This book equips families with the information they need to take
care of their aging family members while taking care of their own
needs for support and rest. It is also intended for professionals,
friends, and volunteers who assist families and for students in the
health care professions. Subheadings and cross-references are plentiful, allowing readers to browse through the text to find areas of special
interest. Suggested resources are presented at the end of each chapter,

offering references for further reading and addresses for contacting organizations directly.

The first five chapters survey the emotional territory of taking care of aging family members, starting with the stresses often experienced by caregivers. The dynamics between partners as caregivers are presented next, followed by an examination of siblings' attempts to share the care and the special considerations arising in other types of family relationships, such as stepfamilies. Chapter Five presents a discussion of dilemmas commonly faced by families:

- Should long-distance family members uproot an older person from her home in order to provide care in their community?
- What can be done when a family is split between those seeking a nursing home for their relative and those wanting to continue providing care at home? What if there are conflicts about how much money is to be spent on care?
- How should end-of-life choices be handled? Are there good ways to bring up these difficult topics?
- What can other members of the family do when an adult son or daughter is exploiting a frail parent, to the parent's detriment financially, physically, or emotionally?

Chapter Six suggests ways to promote the efforts of friends, neighbors, and other helpers. It is followed by chapters on responding to memory loss, physical limitations, and depression. The rest of the book explores publicly funded programs, community long-term care services, living together in the caregiver's home, alternative living situations, and extending family caregiving into the nursing home.

The book concludes with a detailed index, allowing family members and professionals to locate specific issues or to follow topic areas which are discussed from several points of view. For example, elder abuse is examined from several perspectives:

- older people who abuse their caregivers (pp. 27–31)
- exhausted caregivers' self-neglect (pp. 36–41)
- caregivers addicted to drugs or alcohol (pp. 36–38)
- parents accepting abuse from adult children (pp. 117–123)
- friendship verging on exploitation (pp. 133–136)
- older people committing slow suicide by self-neglect (pp. 189–192)
- in-home workers exploiting frail older people (pp. 244–246)

Throughout the book, the word "family" is defined more broadly than as blood ties, rather encompassing anyone who plays a family-like role in an older person's life. Older people without biological family, those estranged from family members, and those who live at a great distance from relatives often receive family-like support from friends, neighbors, and other helpers. When the term "family member" is used, these family-like helpers are implicitly included.

To simplify reading and avoid both awkwardness and sex stereotyping, masculine and feminine pronouns are alternated throughout the text. Case illustrations are presented in the gender most appropriate to the issues under discussion, or for ease in pronoun references. When gender differences are important, they are explicitly acknowledged.

This introduction sets the stage for the chapters ahead. First, the opportunities for personal discovery and satisfaction in caregiving are illustrated. Then, cultural differences among families are explored to encourage respectful dialogue between professionals and families and to ensure effective service delivery. Finally, the demographics of caregiving and aging are presented to demonstrate that taking care of aging relatives is one of the major issues facing families in the 1990's.

WHY TAKE CARE OF AGING RELATIVES?

Long-standing patterns within families tend to limit what people do and say. Outside their families, many people move beyond these patterns of relating, only to resume them in the presence of parents and siblings. For instance, a daughter who easily hugs her friends may find that a deeply established custom of reserve within her family prevents her from hugging her mother. Similar constraints can keep important topics off-limits for years, with family members feeling at a loss about how to start conversations that would break through these barriers.

Caregiving can be an opportunity to change family patterns. In the midst of working together for the sake of aging relatives, family members often develop better relationships and discover new strengths in each other. There may be conflicts and tense moments along the way, but the whole enterprise of trying to ensure good care for someone loved in common can be a powerful force of unity and satisfaction for a family.

Adult children and their aging parents find that giving and receiving care is rich with opportunities for closeness. The touching involved in personal care almost always makes family members speak more tenderly and intimately than would otherwise be possible between them. A daughter who helps her mother button her blouse each morning while recovering from a stroke may talk more personally than she has ever previously ventured with her mother. It is difficult to hold onto past anger or resentment while buttoning someone's clothes or helping someone to the bathroom. The sight of a parent unable to get out of a chair or into a nightgown without assistance is emotionally moving to even the most embittered adult children, often inspiring conciliatory gestures that have been absent for years.

Discovering new appreciation for siblings is another insufficiently heralded component of taking care of parents. Siblings are irrevocably linked with each other through their parents, a connection that re-asserts itself most intensely when parents become ill in later life. Needing to deal with adversity outside themselves, siblings who unite to battle the physical and practical encroachments on their parents' in-dependence often come to respect each other in fresh ways. For exam-ple, a daughter may be compelled by exhaustion to allow her historically unreliable sister to take over their mother's care on week-ends. In doing so, she may find that her sister has overcome many past failings. For her sister, taking care of their mother may be a chance to redeem herself in the eyes of family members who live too far away to see how she has grown and changed.

In many families, comfortable ways for individual members to ob-tain time alone with each other are scarce, unless pretexts arise in the natural course of events. Caregiving provides many pretexts for having one-on-one time, without worry about hurting others by excluding them. A son may have spent most of his adult life visiting his mother in the company of his wife. While performing the most mundane chores, such as driving his mother to the pharmacy to pick up a prescription, he may find chances to be alone with her. The kind of conversations which require open-ended time and freedom from interruptions may occur during longer errands, such as accompanying a parent to the doctor. People who are unable to have face-to-face intimate conversa-tions often lapse into them while riding in a car or doing some other activity alongside a family member.

The sheer fact that adult children will take time out of their lives to help often moves parents to express greater warmth toward their chil-dren. A son who devotes two successive weekends to building his fa-ther a wheelchair ramp may receive the thanks and recognition from his father that he has yearned for all of his life. The appreciation may then instigate a spiral of good experiences between them, as the son is spurred on to complete other vital projects and his father reacts with increasing warmth. Seeing each other more often under the guise of working on these projects can itself promote closeness, heightening their interest in each other's lives. Acts of helping have more power as communicators of love and respect than the most costly gifts sent in the mail or the most ardent claims of affection over the phone.

Parents are commonly reluctant to grant their grown children equal footing with them as adults. This delay can persist long into later life, especially if geographic distance prevents parents from witnessing their children's success in jobs or relationships. More decisively than most life experiences, illness can cause a change in such a relationship by forcing parents to accept help from their children. A father who decides to rely on his son to do his banking, for example, implicitly affirms his son's capacities as an adult. Such reliance conveys a trust that may be deeply satisfying to the son. By allowing his son to be a provider of help, the father actually gives emotionally more than he receives practically.

Similarly, adult children may have difficulty seeing their parents as people. Many do not attain this perspective until they become parents themselves. Making mistakes with their own children, they begin to see how it might have been for their parents: "Mom, now I see what you went through." Remarks like this may open up discussion of what took place for the parent during the family's earlier years. Instead of harboring longstanding resentments, adult children can often liberate themselves through a willingness to look at the circumstances in a parent's life that may have contributed to poor parenting. Parents who feel forgiven and understood are much more likely to speak honestly about the past than those who detect that their grown children still deprive them of the right to be fallible human beings. Toward the end of their lives, parents often find it a relief to express their regrets—and their wisdom—when they sense this kind of reprieve from their children.

In some families, early life issues are difficult to resolve through this means. Adult children who were physically or sexually abused as young children may have chosen to establish totally separate lives as adults. Their way of coping with painful memories may be to avoid contact with their parents or to keep communication to a controlled minimum. In such situations, indirect helping tasks may allow estranged adult children to satisfy their sense of personal decency while still protecting themselves.

Confronting serious illness tends to accelerate the pace of change between adult children and their parents. Each realizes that time is running out, with no further chances to reach understandings. The sight of a parent in a hospital bed is a frequent catalyst for sons and daughters to put aside their hesitations and broach topics they have long wished to discuss. Parents' own confrontations with illness and dying often provoke a receptivity to such conversations, to a degree sometimes astonishing to their children. Previously intractable conflicts may become amenable to compromise; family secrets that have gone unexplained or unspoken for years may be exposed and put to rest. From this perspective, participating actively in the last months of a parent's life can be a blessing.

CROSSING CULTURAL BOUNDARIES

A framework for approaching ethnic and racial differences is next offered, since professionals and family members often have to cross cultural boundaries in the course of providing or receiving services. These insights may enable professionals to cross these boundaries in a respectful manner and may help ethnic families put their private struggles into words. Talking about these issues is not easy. Meaningful discourse begins with having terms for experiences which elude description, no matter how sensitive or complex these matters are and how insufficient words can be when true understanding is at stake.

THE CONTINUUM OF ETHNICITY

Historically, maintaining an ethnic identity in America has not been compatible with social or professional advancement. Discrimination against those who are not part of the mainstream has been a recurring blight in American history. By suppressing their differentness, ethnic individuals have sought to avoid discrimination and make it easier to get ahead. To this day, the more assimilated a person becomes, the easier that person moves in circles of power and achievement. Assimilation can mean a host of superficial changes, such as shedding a foreign accent and changing one's name, or it can mean more subtle, inner shifts of identity. The social and financial rewards of assimilation are often so great that an ethnic identity may begin to feel like a burden rather than a privilege.

The continuum of assimilation can be divided into three parts: traditional, bicultural, and assimilated. These categories are not necessarily stages through which an individual passes, yet they often function in this way. Some people move back and forth between these phases. These categories can also represent three generations of a family, from the first to immigrate, to their bicultural children, to their assimilated grandchildren. There are different degrees of assimilation, just as there are variations in traditional ways of life. Finally, these categories can also depict the conflicts raging internally for an individual. Inside one person there can be simultaneously a traditional self, a bicultural self, and an assimilated self. The following chart summarizes the differences along this continuum.

THE CONTINUUM OF ASSIMILATION

Traditional	Bicultural	Assimilated
Has strong ethnic identity	Has partial ethnic identity	Has slight ethnic identity
Prefers to live among own people	Lives well with own people or with outsiders	Prefers to live with outsiders
Maintains all traditions	Maintains many of the traditions	Maintains few traditions
Is uncomfortable with outsiders	Moves easily among outsiders	Feels awkward among own people

From Wendy Lustbader and Nancy R. Hooyman, *Taking Care of Aging Family Members* (New York: The Free Press, 1994). Copyright © 1994 by Wendy Lustbader and Nancy Hooyman; copyright © 1986 by The Free Press.

Traditional

A strong ethnic identity reflects self-esteem. It can also serve as a form of self-protection. Rather than risk the intolerance of the outside world, people with a traditional orientation choose the survival strategy, "Stick to your own kind." Those who feel uncomfortable with outsiders may find it hard to accept services from people from other cultures, especially in their own home. They may prefer to live within a particular neighborhood or section of a city where their language is spoken and where their traditions can be practiced without fear of bigotry or ridicule.

People who identify solely with their own culture feel separate even when seemingly participating in the mainstream. Inwardly, they sustain the division between "us" and "them," between members of their group and others, usually with a derogatory word for everyone else. Feeling superior to outsiders is common to almost all cultures and is one of the defining characteristics of belonging to an ethnic group. This sense of superiority becomes a bulwark of cultural self-esteem.

Marrying within the group is an expectation that parents with a traditional orientation often convey to their children. Some consider marrying outside the culture a betrayal, because they fear that the children of such a union will not maintain the traditions. Keeping the customs alive is central to ethnic identity. If an older man watches his children intermarry and have children who do not care about "the way things are done," it is equivalent to facing two kinds of death: his personal death, and the death of his traditions. He knows that his grandchildren may become outsiders, estranged from him and all that he cherishes. Dread about the eventual disappearance of traditions is common to all ethnic cultures in America due to the overwhelming pressures toward assimilation.

Bicultural

In contrast to people who chiefly identify with their ethnicity, bicultural people have a foot in both worlds. They respect their traditions and teach the customs to their children, but they also encourage their children to learn the ways of the mainstream and to speak the mainstream language. Bicultural people often become bilingual to the degree of mastering the nuances of mainstream speech, adopting mannerisms and phrases that convey this fluency. When back among ethnic family and friends from their culture, some feel embarrassed when they find they cannot rid their speech of signs of having commingled with outsiders.

Ethnic pride remains strong in bicultural people. They know how to suppress their ethnicity when it is wise to do so, but this suppression is accomplished out of prudence rather than any kind of shame. They feel enraged inside when someone from the dominant culture praises them for "being like us" or for representing a fortunate exception to the supposed rule of their group's characteristic in a particular area: "You sure don't talk like a Black person." Promotions and social acceptance may come at the price of putting up with patronizing compliments from colleagues who are trying to show that they are accepting.

Experiencing an inner split in their identity, some bicultural people do not feel entirely at home in either world. They feel comfortable back in their ethnic neighborhood, but they can only express part of themselves around their own people. Their daily life is taken up with the mainstream, but they are most at ease around others who move between cultures and who live with a similar sense of duality. At times, they may feel they belong everywhere and nowhere.

To be bicultural is to become an instrument of cultural change both within the mainstream and the culture of origin. People from both worlds ask questions of bicultural individuals, probing for understanding and hoping to make sense of cultural differences. The ability to move smoothly through the mainstream and the culture of origin means that bicultural people see each world more clearly than those who are encased in one way of life.

Assimilated

People trying to maintain their traditions often experience a wearing-away of their ethnic identity. Rather than severing themselves intentionally, they find that one compromise after another diminishes their traditional self until it is barely discernable. They may first change their last name to sound less foreign, then cease observing ethnic holidays or practices which intrude on their employment. Over time, these surface adaptations contribute to an internal shift, as assimilated people gain more and more acceptance from people in the mainstream.

Many assimilated people become apologetic about their ethnic background, rejecting any linkage with "those people" who make a "fuss" about cultural differences. They may find themselves feeling ashamed when relatives with a strong ethnic identity display their cultural allegiance rather than attempting to conceal it. Some feel ashamed of their shame, realizing that they have somehow absorbed the dominant culture's scorn for their own people and turned it into a kind of self-hatred.

Those who were once strongly ethnically identified tend to feel differently about becoming assimilated than those who never fully identified. Those who began with a strong ethnic identity in childhood achieve assimilation only through an inner wounding. To fit well into the mainstream, they amputate part of themselves. They may go for years mistaking this hollow place inside themselves for ordinary discouragement, not realizing that their bad feelings result from their cultural severing. If they later make the shift back to being bicultural, they often find that a sense of wholeness resumes along with their ethnic reengagement. In contrast, those who never identified with their ethnicity may feel no such wounding, or they live with a hollowness without being aware of it.

Individuals whose skin color or facial features mark them as different from the mainstream can never fully assimilate. Regardless of how they feel inside, people from the mainstream will first react to them as members of an ethnic or racial group. They will continually face mainstream people who make assumptions about them based on their appearance rather than their individual life experience. Lacking the option of hiding, however, they are also spared some of its complications.

ETHNIC CONFLICT WITHIN FAMILIES

Taking care of an aging relative calls upon a family to work in unison for the person's welfare. Unfortunately, the tensions portrayed above are often acted out among siblings. For instance, if one daughter has maintained a strong ethnic identity and another has become assimilated, the two sisters may have utterly different attitudes about their mother's accepting help from a visiting nurse from another culture. The ethnically identified daughter may insist that problems with their mother's care be kept within the family and not be exposed to the scrutiny of outsiders. In contrast, the assimilated daughter may have no trouble relying on professionals from other cultural or racial backgrounds, as long as she gets to meet them and assess their capability firsthand. Family wars on this issue can leave an older adult without vital services while the siblings argue back and forth.

In the rush to provide services, professionals unfamiliar with these dilemmas occasionally get caught in an alliance with the more assimilated family members against the more ethnically identified family members. Gravitating naturally toward the part of the family which readily answers questions and accepts their help, these professionals may inadvertently widen the split that is hurting a family's ability to provide care. For instance, one brother may accuse another of betraying the family: "I can't believe you told that social worker about Mom's drinking. They already think we all drink too much." The professional's assessment may be more thorough as a result of allying with part of the family but may leave added bitterness in its wake, especially if the professional's solutions conflict with the worldview of the older person or the other siblings.

In these situations, it is preferable to sacrifice a perfect assessment for the sake of promoting family unity and devising culturally acceptable solutions. Holding back from asking intrusive questions may mean leaving parts of an assessment form temporarily blank but may increase the family's level of comfort during the interview. Self-disclosure by the professional is also helpful, such as revealing where one's parents and grandparents are from or how long one has lived in the area. Several sessions may be necessary to give the less trusting side of the family the opportunity to judge the professional's trustworthiness and reliability: "This social worker seems OK. I think she really wants to help us."

A good rapport with the family is essential before any services are provided. Siblings with different attitudes about how the outside world is to be handled are thereby spared painful battles, since all are granted the time to determine whether the professional is someone who can be trusted. The additional time invested may be worthwhile, giving the family a harmonious and successful experience in crossing cultural boundaries. It may also provide a professional a chance to develop an appropriate approach to care.

REMOVING BARRIERS TO SERVICES FOR CULTURALLY DIVERSE FAMILIES

Ethnically appropriate outreach is one of the fastest ways to solve the problem of crossing cultural boundaries. In this approach, the person who first introduces a family to services from outsiders is someone from the family's culture who is also skilled at interfacing with the outside world. This person then serves as a bridge, explaining and interpreting when cultural misunderstandings arise. Over time, the trust conveyed to the outreach person may carry over to service providers from other cultures.

When an outreach person from the family's ethnic or racial group is not available, a professional from another culture should allow the family the time they need to build trust. Asking personal questions too quickly, when one is not an insider, violates boundaries which ethnically identified people feel they have to preserve for the sake of survival. To promote trust, a professional in this situation should realize that it is she who is being interviewed while conducting an initial assessment. An open, conversant approach is much more likely to win trust than a rigid, formal interview with an assessment form as a physical and symbolic barrier. Putting the form down on one's lap or on the table, within easy view of the family, helps reduce divisions.

Acknowledging unfamiliarity about the family's culture also promotes an atmosphere of exchange rather than interrogation. Specifically granting the family an instructional role is the most respectful position to take in situations of cultural difference. To adopt a learning position, a professional must be willing to make herself vulnerable: "Mrs. Chang, I don't know very much about the Chinese culture. Can you help me understand why your husband is refusing to follow the doctor's advice?" When a professional is humble, trust increases rather than diminishes. The family may feel liberated to speak up about misunderstandings they had been afraid to mention, once they are assured that they are not being disrespectful in correcting a professional's mistaken assumptions: "It's not because we don't have faith in the doctor. We are ashamed we can't read the labels on the pill bottles."

Realizing that shame may be the greatest barrier may help a professional ease its force. For instance, when English is not someone's mother tongue, the person is likely to have difficulty understanding medical terms and may be too embarrassed to ask the doctor to repeat instructions in simpler terms or to rewrite medication labels in a clearer fashion. People who had been illiterate in their own language often carry an extra measure of shame in this regard. By offering to review the doctor's instructions as part of services offered to everyone, a professional can spare people the indignity of admitting their confusion: "Many people have trouble with medical words. Let's go over what the doctor said. I may not understand it all myself, but we'll write down your questions so you can give the list to your doctor the next time." If significant gaps in understanding are discovered in this process, the professional can then alert the doctor immediately.

In addition, shame about pronunciation problems may keep someone from phoning for vital services, even after a professional has thoughtfully supplied a list of phone numbers and explained application procedures. Making oneself understood over the phone can be much more strenuous than in person, when gestures amplify spoken communication. Shyness about telephone use may be compounded by sheer inexperience. One empowering approach is for a professional to dial the number, get the right person on the line, and explain the basic situation before handing the phone over to the reticent person. This allows the person to gain experience without having to conquer all the barriers at once.

Crossing boundaries successfully may inspire a family to try other services which are culturally unfamiliar or which require their passing through bureaucratic hoops. Conversely, a negative experience may close the door on future ventures outside ethnic boundaries. For these reasons, both professionals and assimilated family members must maintain a high level of sensitivity to feelings and nuances when a family has to cross cultures to obtain services. Giving care to an aging relative is already difficult enough without having to bear insensitivity from those who presume to help.

TRENDS AFFECTING FAMILY CAREGIVING

Demographic data to put family caregiving into a larger societal context are presented in the following chart. The number of families providing long-term care to older relatives is expected to increase substantially in the next few decades. Among people between the ages of forty-five and fifty-five, over 80 percent have at least one living parent, compared to fewer than 50 percent at the turn of the century. Even among those in their early sixties, 20 percent have a surviving parent. Since people aged eighty-five and older comprise the fastest-growing population group and the prevalence of disability in this group is 58 percent, giving care to aging family members is a challenge that more and more people are facing.[1]

The chart summarizes several demographic and social trends. A review of the data reveals that family members continue to provide the majority of care for older people, and that this role falls primarily to women. Since women are entering the work force in growing numbers, they are increasingly feeling the strain of dividing themselves between duties at home and on the job.

This book cannot begin to do justice to the diversity of situations which arise when families take care of aging relatives. In addition to ethnic, racial, class, and regional variations, each family can be said to evolve its own culture with distinct rules about what can and cannot be said, ways that affection can be expressed, and how major decisions are to be made. Yet despite these differences, there are sorrows and victories held in common. This book seeks to illuminate the universal aspects of giving care, while acknowledging and taking wisdom from all that is distinctive in this most personal of undertakings.

THE DEMOGRAPHICS OF CAREGIVING

Who gives care to aging family members?[2]	Nearly 80% of caregivers are women, who provide the majority of hands-on care
	Among adult children who are primary caregivers, daughters outnumber sons 3 to 1
	80% of family caregivers provide an average of 4 hours of care a day, 7 days a week
	One-third of caregivers are age 65 and older
	Women today can expect to spend 18 years of their lives helping an aging parent and 17 years caring for children
	Less than 10% of caregivers report the use of paid services
	Almost 75% of caregivers live with their disabled elderly relative
Who resides in nursing homes?[3]	Less than 5% of those 65 and older live in nursing homes, but more than 25% will be in a nursing home at some point during later life
	25% of placements are precipitated by the caregiver's illness or death
	Almost 10% of older people living in private homes would require nursing home placement if family support were withdrawn
	Nearly half of the elders in nursing homes have no close relatives
	Over 70% of nursing home residents are women
Where do older people live?[4]	43% have lived in their present home for over 20 years
	5% live in retirement communities
	Almost 30% live alone (32% of women, 22% of men)
	33% of men and 50% of women over age 65 who are widowed, separated, or divorced live with adult children or other family members

From Wendy Lustbader and Nancy R. Hooyman, *Taking Care of Aging Family Members* (New York: The Free Press, 1994). Copyright © 1994 by Wendy Lustbader and Nancy Hooyman; copyright © 1986 by The Free Press.

NOTES

1. U.S. Senate Special Committee on Aging, *Aging America: Trends and Projections* (Washington, DC: U.S. Government Printing Office), 1992.

2. Majorie Cantor, "Family and Community: Changing Roles in an Aging Society," *The Gerontologist* 31 (1991): 337–340. Robyn Stone, Gail Cafferata, and Judith Sangl, *Caregivers of the Frail Elderly: A National Profile*, (Washington, DC: U.S. Department of Health and Human Services), 1987; Older Women's League, "Failing America's Caregivers: A Status Report on Women Who Care," Washington, DC: The Older Women's League, 1989. U.S. Senate Special Committee on Aging. *Aging America: Trends and Projections* (Washington, DC: U.S. Government Printing Office), 1992.

3. Richard Morycz, "Caregiving Strain and the Desire to Institutionalize Family Members with Alzheimer's Disease," *Research on Aging* 7 (1985): 329–361; U.S. Senate Special Committee on Aging, op. cit., 1992.

4. American Association of Retired Persons, *Understanding Senior Housing for the 1990's: An AARP Survey of Consumer Preferences, Concerns and Needs* (Washington, DC: AARP), 1990; AARP and Administration on Aging, "A Profile of Older Americans," Washington, DC: U.S. Department of Health and Human Services, 1990.

SUGGESTED RESOURCES

Articles

Burton, Linda, Peggye Dilworth-Anderson, and Verne Bengtson. "Creating Culturally Relevant Ways of Thinking About Diversity and Aging," *Generations*, 25, 4 (1991), 67–73.

Highlights some of the implications of the increasing diversity among the elderly for existing research, policy and programs.

Capitman, John, Winnie Hernandez-Gallegos, and Donna Yee. "Diversity Assessments in Aging Services," *Generations*, 25, 4 (1991), 73–77.

Suggests practical ways for organizations to assess how well they are addressing diversity and multiculturalism in serving the elderly.

Lockery, Shirley. "Caregiving Among Racial and Ethnic Minority Elders: Family and Social Supports," *Generations*, 25, 4 (1991), 58–63.

Challenges widely-held assumptions about the strengths of social supports among ethnic minority families. Examines the diversity within and between different groups that can affect the degree and meaning of support both for the elderly and their caregivers.

Books

Barresi, C., and D. Stull, eds. *Ethnic Elderly and Long-Term Care* (New York: Springer), 1993.

Discusses how ethnicity may influence delivery of care and individual adaptation. Explores both policy and practice implications.

Bass, Scott, Elizabeth Kutza, and Fernando Torres-Gil. *Diversity in Aging: Challenges Facing Planners and Policymakers in the 1990's* (Glenview, IL: Scott Foresman Professional Books), 1990.

Provocative overview of the challenges facing our increasingly diverse society, including how to develop services that are sensitive to the cultural traditions of different ethnic groups.

Jackson, James, ed. *Aging in Black America* (Newbury Park, CA: Sage), 1993.

Provides a life span perspective that recognizes the considerable variability among older African Americans.

Root, Maria, ed. *Racially Mixed People in America* (Newbury Park, CA: Sage), 1992.

Contains well-written and insightful studies pertaining to the experience of racially mixed people in America.

Organizations

National Asian Pacific Center on Aging. 1511 Third Avenue, Suite 914, Melbourne Tower, Seattle, WA 98101. (206) 624–1221

Sponsors employment programs and develops strategies to increase accessibility of federal programs for low-income Asian-Pacific elderly.

National Association for Hispanic Elderly. 3325 Wilshire Blvd., Suite 800, Los Angeles, CA 90010. (213) 487–1922

Provides social services and employment programs for low-income Hispanic elderly. Offers information and referral for SSI eligibility. Produces documentaries and public service announcements.

National Caucus and Center on Black Aged. 1424 K Street, N.W., Suite 500, Washington, DC 20005. (202) 637–8400.

An advocate organization working on behalf of the Black elderly. Publishes a newsletter, conducts research, and disseminates information on aging Blacks.

National Indian Council on Aging. City Center, Suite 510 West, Albuquerque, NM 87110. (505) 888–3302

Purpose is to improve the lives of Indian and Alaskan Native elders through specialized activities. They maintain a cooperative relationship with a number of federal agencies, conducting research on aging and issuing reports on the needs of Indian and Alaskan Native elders.

1

Taking Care of the Caregivers

Giving care to an ill relative can be one of the most lonely and thankless experiences of a person's lifetime. It can also be one of the most moving and satisfying. In some instances, caregiving is lonely, thankless, moving, and satisfying all at the same time. This chapter identifies common sources of distress in caregiving, offering ways for caregivers to lessen their feelings of resentment without adding to their guilt. Learning how to accept help is a central aspect of self-care, as is paying attention to one's physical and spiritual needs. The chapter concludes with a look at the detrimental effects of alcohol and drug usage on caregiving, as well as the consequences of trying to give care while feeling overwhelmed and exhausted.

THE DANCE BETWEEN GUILT AND RESENTMENT

Feeling guilty, caregivers tend to give more than they should to the person in their care. When they then become overburdened and exhausted, they feel resentful. Responding to this resentment, they set limits on what they are willing to give. They maintain these limits for a while, but soon begin to feel guilty about all that they are not doing for their relative. Responding to their guilt, they start again giving more than they should. This dance between guilt and resentment goes round and round, until caregivers recognize this cyclic process and take steps to halt it.

Coping with a Relative's Loneliness

Family members frequently adopt maxims such as "If I spent more time with Mom, she'd be less lonely." Bearing a pervasive and unending sense of responsibility for their relative's needs, they impose burdensome requirements on themselves for frequent calls and visits as a way to remove the loneliness. They contrast their busy lives with the older person's relatively empty hours and feel guilty, as if the fullness of their lives were a resource which could be shared.

A son or daughter cannot take away a parent's loneliness. Responding to his widowed mother's complaints of long, lonely days, a son may start taking her on outings more often and trying to devise activities to do together. He may take time away from other relationships and interests, spending more time with her than he can give freely. Despite his efforts, he is likely to find that the hours of companionship he provides go quickly for her and that her empty hours still pass slowly. The truth is that nothing he does can diminish the sting of the times when he is not available to her, and he cannot merge his life with hers like a spouse or a young child.

Caregivers in such predicaments may reach a point at which they believe that they lose no matter what they do: doing less for the older person seems to yield nothing but guilt and worry, and doing more only seems to increase their weariness and stress. Imagining what lies ahead, they miss the gray areas of compromise in which workable solutions lie. Instead, all-or-nothing options seem to loom, such as, "It's my personal life or my mother; I can't do both."

The crux of the matter is that no amount of contact from family members can compensate for the deaths of lifelong friends and companions, the reduction of meaningful activities, and the other losses which often accompany aging. The recognition that their devotion has considerable but limited value and that they do not need to assume total responsibility is one of the most liberating insights family members can have.

Families best help their relatives cope with loneliness by creating routines which do not burden their own lives. It is better to do less for someone and enjoy spending time with that person than to give too much and feel resentful. The feeling of being enjoyed by family members means more in the long run than any number of obligatory, guilt-inspired visits and calls. When family members cease imposing inconvenient schedules on themselves, they open up the potential of having good times with their relative.

Further wisdom can be drawn from the common situation in which a daughter feels pressured by her mother's frequent phone calls throughout the day. The more her mother phones, the less warmly and attentively the daughter responds to the calls. With her needs for warmth and attention still unsatisfied, her mother may then phone more often and complain more urgently about her loneliness. Feeling crowded, the daughter may try to fend her mother off with curt statements and a distant tone of voice. Stopping this negative spiral is beneficial to both of them. In return for her mother's agreeing not to call her, the daughter could offer to call her mother twice a day, at designated times when she would concentrate her caring. The daughter would feel less invaded, and her mother more satisfied. The worth of conversations should be measured by the feelings they generate rather than how often they occur and how long they last.

Surviving Full-Time Employment While Caregiving

Handling such dilemmas in a balanced way becomes especially urgent when caregivers are combining full-time employment with care tasks. A son who prepares dinner for his mother on the way home from work every evening, week after week, may feel increasingly exhausted. In addition, he may feel pressured on the job by needing to leave at a set time each day, thereby depriving himself of the option to stay late to finish up his work. The costs of this kind of daily routine in fatigue and job stress can be high, but people often go on making these sacrifices without weighing the consequences against the benefits.

Similarly, a daughter may repeatedly use her paid sick time to handle her father's incidental needs, such as driving him to the doctor. When she has a cold or other minor illness, she is likely to force herself to go to her job instead of taking vital rest. She may also feel pressured to refuse promotions which would increase her work hours and take away time from caregiving. Faced with what seems to be a starkly defined choice, advancing her career or assisting her father, she may feel trapped between conflicting aims of equal value.

Family members caught in a bind between their jobs and their care tasks may benefit when professionals prompt them toward reaching realistic compromises. The son portrayed above could cook for his mother on the weekends, letting her reheat these meals on weekday evenings. Instead of stopping by daily, he could phone her after arriving home. The reheated meals and phone calls may not be as pleasing to his mother as freshly cooked meals and daily visits, yet may relieve the son's workday stress considerably. Also, their weekend mealtimes are likely to be more pleasurable to both of them when he is feeling relaxed and happier to see her.

Likewise, the daughter in the example above could pay for a cab to take her father to the doctor, thereby conserving her sick days for her own illness or more pressing care tasks. She can ask the doctor or nurse to phone her at work after the examination to report on changes in medications or to confer on medical decisions, thereby maintaining continuity in her relationships with medical providers. Accepting a promotion could give her the funds to afford other services for her father, as well as give her increased job satisfaction. Her duty to her father does not have to conflict with her desire to make a good life for herself.

Bearing the Tedium of Daily Care Tasks

Caregivers often find basic care tasks to be relentless and repetitious. The only observable result from their exertions may be the older person's further decline, thereby thwarting the human desire to see improvement in response to effort. Spending a portion of each visit on meaningful projects helps remedy this sense of futility and tends to be worth the additional time expended.

For example, mounting photos in a family album with the older person's assistance, sorting through old papers together, or taping reminiscences of family history may be accomplished in small increments. Adding fifteen minutes to each visit for this purpose may quickly pay off as something to anticipate once care tasks are completed. Making progress on a project directly counters the helplessness and discouragement of losing ground with a progressive illness.

The older person also gains by being able to focus on something other than physical decline. Both caregivers and those receiving care can feel overwhelmed by the tedium of bathing, getting dressed, eating, getting undressed, day after day, especially when each of these activities requires adaptation for a disability. A stroke's damage may turn a previously talkative man inward, leaving him with a withdrawn exterior bearing little resemblance to his former personality. He may allow intrusive forms of help without complaint, becoming a "good patient" but forgoing aspects of himself which made him beloved to his family. In such instances, family members may find that adding meaningful projects to their care tasks may stimulate a welcome reawakening of their relative's former self. The memories evoked by such projects may generate discussions with more animation than would occur if the family's contacts remained limited to meeting basic care needs.

SELF-CARE AS A NECESSITY

Self-neglect by primary caregivers is one of the most common ways that families encounter trouble caring for relatives at home. Some refuse to accept help from other family members or decline professionals' offers to locate supportive services for them in the community. Many have no idea what they would do with time off from caregiving if it were available, having long ago given up on having a life of their own. Some allow the person in their care to abuse them, enduring verbal tirades or excessive demands because they do not know what else to do in these situations. Over time, many neglect themselves spiritually and physically to such an extent that the quality of the care they provide begins to suffer or they become seriously ill themselves.

Learning to Accept Help

Some family members turn down offers of help at the same time that they complain about their exhaustion. When others try to relieve them of tasks, they find excuses to keep getting everything done on their own. Socialized to be nurturing and responsible, female caregivers are especially prone to this pattern. Women often believe that they should be able to do everything themselves, as proof of their love, competence, or marriage vows. Accepting help is experienced as an admission of weakness or failure. Some further believe they should not have to ask for help, resenting family members who do not automatically know their needs and volunteer aid.

Others believe that no one else can do the work as well as they can and that their relative will suffer under someone else's care. They perceive help as intrusive and deficient at best. For example, a daughter may have difficulty accepting a hired house cleaner, presuming that the worker would disrupt her way of organizing the household. She may also reject her sister's offer to help with their mother's needs, recalling childhood lapses in her sister's reliability and believing that inferior care would result from a joint effort. She may then feel embittered that her mother's care is falling entirely on her shoulders, going so far as to complain to the very sister whose assistance she rejected.

Family caregivers caught in such binds often need strong statements from professionals in order to adopt a more flexible approach and stop neglecting themselves. It may help to hear a professional say, "To take care of yourself is to take care of the person you are helping," or "A rested caregiver is a good caregiver; an exhausted caregiver isn't good for anyone." To jolt a tired caregiver into tending to her own needs, it may be necessary to arouse a basic fear by asking, "What do you think will happen to your mother if you keep going like this and get sick?" The caregiver may realize that she is endangering her relative by neglecting herself.

Learning about the specific signs of caregiver stress and depression may further help a caregiver perceive the long-range consequences, both to herself and her relative, of continuing to refuse help. The following chart depicts the most common signals that improved self-care is needed. Unless these signals are heeded, problems can fester and may eventually translate into neglectful or abusive care. After reviewing this chart, a caregiver may be willing to accept a hired helper on a trial basis, with the professional urging her to notice the ways in which her stress is relieved and her depression is lessened. She may find that minor imperfections in the helper's care are well worth her getting some relief.

Obtaining Fruitful Rest

No two people rest in the same way. What is relaxing and gratifying to one person may have no positive effect on another. For this reason, professionals may need to summon individual caregivers to produce a list of activities they regard as restorative. Personal forms of renewal, whether comprised of a long walk, time with a supportive friend, or a bridge game, allow a person to focus on aspects of life other than those which have been draining. Even when a weary caregiver is unable to leave the premises, sitting out on the front steps, watching a sunset, reading a novel, soaking in a hot bath, or finding a quiet place in the house to take a nap may be revitalizing.

Pleasurable activities, however briefly enjoyed, can place sacrifices back into the context of life as a whole, from which they derive their meaning. For instance, a woman caring for a bedbound husband may find that working in a flower shop a day or two each week helps keep her in touch with the outside world and with herself, even though the money she earns barely pays for half the cost of substitute caregivers. Handling the flowers and dealing with customers may take her so completely away from the world of illness that she arrives home refreshed and ready to go on with the care.

THE WARNING SIGNS OF STRESS AND DEPRESSION

Sleep disturbance: difficulty falling asleep or remaining asleep; waking up early in the morning feeling anxious or irritable; unable to stop worrying or ruminating

Appetite changes: unusual over-eating or loss of appetite; significant weight gain or loss

Increased medication or alcohol usage: Overuse of sleeping pills, painkillers, alcohol, or caffeine

Mood changes: uncharacteristic short-temperedness, crying, or agitation; expressionless face or flat tone of voice; recurrent thoughts of death or suicide

Physical problems: decreased resistance to illness; delay or neglect of vital physical needs; poor nutrition

Chronic fatigue: loss of energy; decreased motivation, concentration, and attention; unending sense of tiredness

Rough handling: marked impatience when giving care; hitting, pushing, or yelling when frustrated or angered; neglecting vital care tasks

From Wendy Lustbader and Nancy R. Hooyman, *Taking Care of Aging Family Members* (New York: The Free Press, 1994). Copyright © 1994 by Wendy Lustbader and Nancy Hooyman; copyright © 1986 by The Free Press.

By alternating intervals of exertion with periods of rest, caregivers can greatly improve both their morale and their stamina. They can pace themselves while looking ahead to scheduled time off. Professionals should urge caregivers to follow through with promises to themselves, such as setting a goal of at least one outing per week and designating its day and time. Arranging for someone to stay with their relative may require so much effort that such outings will not occur unless firm commitments are made in advance.

A major problem with outings arises when the ill person protests at being left behind. The caregiver may then be tempted to cancel her plans out of guilt and sympathy. An effective response in such instances is the truth: "Mom, I know you hate being left with a stranger, but I've got to get out or I'll be too irritable with you." It may help also to remind the person that the substitute helper will be a stranger only the first few times and may actually break up the boredom of always seeing the same family members.

Out-of-town vacations are particularly effective for renewing a caregiver's spirits, but are often the hardest kind of respite to carry out. Families may repeatedly postpone their vacation plans because they feel guilty about the prospect of having a good time while their relative stays home. When families turn their lives over to caregiving, taking time for themselves on a vacation can seem frivolous compared with the daily reality of care needs. Their guilt may be especially intense if the vacation is to a place which their relative cherished or had planned to visit prior to becoming ill.

Some families arrange to have neighbors check on their relative or hire helpers through an agency, only to cancel their plans at the last minute out of worry that something might happen while they are away. The question, "What is the worst possible thing that can happen while you're away?" may help families begin to contend with the worst. Their anxieties can be addressed through advance discussion of an emergency plan with the substitute helpers, thereby preparing for what they fear. An emergency plan may include a notebook listing critical phone numbers, medications, daily routines, and idiosyncratic needs. Caregivers can be encouraged first to try small vacations, such as weekends away. During these trial periods away, they may discover that they gain so much more patience and enthusiasm for the care that vacations are worth the worry.

Heeding Physical Needs

To endure in the long run, caregivers must pay careful attention to maintaining their physical health. Proper diet and exercise are as essential as rest, yet many caregivers feel so busy taking care of their relative that they fail to take care of their own health. A daughter cooking low-salt meals for her father may grab highly caloric snacks rather than preparing meals for herself. A wife caring for her bedridden husband may so dislike having meals alone that she goes for days without eating. Professionals can help by questioning caregivers about their nutrition, pointing out deficits, and prodding them to devise ways to improve their eating habits.

Caregivers may regard exercising as one more demand to fit into their already crowded schedules. A caregiver who has difficulty getting out of the house may benefit from a stationary bike, aerobic tapes or records, or tension-releasing exercises which can be done while their relative is sleeping. Many exercises can be performed while sitting in a chair, talking on the phone, or watching television. After a caregiver begins to incorporate exercise as part of her daily routine, the benefits of feeling more energetic and less tense tend to outweigh the time taken away from other duties.

A major health problem for many caregivers is interrupted sleep. During the night, their relative may require changes of bedding, pain medication, help getting to the bathroom, or repositioning in bed. A relative's wandering or pacing may also cause sleep disturbance. Over time, unrelieved fatigue produces discouragement and moodiness, yet most caregivers cannot afford to hire overnight helpers. Finding family members or friends willing to spend the night tends to be difficult at best.

Generally, sleep deprivation cannot go on for long without the caregiver becoming ill or the quality of the care becoming seriously compromised. Professionals should regard such situations as top priority for intervention. Unless rest for the primary caregiver can be obtained through substitute helpers or sleep medications, placing the older person in another setting may be the only realistic solution. (See "Recognizing the Red Flags for Nursing Home Placement," pp. 317–319.)

Setting Limits with Abusive Older People

Many people abuse their caregivers. The apparent powerlessness of physically fragile older people can be deceiving. Bearing the travails of illness, some focus exclusively on themselves and try to exert control in ways destructive to their relationships with their caregivers. Those who have had lifelong difficulties with being considerate may become still more self-centered and insensitive. Some take out all of the rage from their infirmities on the nearest target, the caregiver who spends the most time with them.

Ways to inflict harm without physical strength are abundant in the close quarters of caregiving. Occasionally, abusive behavior develops so gradually that caregivers tolerate it without naming it, knowing only that they feel continually angry and frustrated with the person in their care. The following chart may help caregivers identify the basis for their feelings.

The goal of limit-setting with abusive people is to prevent caregivers from becoming resentful. Firmly holding to limits protects the relationship and is therefore an act of caring, not heartlessness. A daughter who succumbs to her mother's demands to run up and down stairs several times an hour for unnecessary tasks will eventually detest the sound of her mother's voice. Similarly, a health-care professional who allows an older patient to prolong appointment times excessively will dread that person's visits. Awareness of abuse and ways to respond constructively are vital for caregivers and professionals wanting to promote a secure and balanced relationship with the person they are helping.

A firm belief in the importance of setting limits must precede any attempt to contain abusive behaviors. A daughter who feels it is "cruel" to limit the number of times she will run upstairs to wait on her mother will not be able to heed her own tiredness. If she instead assures herself, "It's more loving to stay downstairs and keep from resenting her," she might be able to hold to reasonable limits on the number of trips she makes. In the same way, a health professional must be certain that interrupting a nonstop talker in order to end appointments on time is ultimately respectful rather than rude.

The next step in setting limits is to define them clearly. The daughter in the above example could announce to her mother that she will come upstairs only three times each morning. She could say to her mother, "Mom, be careful not to use up one of my trips on help you do not really need." This would be a caring way to convey an unbending attitude toward this restriction. The daughter could also advise her mother to "save up" small tasks that can be delayed, grouping them along with more urgent needs later in the morning.

With nonstop talkers, it is helpful to state at the beginning of a discussion when it will end: "In about fifteen minutes, I'm going to have to go." Midway through the time period, a reminder should be offered: "We only have half our time left, so I hope you've gotten to the things you most want to tell me." Five minutes before the end, concluding phrases should be inserted, no matter how little conversational space the person permits: "We have to end in a few minutes, so I'd like to finish up this one piece of business with you." Talking above the person's voice may be imperative for those who do not pause between sentences. Finally, a minute before the ending, standing up and moving toward the door conveys that the conclusion is imminent. In many instances, it is necessary to say goodbye and walk out the door while the person continues to talk.

The next phase of limit-setting is the most difficult. People subjected

ABUSE OF CAREGIVERS BY ILL PEOPLE	
Financial	Demanding hired help when it is a luxury, not a necessity
	Turning up heat beyond reason or prudence
	Giving away resources promised to family members
	Demanding excessive long-distance phone calls
	Spending funds on alcohol or drugs, not care
	Refusing to spend money on essential services
Emotional	Complaining bitterly about unavoidable situations
	Finding fault with errors made in good faith
	Feigning symptoms to get extra attention
	Berating caregivers for setting reasonable limits
	Blaming others for problems caused by themselves
	Prolonging conversations through nonstop talking
	Yelling at caregivers for small mistakes
Physical	Waking caregivers thoughtlessly during the night
	Asking for help out of whim rather than need
	Refusing devices that would ease care tasks
	Pushing, scratching, hitting, biting caregivers
	Demanding help beyond the caregiver's capacity

From Wendy Lustbader and Nancy R. Hooyman, *Taking Care of Aging Family Members* (New York: The Free Press, 1994). Copyright © 1994 by Wendy Lustbader and Nancy Hooyman; copyright © 1986 by The Free Press.

to limits for the first time tend to test the boundaries by acting out. In this regard, it is helpful to imagine in advance exactly how the person is likely to challenge the limit-setter's will. The daughter described above could reasonably anticipate that her mother will use up her three requests for relatively trivial purposes, and then will claim an "emergency" when she calls out the fourth time. After the second request, a preventive strategy is to predict this behavior: "Mom, you'd better save the last request in case something really urgent comes up, because I've got to stick to what I said."

During the acting-out phase, being candid about how hard it is to adhere to limits can sometimes reduce the intensity of the person's challenges: "Mom, I worry about you all the time, so it's hard for me to resist coming upstairs when you call." Such comments help break the person's habit of trying to obtain reassurance through excessive demands. Openness about the overall purpose of setting limits also helps halt this pattern: "Mom, if I stay downstairs and get my other work done, I'll be able to come upstairs later and enjoy my time with you. Otherwise, I get too tired and stressed out."

When nonstop talkers sense the approach of an ending to a conversation, they tend to test the limit by earnestly detouring from the immediate topic. Some begin crying or suddenly bring up something of great emotional import: "Doctor, I've never told this to anyone before." A helpful response in these instances is, "I wish this hadn't come up just as we've run out of time, because I want to talk about this in depth with you. Let's be sure to start our next conversation with this." Both parties' feelings of abruptness can be smoothed by using touch to convey caring, while urging the older person through the door.

A caution for family members wanting to limit a relative's troublesome behaviors is to avoid trying to change too many at once. Holding to limits requires considerable mental energy best applied to a few target behaviors at a time. Another wisdom is to integrate rewards into any limit-setting attempt, such as performing extra services when a person becomes less demanding. It is helpful to ask the person to make a wish list of tasks which are not necessary but which the person would like accomplished when time allows. These tasks can then be used to thank the person for respecting the limits.

A caution for professionals is to avoid being charmed by older people who are abusive to family members behind the scenes. Some people maintain a lifelong pattern of friendliness toward the outside world and maliciousness toward family members. A nurse may sympathize with an older person's complaints about supposedly neglectful family members, not bothering to check with the family about their perceptions of the situation. She may then allow these stories of familial neglect to color her responses to family members during phone calls and conferences. The family may actually be exerting considerable effort toward keeping their difficult relative at home and may be weary of professionals who do not look below the surface.

A related error is for professionals to grasp at presumed sources of support without taking the time to investigate the family history. A hospital discharge planner may pressure a daughter to allow her father to stay in her home until he completes his recovery. If the discharge planner is unaware that the father sexually abused his daughter earlier in life, attempting to tap a relationship scarred by this kind of pain can be severely detrimental to the daughter. As a standard precaution, professionals should heed hesitation or reluctance expressed by adult children. Nonfamilial options are preferable to forcing adult children to tolerate emotional strain of this magnitude.

Some families are able to set limits with difficult people only after professionals label what they are experiencing as abuse. For this reason, professionals should be alert to families' need for the situation to be framed in these terms. The word *abuse* is a powerful tool for professionals to help families change or get out of destructive caregiving situations. The word conveys the concept that behaviors are occurring which should not be tolerated, often freeing overly kind and selfless people to recognize healthier boundaries.

Heeding Spiritual Needs

For caregivers, finding inner strength is a matter of daily necessity. Their ability to endure often depends on having a solid awareness about why they are doing what they do. There are too many sacrifices and disruptions to go on for long without good reasons. Yet putting such purposes into words is not easy, especially for families who are not members of an organized religion or a traditional culture.

In large measure, spirituality is comprised of explanations: reasons for being alive, assurances for choosing one life course over another, and narratives which help people make a connection with something greater than the material world. The stories people tell themselves to make sense of their choices are particularly important for caregivers: "I'm showing my children what it means to 'honor thy father and mother,'" or "I couldn't live with myself otherwise. It's the only decent thing to do." Reaching for a spiritual view enlarges the day-to-day struggles of caregiving, placing them in a context in which it is possible to find meaning.

Professionals in the field of aging are often surprised by the concerns which caregivers raise in these situations: "Doctor, does it mean that I'm a bad person that I keep hoping my mother will die soon? Do you think God will punish me?" Many doctors, nurses, and social workers try to change the subject when such questions are brought up, or they tolerate the conversation while feeling increasingly uncomfortable. In the health professions, there is little training in spiritual discourse. On the contrary, references to God and to religious frameworks for making sense of suffering tend to be entirely omitted in the effort to remain religiously neutral. This dedication to neutrality has led to speechlessness for many professionals in arenas where caregivers crave dialogue.

Giving a caregiver a chance to speak her spiritual questions and beliefs out loud may contribute significantly to her endurance. Such expression tends to enhance someone's strength, whereas cutting off spiritual dialogue may leave a person feeling more alone and less able to face her circumstances. Rather than trying to provide answers, professionals should offer responsive listening and commentary: "I don't know what God would feel about your situation, but I can tell you I respect the way you're approaching this." Since voicing questions in itself often leads to clarity, the listener's contribution is to be there in an openhearted way.

Language is often a barrier when spiritual dialogue is attempted, especially when people do not share the same set of beliefs or points of reference. Words like "blessing" or "forgiveness" come laden with various meanings, depending on one's religious background. Professionals can respectfully join a caregiver in using such words, without divulging or imposing their own religious views: "I can see the meaning of this blessing for you." Speaking someone's language often provides deep comfort in ways that it is most needed.

Family caregivers may face a similar awkwardness when they attempt to comfort their relatives. Members of the same family often do not hold the same beliefs or even follow the same traditions. Also, the questions which assail people facing death or frailty may feel threatening to those who have not yet arrived at this juncture: "What is the meaning of my life? Why do I have to suffer? Will I be remembered? Is there life after death, or is this all there is?" Caregivers may try to change the subject when these concerns are brought up, or they may permit the conversation to go on while wishing it would end.

In some instances, teaching family caregivers how to listen responsively to spiritual questions becomes a professional's most important role. Caregivers may need assurance that listening to their relative's beliefs does not imply agreement, but rather respect for someone's right to see the world in their own way. Many benefit from reminders that reciting their own beliefs is unnecessary and that there are ways to deflect probing questions without being disrespectful: "Mom, I'm not sure where I stand on all this, but it is good to hear your reflections." The key is to listen and to encourage expression, and through this process to try to understand how someone is bearing their circumstances.

One valuable sensitivity is to determine how strongly someone is affected by the power of prayer. Some people pray or meditate every day and find that it helps them renew their spirit for the day ahead, whereas others experience their spirituality keenly without a daily ritual. By encouraging someone to speak freely about their practice of prayer, professionals and family members may open up broad realms for discussion. A statement like, "Praying can be a real lifeline when you're afraid or frustrated," may liberate someone to talk about the ways in which prayer is helping her bear her difficulties. Talking about spiritual practices tends to enhance them.

Family members often discover that it is in the gray areas of caregiving that their spiritual beliefs are most sorely tested. A prior sense of certainty in these matters may vanish in the face of questions like, "How much of my life should I give up for my mother?" or "How many sleepless nights do I owe to my husband?" In such situations, a caregiver who thought she knew where she stood may find herself wishing someone would tell her what to do. She may grope desperately and widely for outside guidance, looking to religious traditions and professional helpers for answers which keep eluding her.

Spiritual agony can be more intense in its impact than physical suffering. Such questions may require more extended listening than a health care professional has time to supply. Linking the caregiver with clergy or with a pastoral counselor is sometimes the best course of action. For those who do not identify with a particular religion, counseling agencies sponsored by religious groups may nevertheless yield the right kind of help. Such agencies often employ nondenominational counselors who do not preach but rather assist people on their own terms. This can usually be determined through a direct inquiry as to the nature of the services offered and whether a particular religious orientation is expected by the agency.

Attending Caregiver Support Groups

Family caregivers often feel that no one except those in the same situation can understand the toll of caregiving on their daily lives and relationships. Such feelings are intensified when friends question their sacrifices or urge them to consider using a nursing home. At the most basic level, support groups composed of family caregivers provide an opportunity to talk with others who are capable of understanding their choices. The chance to commiserate about painful aspects of their lives and laugh at humorous incidents relieves what is often a deep isolation.

Support groups also encourage an active stance toward problems. When participants offer each other suggestions of favorite physicians or information about financial benefits, their awareness of community options grows. Even when appropriate community resources do not exist, group problem-solving can often generate creative solutions. Families share practical caregiving tips, equipment, and supplies. In this exchange process, members find that giving help can be as beneficial as receiving it. Sharing their insights to help solve others' problems, they become aware of the competence they have achieved as caregivers.

Even if a specific problem cannot be solved, the caregiver may feel better about the situation as a result of the group discussion. Simply giving voice to a difficulty often diminishes its weight. For example, a woman upset about yelling at her husband for repeatedly forgetting information may feel less self-loathing when others confess to the same impatience. A man feeling guilty about deciding to place his mother in a nursing home may listen with relief as others describe their wrestling with similar decisions. By hearing others tell their stories, support group members come to recognize the universality of their struggles and that they do not have to be "perfect."

Although support groups are not conducted as therapy sessions, the process of expressing feelings and listening to other people's dilemmas has therapeutic effects. Members can express negative emotions, such as anger and resentment, without fearing that they are being judged for feeling this way. Since group members are not part of their regular circle of friends, participants are liberated from social pressures. They do not have to maintain a strong exterior or feign certainty regarding issues about which they feel confused or ambivalent. They can also bring up embarrassing questions, such as a husband asking others in the group what to do about his wife's nighttime incontinence.

The sense of support and active mastery can extend beyond the group meetings. Members generally watch out for one another, expressing concern when individuals are absent and monitoring their weekly coping efforts. Sometimes members form phone reassurance networks, calling regularly to check on one another. Those able to get away may meet for lunch, share a potluck dinner, or provide respite and other kinds of assistance for one another. Members may sponsor a newsletter as a way to provide information and strengthen their sense of belonging. Support groups also serve a consciousness-raising function, increasing members' awareness of gaps in public funding for vital services. Caregivers may then become involved in public education, advocacy, and legislative action.

Despite these advantages of participation, a number of barriers can prevent family caregivers from attending support groups. Finding someone to stay with their relative while they attend the meetings is often the chief difficulty. Even when such a person is located or hired, the older person may protest so strongly that the caregiver finds it easier to stay home. For exhausted caregivers, attendance at a support group meeting can seem to be one more demand on their time. They simply may not have the motivation to make the necessary arrangements, particularly if transportation is a problem. Many caregivers, especially older spouses, may be unaccustomed to revealing their personal feelings and concerns to strangers. They may equate support groups with the stigma of "mental health services" or believe that admitting problems to others is a sign of weakness.

These barriers can be most readily addressed by support group facilitators. A list of group members willing to give rides to others can be maintained, and phone trees can be coordinated to remind members of meetings. The chosen meeting place should be accessible to disabled participants, have phones available, ample parking, and nearby bus routes. The meeting time may need to be negotiated, with retired caregivers preferring daytime meetings to avoid night driving and employed caregivers preferring the evenings. Saturday mornings may be an acceptable compromise.

Outreach visits by current support group members may help to motivate caregivers who are reluctant to reveal their feelings to others or who have been too tired to make the effort to attend. By taking the trouble to visit the caregiver at home, the group member conveys the group's importance. The chance to talk one-on-one may help a caregiver both release suppressed feelings and experience the value of doing so. The assurance of already knowing one participant may further inspire the caregiver to give the group a try. Once people observe the benefits of a support group for themselves, they have an easier time telling their ill relative why they have to go: "Mom, the group gave me so many good ideas about how to take good care of you that I'm planning to go every month. I know you feel nervous when I'm gone, but this will help both of us in the long run." Over time, the ill person is likely to see what a positive difference it makes.

WHEN SELF-CARE FAILS: ABUSE AND NEGLECT

Despite encouragements to take care of themselves, some caregivers turn to ineffective ways of coping. They try to alleviate their stress with alcohol or drugs, or they allow themselves to become so exhausted that they neglect the ill person's basic needs. In other instances, past family problems resurface and lead to abuse and neglect. Those who recognize that they are providing poor care to their relative are often at a loss as to how to stop their harmful behavior or how to improve their situation. Shame about what is going on behind the scenes may be a major barrier to their accepting help from other family members or professionals.

Using Alcohol or Drugs While Giving Care

Stressed by all the demands, caregivers may begin using alcohol or prescription drugs to quell their anxieties or to forget their worries when they do manage to get time away from their duties. They may feel entitled to a small nip in the morning "to get going" and throughout the day for "a little pleasure" in an otherwise tedious existence. Professionals who work with families must remain alert to the possibility that alcohol or drug abuse is playing a deleterious role in the care situation. Others in the family may attribute signs of poor care to the caregiver's physical exhaustion, low mood, or inadequate sleep. Family members who feel guilty about their failure to assist the primary caregiver may look the other way at obvious warning signs, such as several empty liquor bottles in the trash.

Alcohol and drug problems arising for the first time, in response to being a caregiver, differ greatly from longstanding problems with substance abuse. Those with recent onset can usually be helped with self-care techniques, supportive services, and other measures discussed throughout this book. In itself, the step of admitting that alcohol or drug dependence has become a problem often enables caregivers to take constructive measures, such as attending a support group or consulting their family physician for advice on other ways to handle their distress.

Those with longstanding problems with alcohol or drugs should be urged to seek appropriate treatment. Caregiving pressures often make existing addictions worse, because the individual has even fewer alternatives than before for coping with difficulties. The following chart depicting the negative effects of substance abuse by caregivers may help motivate someone with a longstanding problem to seek professional help. It is also useful to review the chart with an older person who is in the care of someone with an alcohol or drug problem, as it describes conditions which the person may be too ashamed to reveal. Seeing a printed list may prove to the person that such problems are common and that they can be discussed openly.

NEGATIVE EFFECTS OF SUBSTANCE ABUSE BY CAREGIVERS

Oversleeping in the morning: neglecting early-morning care needs and medication dosages; leaving the older person in bed an excessive length of time; failing to change incontinence pads promptly

Medication errors: miscounting dosages; mixing up medications; forgetting to give medications on time

Risk of injury: impaired judgment and coordination when lifting the person or assisting in the bathroom

Sleeping through cries for help: inability to be aroused from a stupor during an emergency or other urgent need

Loss of emotional inhibitions: releasing uncontrolled anger; making abusive remarks to the older person that would not be made while sober; hitting, bruising, or sexually assaulting the older person

Keeping the older person awake at night: loud partying near the older person's bedroom; disruptive guests

Neglecting basic needs: failing to assist the older person with personal hygiene and meal preparation; leaving the person in bed all day

Misuse of money: inadequate funds left for food, medicine, rent, phone, heat, and transportation—all of which affect the older person's daily comfort and health

---

From Wendy Lustbader and Nancy R. Hooyman, *Taking Care of Aging Family Members* (New York: The Free Press, 1994). Copyright © 1994 by Wendy Lustbader and Nancy Hooyman; copyright © 1986 by The Free Press.

Substance abuse is almost always present in situations of elder abuse and neglect. Other warning signs include the older person's emotional distress, unexplained bruises, unclean hair or clothing, or discontinuity with health providers, and caregivers' resistance to other people having regular access to the older person. Guarded caregivers who do not allow professionals to be alone with the older person usually have something to conceal. When encountering such resistance, professionals should become all the more determined to obtain time alone with the older person. One strategy is to enlist the help of a second professional who can occupy the caregiver long enough to allow the other professional to have privacy with the older person. Another is to state that private time is a mandatory part of the professional's service to the older person and to insist courteously but firmly upon obtaining it.

Mismanaged funds or physical striking more readily come to professional attention than abuse which leaves no tangible evidence. For example, the fact that an older person is left alone for long periods of time, yelled at for spilling foods and wetting the bed, or deprived of a quiet environment at night may emerge only after a careful series of interviews in which the professional checks on these more concealable forms of abuse. Fearing nursing home placement or charges filed against loved ones, the older person may deny that there are any problems unless the professional provides assurances that the older person will remain in control of these choices: "I'd like to help you stay at home or get what you want for your health and safety." Emphasizing that getting help for the caregiver is a top priority may also reassure the older person that talking about these problems is in her family's best interest.

Giving Care While Exhausted

Poor care can also result from family members' physical exhaustion. For example, an older man may refuse to get up at night to help his wife to the bathroom, reasoning that interrupted sleep makes him too tired the next day: "If I have to help her all night, how am I going to be able to help her all day?" He may feel badly about his wife's discomfort and humiliation from being forced to urinate into protective pads during the night, but regard it as a worthy trade-off for his obtaining rest. Unable to meet all her needs, he may choose to overlook the fact that her bedsores become worse as a result of nightlong contact with urine.

Perceiving a situation as abusive often depends upon context and point of view. The wife in this example may feel that her husband is cruel in refusing to help her during the night, no matter what his justifications. She may complain to her visiting nurse that her bedsores "ache all night" after she urinates in the pad and that her husband is "insensitive and selfish." From a medical point of view, the nurse would be correct in informing the husband that his failure to assist his wife during the night is hastening her skin's deterioration. Unless the nurse also offered a solution to his need for rest, however, this information would only intensify the bind he faces between his need for rest and his desire to give his wife the best possible care.

Similar to many situations of abuse, the lack of substitutes to provide relief to the primary caregiver is the cause of harm in this example. The problem in not inherent in the husband as a caregiver, but rather in the nature of the demands on him and his lack of resources to cope with them. Another example of how limited options can result in abuse is a daughter who virtually drops her father into his wheelchair instead of transferring him smoothly. Her aching back and suppressed anger at confinement by the care tasks combine with her lack of training in transfer techniques to produce her rough handling of her father. If a physical therapist from a home care agency provided her both with this training and a Medicare-covered home health aide to allow her time off from care demands, the daughter would probably stop harming her father in this way.

In situations with overwhelmed caregivers, professionals should convey an attitude of gathering information for the sake of improving care, rather than that of a detective seeking to uncover weakness or blame caregivers for malicious intent. Caregivers may already be condemning themselves for yelling at the ill person when no one else is around or for pushing or slapping the person in moments of extreme fatigue. The following questions do not have to be asked directly, but they can serve as a guide during the assessment process. When the care situation is difficult, the availability of extra help and professional support become critical factors in family members' ability to provide good care.

Resuming Family Problems from the Past

Past family conflicts, difficult care needs, and current life stress can merge into an abusive situation. When forced to be caregivers, family members with unresolved resentments may consciously or unwittingly use care predicaments to get back at the parent. For example, a daughter who had been sexually abused by her father as a child may choose to stay in bed while her father cries out for pain medication during the night. She may reassure herself, "I'm entitled to get some rest," yet may also be fulfilling an old need for retaliation now that her father is

---

ASSESSING THE NEEDS OF OVERWHELMED CAREGIVERS

1. How much rest are caregivers getting?
2. What personal sacrifices are caregivers making in order to serve the person's needs?
3. Are caregivers neglecting their own health?
4. Is constant surveillance required as part of care tasks?
5. Have caregivers turned to alcohol or drug abuse in their distress? Has substance abuse been lifelong?
6. How drastically has the older person's personality changed in response to illness?
7. Are caregivers receiving verbal or physical abuse from the person in their care?
8. Is the primary caregiver overwhelmed by demands from several dependent people at once?
9. Are financial constraints interfering with the caregiver's ability to follow medical advice?
10. Are problems from the family history resurfacing and contributing to abuse or neglect?

From Wendy Lustbader and Nancy R. Hooyman, *Taking Care of Aging Family Members* (New York: The Free Press, 1994). Copyright © 1994 by Wendy Lustbader and Nancy Hooyman; copyright © 1986 by The Free Press.

as vulnerable as she once was. Since acting out pain from the past in this manner tends to worsen a person's self-esteem, caregivers in these situations should be urged to seek professional help. In these instances, it may be better for both the family member and the older person to find another caregiver or another care setting.

The power to provide or withhold vital help to a physically dependent parent offers adult children a position of superior strength through which many conflicts can be expressed. Often, there is a need to triumph over previously dominant siblings by taking charge of the parent's care and controlling siblings' access to information about the situation. Assuming control of the parent's financial resources is a particularly potent weapon in sibling battles of this nature. Professionals can sometimes help by hearing out a caregiver's resentments, both historical and contemporary, toward siblings and then pointing out the ways in which these emotions are detracting from the family's ability to provide good care. After feeling heard, the caregiver may be better able to consider others' points of view, or may be willing to accept a referral to professional counseling to deal with unfinished business about family relationships. (See further discussion of these issues in Chapter 3, "Siblings Sharing the Care")

Professionals encountering abuse within families should recognize that they can easily make the situation worse if they cannot offer better alternatives. The most common professional error is to move too quickly from detecting the abuse to confronting the caregiver. When the family has been caught in a cycle of violence in successive generations, the emotional complexity may far exceed the time and expertise the professional can offer. To be beneficial, interventions must be preceded by a careful effort to understand why the abuse is occurring, why it is tolerated, and what realistic alternatives can be provided.

Without such forethought, interventions tend to produce destructive consequences. Outside helpers may be prevented by either family members or the older person from having further access to the household. The caregiver's anger at being confronted may translate into a worsening of the abuse or neglect. Family members and the older person may feel demeaned by their awareness that people outside the family know about the situation. Finally, the caregiver may fend off assistance that might have led to improved care for the older person.

No matter what the circumstances at home, older people generally prefer care from family members over placement in other settings. For most elders, the known seems better than the unknown, even if their situation appears unacceptable to outside observers. Supporting family caregivers and encouraging them to take care of themselves is therefore often the best way for professionals to serve older people.

Family caregivers face a host of dilemmas: "How can I know when I've done enough? When is it OK to take care of myself? How can I get other members of the family involved?" They may wonder how long they can go on, and yet may not know how to begin to get help. Those who find themselves neglecting someone they love or doing harm may feel too ashamed to accept supportive services or to consider other options. The next two chapters examine how caregiving affects partners and siblings; later chapters move from family relationships to specific physical and mental problems, and various service and living options. There are no simple answers to families' dilemmas, but knowledge does create choices.

SUGGESTED RESOURCES

Articles

Gallagher, Dolores, Jonathan Rose, Patricia Rivera, Steven Lovett, and Larry Thompson. "Prevalence of Depression in Family Caregivers," *The Gerontologist*, 4 (1989), 449–456.

> Caregivers who sought help to increase their coping skills were found to be less depressed than those who did not seek help. Women were generally more depressed than men. No differences in depression were found among those who cared for more impaired persons.

McFadden, Susan, and Robert Gerl. "Approaches to Understanding Spirituality in the Second Half of Life," *Generations*, 14, 4 (1990), 35–39.

> The authors review the ongoing process of spiritual integration and the contextual approach to spirituality in old age.

Missinne, Leo. "Death and Spiritual Concerns of Older Adults," *Generations*, 14, 4 (1990), 45–47.

> The author emphasizes the need to distinguish spiritual from psychological needs and how caregivers can assist older people with achieving spiritual integration.

Books

Barusch, Amanda. *Elder Care: Family Training and Support* (Newbury Park, CA: Sage), 1991.

> Provides practical advice on how to develop, implement, and evaluate training and support programs for family caregivers.

Fischer, Kathleen. *Winter Grace: Spirituality for the Later Years*. (Mahwah, NJ: Paulist Press), 1985.

> Describes spirituality not as a separate compartment of life, but as a dimension beneath all experience. Helpful to caregivers and to those receiving care.

Greenberg, Vivian. *Your Best Is Good Enough* (New York: Lexington Books), 1989.

This book sensitively addresses the complex emotions—anger, guilt, frustration, and sadness—that adult children often face when caring for aging parents. Emphasizes the importance of setting limits and reducing unrealistic expectations.

Organizations

American Association of Retired Persons (AARP). 1909 K Street N.W., Washington, DC 20049 (202) 728–4200.

This nonprofit organization works to meet the needs of older people throughout the nation. They offer a wide range of publications and services for people over fifty-five.

Caregiver Education and Support Project Extension Service, Oregon State University, Milam Hall 161, Corvallis, OR 97331. (503) 737–3211.

This project has developed educational pamphlets for family caregivers, providing information in an easy-to-read fashion. Videos and other educational tools are also available for national distribution at cost.

Elder Care Locator. (800) 677–1116.

This national toll-free number is designed to help identify community resources for seniors anywhere in the United States. The name, address, and zip code of the person needing assistance allows the Elder Care Locator to identify the nearest information and assistance sources in that person's community. Call between 9:00 A.M. and 8:00 P.M. Eastern Time.

Gray Panthers. 2025 Pennsylvania Avenue, N.W., Suite 821, Washington, DC 20006. (202) 466–3132.

This coalition of intergenerational activists works to promote the concerns of older people, often organizing around issues that cross age groups.

National Council on the Aging (NCOA). 600 Maryland Avenue, S.W. West Wing 100, Washington, DC 20024. (202) 479–1200.

A private, nonprofit group serving as a central resource for information, technical assistance, training, planning, and consultation in gerontology.

National Council of Senior Citizens (NCSC). 1331 F Street, N.W., Washington, DC 20004. (202) 347–8800.

Composed of representatives of senior organizations throughout the nation, this group focuses on education and social action.

National Resource Center on Health Promotion and Aging. 601 E Street, N.W., Suite B5, Washington, DC 20049.

Publishes a bimonthly newsletter, "Perspectives in Health Promotion and Aging," containing updates on health issues of interest to caregivers.

Older Women's League (OWL). 730 11th Street, N.W., Suite 300, Washington, DC 20001. (202) 783–6686.

OWL's national membership is committed to helping meet the special needs of middle-aged and older women, especially in areas such as Social Security, pension rights, health insurance, and caregiver support services.

2

Partners as Caregivers

Partners are the most common caregivers. Adult children and other family members generally assume care responsibilities only when a partner is absent. Most frequently, an older wife is caregiver to a disabled husband. Care pressures are intensified when a partner is coping with her own health problems as well as the stresses of medical expenses. The questions below suggest critical factors to be considered when partners give care, whether in the context of a lifelong marriage, a late-in-life marriage, couples living together without marrying, and gay and lesbian couples. This chapter examines the effect of caregiving on intimate partnerships, identifying problem areas and suggesting solutions that can be adapted to individual circumstances.

IN SICKNESS AND IN HEALTH?

Couples facing a debilitating illness quickly discover the nature of their commitment to each other and the strengths and weaknesses of their union. Each partner grapples with changes in roles, self-image, and in the balance of the satisfactions and sacrifices experienced in the relationship. The upheaval may emerge gradually or come on suddenly, but reorganization of the partnership's terms becomes necessary when illness dominates a couple's life.

FACTORS TO CONSIDER WHEN PARTNERS BECOME CAREGIVERS

1. What was the length of the relationship prior to the illness? Has there been a long shared history?
2. Is this a union of convenience or a deep bonding? Do both people believe that care during illness is an essential part of the commitment?
3. How conflictual was the relationship prior to the need for caregiving? Has there been a history of battering or verbal abusiveness?
4. What is the health status of the caregiver? Is he or she healthy enough to meet the care demands without sustaining physical harm?
5. What is the timing of the illness relative to the couple's retirement plans? Does the healthier partner feel cheated as a result of missed plans?
6. What is the nature of the sexual adjustment entailed by the illness? Has the illness made sexual activity frightening or painful?
7. What is the impact of the illness on the couple's financial resources? Is there added stress from medical expenses or the need to hire extra help?
8. How adaptable is the couple's residence? Can adjustments be made to accommodate the care needs?
9. To what extent is the couple receiving help from family members, friends, and community services? Is the couple isolated from these sources of support?
10. What are each person's cultural or spiritual attitudes toward adversity? Has the couple faced past hardships in a unified or divisive way?

From Wendy Lustbader and Nancy R. Hooyman, *Taking Care of Aging Family Members* (New York: The Free Press, 1994). Copyright © 1994 by Wendy Lustbader and Nancy Hooyman; copyright © 1986 by The Free Press.

Unearthing Beliefs

There are all kinds of unions. People commit themselves to each other for a wide variety of reasons, some of which have little to do with the notion of being in love. Among these are the desire for children, physical attraction and sexual need, parental and societal pressures, economic security, unmet dependency needs, and the desire for compan-ionship. The meaning of commitment for particular couples can range from, "I'll stay with you so long as you enhance my life and meet my needs," to "I'll stay with you through sickness and health, till death do us part."

In some relationships, money and freedom are much more impor-tant than loyalty. Caregiving is acceptable in these instances only if it does not interfere with the healthier person's life plans. For example, a woman in later life may marry a man because he has ample income and is a good traveling companion. If he has a stroke a year later, she may resent her resulting confinement as well as the costs of hiring aides to assist with his care in their home. Deciding to place him in a nursing home and seek a divorce, she may feel entitled to reclaim her freedom: "Look, I didn't marry him to take care of him."

In other types of relationships, loyalty is supremely valued. The per-sonal sacrifice required by caregiving is seen as a meaningful way to express gratitude for years of devotion. The healthier partner tends to regard nursing home placement as a failure to live up to their mutual commitment, no matter how seriously placement is warranted by the nature of the care. In these instances, partners often need help relin-quishing their role as caregiver when it has become detrimental to their own health.

Partners rarely put their beliefs about commitment into words until challenged by a major life event. For this reason, partners with contrasting beliefs often recognize these differences only in the midst of a crisis. A person who believes that giving care during times of ill-ness is fundamental to a committed relationship may learn after he has a stroke that his partner regards individual life enhancement as more important.

Learning New Roles

Partners tend to evolve a division of labor in which each has responsi-bility for different areas of their mutual life, such as one person han-dling the bill paying and the other taking care of the grocery shopping. Over time, these roles become deeply ingrained, with each individual developing a particular method of getting things done. When an illness upsets these long-standing roles, the strain on a couple can be sub-stantial. In fact, role disruption can be one of the most devastating of all the effects of illness on partners.

The primary source of strain arises when the ill person loses control over a domain of life previously managed without interference. Frustrated by seeing the partner doing the tasks incorrectly, the ill person may harp on trivial errors and details. How neatly clothes are to be folded, the way dishes are to be washed, the degree of exactitude necessary to balance a checkbook, how carefully a car is to be handled, the way a garden is to be maintained—all of these preferences can be infuriating to a person who can no longer carry them out and instead has to watch someone else's haphazard efforts.

For the caregiver, there is the pressure of trying to master the new roles while under the partner's critical scrutiny. Being told exactly how to fold a towel or write out a check can be irritating, and receiving reprimands instead of thanks can be enraging. The disabled partner may repeatedly undermine the caregiver's efforts to become comfortable with new roles such as cook, housecleaner, car mechanic, or financial manager.

Professionals and family members observing this dynamic around role changes can help by regularly supplying the missing appreciation which the ill person is unable to give to the caregiver. Statements like, "You did a great job mowing that lawn," may mean a great deal to someone who hears only about the uneven patches of grass she left behind. Offering supportive suggestions also helps the caregiver master new roles, since trying to learn from a critical and impatient partner is almost impossible. Even after some mastery is attained, the caregiver should still be cautioned to expect outbursts of anger. These explosions tend to have nothing to do with the quality of the effort exerted, but rather stem from the rage of lost control and stylistic differences in the way tasks are accomplished.

Maintaining Physical Intimacy

The degree to which a partner's body image is wounded is an important aspect of a couple's coping with illness. Limb amputation, colostomy, and breast removal are examples of changes in body image which may evoke intense grief or self-loathing. More subtle but still painful shifts in body image may also occur with open sores, severe weight loss, skin problems, and arthritic deformities. People experiencing such changes often try to avoid contact with the altered body part and to prevent others from having direct sight or contact. They may be reluctant to have their partners participate in their personal care out of fear that their revulsion will be shared. To guard further against this vulnerability, they may distance themselves from all forms of physical affection, often to the caregiver's hurt and bewilderment.

If alerted to this tendency in advance, caregivers may be able to avoid interpreting the ill person's aloofness as personal rejection or sheer obstinacy. They may be able to allow their partner time to grieve and to reach acceptance of their new appearance. In some instances, it may be possible for the caregiver to help the ill partner feel less self-loathing by slowly demonstrating their own acceptance. For example, many ill people say that simply being held gives them a profound sense of comfort and encourages them to begin accepting what has happened to their bodies.

Occasionally, however, caregivers do have difficulty accepting their partners' physical changes. Those who had been sexually enthusiastic prior to the illness may experience a dramatic loss of interest. For many people, caregiving and sexual attraction do not mix, especially when stool or urine-soaked clothing must be handled. Using substitute caregivers for such hands-on care tasks, when this is financially feasible, often helps caregivers with their sexual adjustment. In some instances, fears about causing pain or injury may further inhibit a caregiver's sexual expression. (See "Adapting to Sexual Changes," pp. 165–167.)

EXCESSIVE CAREGIVING

Many partners carry caregiving to an extreme. Whether appeasing their guilt or filling a need to feel useful, these caregivers reject chances to rest. They may do too much for the ill person, thereby keeping their partner in the sick role longer than necessary. They may deprive their partner of contact with other people in their need to be a martyr who does it all. They may work themselves into a state of exhaustion, inadvertently harming the person in their care. Awareness of these patterns often helps partners provide better care and preserve themselves.

Appeasing Guilt

Some caregivers feel that to go on enjoying life while their partner is suffering is contrary to the meaning of dedication. As a result, they deprive themselves of out-of-home activities and personal pleasures. Such individuals bear an unrelenting sense that they should be doing more for their partners, no matter how much help they have been providing. They tend to feel guilty when they go out on their own, even if their partner had no interest in coming along. Similarly, they may lose enthusiasm for eating if their partner's appetite is sparse, or they may cease taking walks if their partner is bound to a wheelchair. Unfortunately, these deprivations are often as detrimental to health as they are appeasing to guilt.

Wrongs committed in the past are another common source of guilt. Partners who feel the need to perform acts of penance are especially vulnerable to carrying their caregiving too far. For example, a husband who has been paying emotionally for an affair since early in his marriage may become servile as a caregiver, waiting on his wife hand and foot. He may forgo his own needs entirely, believing that this is fitting punishment for a wrong that could not be righted. If the ill partner participates avidly in this dynamic of guilt and punishment, family members and professionals may find that both partners rebuff any attempt to relieve the caregiver's self-imposed burden.

Another kind of guilt stems from forbidden feelings which a partner tries to suppress. One of the most common of these is anger at the partner for becoming ill. Although the caregiver knows rationally that the person could not help becoming ill, anger can arise in reaction to the immensity of the disappointment. For instance, a couple planning to embark on a cross-country trip in their new camper may find their plans terminated by the husband having a severe heart attack. Providing twenty-four-hour care instead of touring the country, the wife is likely to feel angry, no matter how loving their relationship or how clearly she acknowledges to herself that the heart attack is not her husband's fault. Guilt from suppressed anger is most detrimental when it prevents the partner from obtaining necessary rest or is expressed in subtle hostility.

Dislike for a partner whose personality has changed is another forbidden feeling. Some people become selfish when they get sick. It is deeply upsetting to have loved someone with an expansive personality who has become narrow and constricted as a result of illness. A wife may miss her husband as he used to be, and may try to stifle her dislike of him in his current state. Family members can provide valuable help by acknowledging these unappealing changes and voicing their own aversion. When this secret is out in the open, the partner feels less guilt.

Needing to Feel Useful

Having no other useful activity on which to focus, some partners seize upon caregiving to fill empty time and give their life meaning. The caregiving functions as something to do and talk about in a previously uneventful life. It may also yield appreciation from family members—which had been absent prior to the illness—as well as increase the frequency of their visits and calls. When it bestows a much-needed sense of importance, caregiving can be difficult to contain within reasonable boundaries.

One result is that the caregiver feels threatened when others point out improvements in the ill person's health or functional abilities. It is as if these gains detract from the caregiver's pivotal position. When a family member says, "Dad's walking a lot better this week than he was last week," his wife may retort with an onslaught of evidence to the contrary or a recounting of all the effort she expended for other aspects of his care. This need to focus on hardships rather than gains can be confusing to family members, unless they realize how much satisfaction the caregiver is deriving from displaying her competence and endurance.

A caregiver's need to keep her partner in a sick role can also produce roadblocks to the partner's improvement. Excessive care fosters excessive dependence. By providing unnecessary help, the caregiver takes away opportunities for stimulation, exercise, and practice of self-care skills. For instance, a man recovering from a stroke may have no chance to learn how to button his shirt on his own, if his wife always rushes over to rescue him from the frustration of trying.

Such situations are particularly difficult to unravel if the ill partner welcomes the excessive care. Family members and professionals may encounter determined resistance when they urge the caregiver to try to set limits on what she does and when they challenge the ill partner to try to increase his autonomy. Both partners may become angry at attempts to break the mutually satisfying cycle: "Please butt out. We were doing just fine here on our own."

One strategy is to ask the caregiver to envision what her sudden illness or hospitalization would mean for her partner. This question may help her recognize the degree to which she has encouraged, or at least failed to limit, her partner's dependence on her. She may be able to picture the problems family members would face trying to stand in her shoes: "You're right. No one in their right mind would do for your father what I do for him." She may be able to perceive that pulling back and prodding her spouse to regain as much independence as possible is actually the best way to take care of him.

Learning how to withhold help does not happen all at once. Partners may need to experiment with different approaches. For instance, when a man recovering from a stroke pleads for help buttoning a shirt, forcing him to tolerate his initial frustration requires a great deal of mental fortitude. The caregiver must firmly believe that letting him fumble promotes his rehabilitation. If he yells at her during his struggle, her belief may falter. A helpful technique in such situations is for the couple to agree in advance on a set number of minutes that the disabled partner will attempt to accomplish the task on his own. The caregiver then takes on the role of timekeeper rather than taskmaster. If he still needs help after this defined period of effort, the caregiver can take over without worrying that she is interfering with his progress.

Having Too Much Time Together

Another aspect of illness which affects partners is the frequency of contact required by the care. For couples whose relationships have survived largely on the basis of minimal contact, the addition of disabling illness to retirement can be markedly disruptive. The sheer amount of time spent together in the home may multiply to the point where both partners experience feelings of encroachment. As long-standing boundaries are violated, the losses in solitude and privacy can themselves produce irritability and conflict. The loss of buffers, such as recreational or volunteer activities, may uncover relationship problems previously masked by the couple's ability to avoid each other. Rather than attempting to mediate such conflicts, family members and friends can often do the greatest service by helping such couples recover some of their time separate from one another.

INADEQUATE CAREGIVING

Giving too little care can be just as detrimental as giving too much, but in different ways. Couples sometimes collude in not letting family members know how poorly the person in the caregiver role is functioning or how many risks they are both taking in trying to patch together a livable situation. Also, partners often have trouble talking to each other about death, and this in turn inhibits their ability to make necessary decisions.

Reversing Dependency

In some relationships, the distribution of power is skewed. One person assumes the role of unchallenged decision-maker and the other, that of compliant follower. Over time, the managerial partner establishes a parentlike relationship with the submissive partner, rather than a relationship of equals. This arrangement works successfully to the extent that both people are satisfied by their roles, one enjoying control and the other glad not to have it. If the more dependent person in such a couple becomes disabled, the partners may easily absorb the change into its ongoing pattern of interaction. If the parentlike person becomes disabled, however, the reversal of the dependency and the resulting shift in power can cause chaos in the relationship.

Upon losing the partner's protection, the more dependent person is likely to try to place other family members in the decision-making role vacated by the ill partner. Family members may suddenly find themselves responsible for two older people, one thwarted by illness and the other weakened by years of submitting to another's will. In these instances, it is often helpful if family members can hold back from taking over, despite the dependent person's pleas for them to do so. Caregiving may present a chance for that person to discover competence that had never before been exercised and abilities that were formerly overshadowed by the partner's need to dominate.

At first, the caregiver may experience sleeplessness and anxiety springing from the double tension from the tasks themselves and being in control for the first time. This person may abdicate responsibility when feeling overwhelmed, leaving the ill partner inadequately protected or stuck trying to handle care needs without necessary assistance. Conversely, the disabled partner is likely to suffer keenly the lost control and may insist on doing things which have become dangerous. Family members and professionals should privately allow each partner to vent their complaints about the other, as this may help release tension as one learns to compromise and the other learns to assert.

Facing Simultaneous Care Needs

When both partners need to give and receive care, problems can mount exponentially. Their joint caregiving may become mutually detrimental over time, yet they may be determined to go on making do within their remaining capacities. Older couples in these situations often try to keep their adaptations and compromises out of family members' view, fearing that nursing home placement for one or both of them would result if their true level of dependency on each other were to become known.

The systems of symbiotic helping evolved by couples can leave family members unaware of the extent of their care needs for years. For example, a woman with declining ability to use her hands may employ her intact memory to compensate for her partner's progressive memory loss, giving him step-by-step directives for the tasks she can no longer manage and he can no longer remember how to do correctly. Similarly, a man needing assistance with walking may use his eyes to help his visually impaired partner, while she uses her physical agility to help him get around. A couple's inventiveness in this regard tends to reflect the intensity of their motivation to remain together in their own home.

These interlocking systems may produce a reasonably safe situation, as long as the couple is able to remain together on a daily basis. If one of the partners is told that a week's hospital stay is needed for surgery, for instance, the couple may keep postponing the surgery without giving a sound explanation to family members. Knowing that the partner who stays home could not manage a week's survival independently, the couple may make excuses for the delay that seem stubborn or irrational to exasperated family members. Often, such situations explode when one of the partners has an emergency hospitalization and family members rapidly discover the frailty long concealed.

Another stressful situation for families is learning that the care of one partner is clearly threatening the welfare of the other. In these instances, family members may find it difficult to allow the couple the choice of remaining at home together. A man with cardiac problems may persist in picking his wife up off the floor after her frequent falls, despite his physician's warning against such lifting and his family's pleading not to endanger himself. His willingness to gamble with his health for the sake of keeping his wife home with him may greatly exceed his family's tolerance for these risks: "Dad, we've got to put Mom in a nursing home, or you'll end up having a heart attack."

These situations are worsened when the parent with greater care needs is resented by the adult children. They may become angry at their favored parent for sacrificing himself on behalf of the other: "Dad, what has Mom ever done for you? We're sick of seeing you suffer for her sake." Professional help may be needed for embittered adult children to contain such grievances and employ their concerns constructively, rather than add to the caregiver's distress. Since a parent's refusal to relinquish caregiving can stem from aspects of the marriage imperceptible to adult children, the professional's intervention in such instances may focus on helping them understand these hidden aspects of their parents' relationship.

Worrying About Who Will Die First

The dynamic of care between partners is often powerfully affected by their unspoken worry about what will happen when one dies before the other. Couples may go to elaborate lengths to avoid mentioning each other's death. This silence may in turn impede their ability to make decisions about the care situation and to plan effectively for the welfare of the partner most likely to be left behind.

A primary reason for silence about death is that discussing someone's demise makes the reality of losing that person painfully evident. No matter how sensible it is to explore jointly future possibilities, the need to deny death may be intense enough to stymie all discussion. With some couples, one of the partners repeatedly tries to start conversations about these concerns while the other just as vigorously evades them. With other couples, both partners contribute to the maintenance of the silence. Months can be spent lingering over important decisions, such as a move to a retirement home, which could have been resolved quickly if the essence of their private worries could have been revealed.

A diagnosis of cancer is one of the most common triggers of the need to talk about death. A man confronting a terminal diagnosis may feel urgent about taking steps to ensure his wife's financial and emotional well-being before he dies. With this underlying motivation, he may perceive several advantages to their moving to a retirement home, such as his being able to assist with the sale of their home and to invest the proceeds in order to ensure his wife sufficient income. In addition, he may want his wife to establish secure social routines to help diminish her loneliness after his death. Should the topic of his dying remain unmentionable between them, however, he would be unable to use these persuasive arguments to overcome his wife's resistance to leaving their long-term home.

Worry about having enough money after a partner's death can impede the caregiver's immediate self-care, as well as future planning. For example, a wife may resist hiring extra help, regarding the high hourly rates as too severe a drain on their life savings. When her son pleads with her to spend money to get some needed rest, she may be ashamed to tell him that she is too worried about her own future financial status to do so. Her son's attempts to persuade her, such as pointing out that the quality of care she provides is beginning to suffer, may only serve to isolate her further in her unmentionable fears.

A professional can allude to death without being inhibited by personal grief and may therefore be better able than family members to bring up these sensitive topics. For instance, if home care services are provided after a hospital stay, family members can request that a social worker visit the older couple to hold planning sessions with them. A professional can illuminate unspoken concerns through guided discussion, such as presenting end-of-life medical choices that the couple is likely to encounter. Finally voicing their dread, the couple may face a barrage of pent-up feelings. Allowing them to weep together, without rushing to stop their tears through comforting words, is often the most helpful response a professional can offer. After their emotions are released, the couple may be able to make substantial progress toward resolving their mutual worries.

Discussion of the event of death itself is of both practical and emotional value. A statement such as, "I want to die in my own bed, but it's okay to call an ambulance if you get scared," can release a partner from condemning herself later for her husband's dying in an intensive care unit. If various responses to medical emergencies are explored in depth, each partner's ability to make decisions on behalf of the other during a crisis can be immeasurably improved. Permission not to prolong the other's life through artificial means may especially bring relief. Finally, specific preferences for funeral arrangements can be clarified and the location of vital documents recorded.

Telling each other what they appreciate about each other are among the most important feelings likely to surface when a couple is released from the taboo of discussing dying. A husband may remark in front of his wife, "She gets short with me sometimes, but she's done a heck of a job taking care of me through all this." Such statements can help prevent the guilt otherwise felt for years after the partner dies. During bereavement, caregivers frequently remember and regret moments of impatience that occurred during the long haul of the illness. Similarly, guilt about finding another relationship later can be reduced if partners have the opportunity to express both gratitude for their years together and a hope for the surviving partner to experience satisfying companionship with someone else.

LESBIAN AND GAY COUPLES

Most older lesbian and gay couples have paid a high emotional price for living out their sexual orientation. Siblings and parents may have rejected them, or their families may be split concerning acceptance of their sexual orientation. Friends and employers may also have spurned them. As a result, gay men and lesbians often reach old age with keenly hewn survival skills and may cope with the trials of illness better than heterosexual individuals. They may have developed alternatives to the usual kinship networks, devoting themselves to friendships equivalent to family bonds in loyalty and affection.

Professionals and family members should try to be especially alert to the needs of lesbian and gay couples, since community services tend to be oriented toward heterosexual partnerships. This section surveys the needs of older lesbian and gay couples as caregivers, with particular attention to the problems they confront as sexual minorities.

Coping with Rejection from Families

The absence of family support when confronted with disabling illness can result in extreme bitterness for lesbian and gay couples. For instance, those who expressed their homosexuality after ending a long marriage may be scorned by their adult children. A daughter may refuse to meet her mother's lover, resisting such a profound change in her view of her parent. A son may become antagonistic toward his openly gay father, eliminating all contact or making hurtful remarks when they do see each other. As years pass and older lesbian and gay parents come to need help from their adult children, they may find that the rift has remained too wide and that they do not receive the same advocacy and assistance that other parents do. Rejection during this time of need tends to contain the added pain of bitterness for all the other rejections which may have transpired over a lifetime.

Occasionally, late-life care needs can present families with opportunities to heal these rifts. For example, a son may be forced to get to know his father's partner while sitting in an intensive care unit after his father's heart attack. Clocking many hours together in the waiting room, the two may talk at length for the first time. The son may discover qualities in his father's partner that he respects, as well as come to appreciate the caregiving tasks which the partner will be assuming.

Working together to ensure a smooth transition to home care may then become a unifying experience.

Accessing Resistant Medical Systems

One of the most painful predicaments that lesbian and gay couples encounter is nonacknowledgment by medical professionals when one of the partners is ill. Since such partners are not blood relatives or legal spouses, they are generally not accorded the recognition and support during medical crises extended to husbands, wives, and adult children. Hospital staff may refuse to release medical information or allow special visiting status to a gay or lesbian partner, irrespective of explanations about the nature of the bond with the sick person. Already vulnerable in reaction to the medical emergency, the partner may have difficulty asserting rights to have questions answered and contact assured. In contrast, the ill partner's brother or sister is likely to be allowed immediate access on the basis of a blood relationship, no matter how weak the actual bond between them.

One way that a lesbian or gay person can assure a partner's access to medical information during a future crisis is to sign a power of attorney for health care. This document designates a specific individual to handle health care decisions in the event that the signer of the document becomes incapacitated. In the absence of such a document, next of kin take legal precedence over lesbian or gay partners. Making these arrangements in advance of the occurrence of medical problems is advisable, despite a couple's natural reluctance to facing such choices.

Crossing the Language Barrier

Professionals tend to presume heterosexuality when they interview older people. Questions about marriage, children, and sexual activity are asked within the context of mainstream expectations. Opposite-sex pronouns are used when asking about intimate relationships. In contrast, when professionals omit heterosexual references, gay and lesbian people feel that the possibility for their existence has been allowed.

Using the term "partner," rather than asking about a husband or wife, signals that the professional is sensitive to the concerns of sexual minorities and is likely to act upon this sensitivity. The word "partner" may be foreign to heterosexual older people, but most understand that the term refers to longstanding relationships such as marriage. As a further benefit, avoiding the word "marriage" may allow heterosexual people to talk about living together without legal sanction, another area where people may hide unless the professional cues them that such relationships are acceptable.

Some older people in later-life same-sex relationships do not identify with the term "lesbian" or "gay." An older woman may develop a sexual relationship with a close woman friend, but not perceive herself as a lesbian or feel kindred with the community of sexual minorities: "I am in love with this friend of mine, that's all." Especially in current generations of older people, lifelong scorn toward sexual minorities can be a powerful block against using certain words or categorizing a love relationship as gay or lesbian. Professional tact with the use of labels is crucial when people do not want to define themselves as lesbian or gay. Watching for cues about how an older person defines a relationship is the best strategy for finding the appropriate language during discussions.

Refusing to Be Hated at Home

The personal nature of in-home care makes acceptance of lesbian and gay orientation by these workers more crucial than with other kinds of services. For instance, a man who admits a home health aide to his residence to assist his partner may quickly discover that the aide is repelled by their gay relationship. The aide's coldness or rejection may be so apparent that it becomes aversive for the couple to go on receiving help from this individual: "We'd rather fend for ourselves than to be hated in our own home." Some lesbian and gay couples attempt to conceal the nature of their relationship from potentially rejecting in-home workers, but end up feeling just as violated by having to hide in their own home. Many do without services to which they are entitled.

Professionals can be of concrete assistance by discussing these issues in their training of in-home workers. Providing them with opportunities to ask questions about sexual minorities and to work through any negative feelings is invaluable, given the myths and taboos surrounding homosexuality in American society. A supervisor who has discussed these issues with the staff is then in the position to assign the most tolerant workers when services are requested by lesbian or gay caregivers. A professional's sensitive advocacy in this regard is likely to spare a lesbian or gay couple from the intrusion of prejudiced strangers into their private realm.

Finding and Keeping Relationships

The quest for partners in later life is challenging for anyone whose mobility is compromised by physical problems, but lesbian and gay older people face added constraints. Their numbers are few; convenient meeting places are scarce. For instance, a man accustomed to finding partners in gay bars may be forced to give up this option because of medical prohibitions on his alcohol use and breathing cigarette smoke. Finding a partner in his neighborhood senior center may not be a feasible alternative. In addition, the emphasis on youthful attractiveness in some segments of the gay world may cause an older man to withdraw from social circulation altogether: "Who would want someone like me?" Organizations and support groups for older gays and lesbians are beginning to form in communities with large populations of sexual minorities.

For professionals, it is important to discard stereotypical views of the nature of gay and lesbian relationships. Contrary to commonly held images, the varieties of bonding are the same as within the heterosexual community, ranging from monogamous life-partners and nonmonogamous primary relationships to serial monogamy and episodic liaisons. Lesbian and gay life-partners confront issues similar to those described earlier for long-term heterosexual spouses, such as the disruption of retirement plans by a partner's becoming ill and role changes in response to illness. One positive difference is that same-sex couples may not have instituted separate breadwinner and housekeeper roles to the degree of their traditional heterosexual contemporaries, which can give them more flexibility when one of the partners becomes ill.

Professionals can be especially helpful to long-term lesbian and gay couples by urging them to obtain competent legal advice regarding issues of finances, inheritances, and funeral arrangements. For example, state laws are skewed toward the ability of blood relatives to contest wills when a gay or lesbian person leaves them out of an estate in preference to a partner. Since Living Wills and bank accounts with rights of survivorship are less vulnerable to legal challenge than wills, these options may be particularly attractive to gay and lesbian couples who anticipate familial interference in these matters.

Giving care to an ill partner challenges the coping skills achieved by the most harmonious couples, and can compound the difficulties which plague troubled relationships. When deaths of lifelong friends and losses of meaningful activities are added to caregiving stresses, a relationship can be strained to the breaking point. Professionals and family members should therefore not assume that a partner will provide daily care; rather, many factors which affect a couple's ability to cope with illness should be assessed. The viability of care arrangements should be evaluated when partners first assume these duties, as well as periodically throughout the caregiving process.

SUGGESTED RESOURCES

Articles

Barusch, Amanda, and Wanda Spaid. "Gender Differences in Caregiving: Why Do Wives Report Greater Burden?" *The Gerontologist*, 29 (1989), 667–676.

> Discusses possible explanations for the fact that wives tend to feel more burdened by caregiving than do husbands. Concludes with practice implications.

Cantor, Marjorie. "Strain Among Caregivers: A Study of Experience in the United States," *The Gerontologist*, 26 (1983), 597–604.

> Spouses were the highest risk group among the caregivers studied. All caregivers expressed emotional strain and negative impacts from sacrifices, but spouses in particular expressed a need for relief and respite.

Montgomery, Rhonda, and Edgar Borgotta. "The Effects of Alternative Support Strategies on Family Caregiving," *The Gerontologist*, 29 (1989), 457–464.

> Respite and education were found to reduce feelings of burden and to delay nursing home placement among adult children giving care to parents. In contrast, the same services for spouse caregivers encouraged nursing home placement.

Pruchno, Rachel, and Nancy Resch. "Husbands and Wives as Caregivers: Antecedents of Depression and Burden," *The Gerontologist*, 29 (1989), 159–165.

> Identified gender differences in depression and feelings of burden, with wives experiencing more depression and burden than caregiv-

ing husbands. Findings suggest that the demands of the caregiving role are experienced differently by men and women.

Quam, Jean, and Gary Whitford. "Adaptation and Age-Related Expectations of Older Gay and Lesbian Adults," *The Gerontologist*, 32 (1992), 367–375.

Respondents in the study reported acceptance of the aging process and high levels of life satisfaction, largely because of strong social support. Authors suggest the value of separate services for aging gay men and lesbians.

Wilson, Vanessa. "The Consequences of Elderly Wives Caring for Disabled Husbands," *Social Work*, 53 (1990), 417–421.

Found that wives have lower morale scores than husbands in tasks associated with caregiving. Discusses practice implications for addressing emotional and physical strain entailed by caregiving.

Books

Butler, Robert, and Myrna Lewis. *Love and Sex After Sixty: A Guide for Men and Women for Their Later Years* (New York: Harper and Row), 1988.

A readable guide to normal age-related physical changes and sexuality. Provides useful suggestions regarding new patterns of lovemaking, adjusting to the loss of partners, and the importance of nonsexual forms of intimacy.

Kehoe, Monika, ed. *Lesbians Over Sixty Speak for Themselves* (New York: Harrington Park Press), 1989.

Addresses social, economic and health problems, family and sexual relationships and involvement in the gay community. Based on a sample of over 100 women.

Macdonald, Barbara, with Cynthia Rich. *Look Me in the Eye: Old Women, Aging, and Ageism* (San Francisco, CA: Spinsters Ink), no date.

A powerful and moving series of essays on aging and ageism and how it feels to be an older lesbian in this society which values youth and heterosexuality.

Sommers, Tish. *Women Take Care: The Consequences of Caregiving in Today's Society* (Gainesville, FL: Triad Publishing), 1987.

Written in collaboration with Laurie Shields, her caregiver, the author poignantly describes the burdens and joys of caregiving, as well as the negative economic consequences for women in old age.

Organizations

Senior Action in a Gay Environment (SAGE). 208 West 13th Street, New York, NY 10011. (212) 741–2247.

Provides services to older lesbians and gay men, but in the New York area only. Maintains a list of other groups around the country and provides information for starting groups dealing with lesbian and gay aging. Newsletter available.

The National Senior Citizens Law Center (NSCLC). 1815 H. Street, N.W., Washington, DC 20006. (202) 887–5280

Publishes a pamphlet, "Medicaid Division of Assets and Rules for Long-Term Care," which explains the rules for avoiding spousal impoverishment.

3

Siblings Sharing the Care

Those who work with families are often struck by how vividly issues from early life can reemerge when a family reunites to provide care for a parent. Coming together to face a parent's illness requires a different kind of cooperation among siblings than organizing holiday dinners and family reunions. As they confront difficult decisions, siblings often find themselves replaying the family history with surprising force. This chapter identifies the most common conflicts which interfere with siblings' efforts to collaborate in caring for their parents, and suggests ways to overcome these divisions. The unfairness which frequently arises when siblings share the care can begin to be remedied, once siblings recognize how they may be using care dilemmas as a forum for expressing their old grievances.

SOURCES OF UNFAIRNESS IN CAREGIVING

To a remarkable degree, one person in a family tends to do most of the work in taking care of aging parents. Others may help from time to time, contributing their time and concern, but there is almost always a primary caregiver who shoulders the greatest share of the tasks. Siblings generally follow the path of least resistance, putting the bulk of the care on the family leader, the health care professional in the family, the lone sister surrounded by brothers, the one with the most unstructured time, the one who lives the closest, or the one most interested in protecting the inheritance. Unless such overloads are remedied, primary caregivers tend to become increasingly exhausted. Many become resentful of those not doing their share and yet may be unable to get them to be more involved.

FACTORS TO CONSIDER WHEN SIBLINGS SHARE THE CARE

1. Are worries about the inheritance straining arrangements for care? Are these strains unspoken or out in the open?
2. How geographically spread out are the siblings? Does only one live locally, or are the majority nearby?
3. Does a large financial disparity exist between siblings? Does one have far greater resources than the others?
4. What has been the nature of siblings' adult relationships with each other? Have they had minimal contact or active friendships with each other?
5. How obviously do the parents have a favorite or a scapegoat among the siblings? Have these feelings been carried over into adult life?
6. Is there a natural leader among the siblings? Has one mediated conflicts or consistently helped the others?
7. Is there a health care professional among the siblings? Do the others view this person as the one who should provide the care or make the decisions?
8. Is there a split in the family between those who want to take care of the parent at home and those who prefer to seek nursing home placement?
9. Does the family expect daughters to be caregivers in preference to the sons? Do the women accept this role?
10. What are the other obligations pressuring each sibling? Do some have young children or other relatives for whom they are already providing care?

Burdening the Family Leader

Having served as a mediator or source of guidance in past family crises, the family leader is naturally called into a central role during the crisis of a parent's frailty. If this family leader also happens to be a nurse, social worker, physician, or other health professional, siblings usually expect this person to apply these skills to their parent's care. A nurse may be told by her sister, "You know all about these medications and their side effects, so you drive over there every night and set up Mom's pills." The nurse is likely to collude with her sister's expectations by agreeing to manage the pills, rather than teaching her sister how to handle this task on her own.

A common trap for such caregivers is to end up taking care of other people all day at work and then all night at home. Rarely asking for help themselves, they may not know how to say "no" when family members lean on them too heavily. Because their role in the family is so ingrained, their siblings may see them as an endless source of strength, long beyond the point when outsiders can perceive their strain. Their role as perpetual caregivers may be so tied into their self-esteem that they fail to recognize their own exhaustion and they pass up chances for rest and personal renewal.

Expecting the Daughters to Do It All

Another form of overload occurs when siblings' expectations of each other follow traditional sex roles. A daughter's efforts to involve her brothers with the physical aspects of caregiving may be resisted by claims of unfamiliarity with "women's work." Her brothers may willingly handle tasks such as paying bills or driving the parents to appointments, while expecting her to take care of the daily housework. Sons also may resist helping with personal care tasks, such as toileting or bathing, because of their discomfort with intimate contact with a parent, or because it violates their family's customs about parent-son contact. (See "Women and Men as Caregivers," pp. 81–86.)

Parents often contribute to the maintenance of these roles. An older woman may never ask her son to vacuum her living room but may harangue her daughter for not doing it often enough. If the daughter is employed full time in addition to maintaining her own home and child care, she may feel enraged at her mother for failing to see that she is just as busy as her brother. If her brother takes advantage of their mother's bias and does not offer to do the household tasks, the daughter may deeply resent him for going along with the unfairness.

Spending Money Rather Than Time and Effort

Resentment may also surface when a sibling who has more money than the others prefers to purchase services rather than provide them personally. Those who lack spare money may feel that it is unfair for them to invest time and effort while a financially comfortable sibling simply writes out a check. The wealthier sibling may also try to grant rewards to family members in exchange for tasks: "I'll let you keep our extra car if you take Mom to her appointments with the doctor." Any attempt to substitute payments for hands-on care may be perceived by the others as an unjust escape from their mutual duties.

There may also be a disparity between the kind of contributions siblings can afford to make to a parent's life. A financially successful sibling may be able to take the parent out to dinner once a week, whereas a financially strapped sibling may be limited to scrubbing the parent's bathroom and kitchen weekly. Although the same number of hours may be devoted to the dinner as to the scouring, the sibling who performs the physical labor is likely to feel indignant about the other's capacity to make a more glamorous and enjoyable contribution to the parent's life.

Whose Time Matters More?

Occupational differences among siblings can add further strains around time, money, and status. Negative feelings may resurface about circumstances in the family history which allowed one sibling to advance further than the others: "It's because Dad put you through school that you've got more money than the rest of us." The fact that educational differences produce unequal options may be accepted as a wider social reality, but within the context of a family it may be infuriating.

These differences can lead to painful battles about whose time matters more. For example, a sibling with a higher-status occupation may view another's employment as expendable or adaptable to intrusions, expecting that person to be the one to help the parents with unpredictable daytime needs. For example, a lawyer may prevail upon his brother, a cab driver, to go over and help their mother when she has trouble lifting their father: "Since my time is worth so much more an hour, it makes sense for you to be the one Mom calls on during the day." In reality, the cab driver may have greater need for every hour he can work, because he earns so much less per hour. His anger at his brother may multiply in intensity as past and present resentments merge.

Other clashes about the value of time occur when those who are un-employed or engaged in homemaking are expected by their siblings to do more than their share: "After all, you don't have a job to go to every day. You can do Mom's laundry and take her shopping." Similarly, sib-lings who are self-employed can be vulnerable to claims on their time by those who assume they have full discretion over their work hours. Likewise, those who work at home may find that family members feel free to impose on them more than those protected by formal hours in a separate workplace.

Out-of-Town vs. Local

When out-of-town family members come for a visit, they often subject local siblings to a barrage of suggestions about how the care of their parents could be better managed. They offer ideas like, "Mom's so bored and lonely. Why don't you take her out for dinner more often?" The local helpers may retort with anger: "It's easy for you to come trot-ting into town for a week and tell us what to do, then disappear for months while we're stuck with all the work." Hurt may arise on both sides as the visitors wait in vain to hear that their ideas are useful and the local siblings resent that their efforts are not recognized and ap-preciated.

Guilt from having played a minimal role in their parent's care often feeds out-of-town siblings' need to tell the local caregivers what to do. In addition, shock at their parent's deterioration since their last visit may evoke feelings of helplessness and outrage: "Why didn't you tell us Mom's memory had gotten so bad?" Local siblings may not have no-ticed a decline that occurred gradually, no matter how obvious this change is to visitors. Urgency to "do something" about what has hap-pened to the parent may emerge as accusations: "Why haven't you brought her to the doctor? How could you let her live like this?"

Occasionally, conflicts arise because the older person revives in re-sponse to the visit of a rarely seen son or daughter, failing to display the difficult behaviors and symptoms that will resume as soon as the visitor leaves. Suddenly, the person walks more easily, gets dressed on her own, or retrieves memories more readily. The visitor may then berate the local sibling for having made things sound worse than they are: "Mom's not so bad. You exaggerated to make me feel sorry for you." It may be impossible for local relatives to persuade visitors that they are not seeing how arduous it has actually been to take care of the parent.

Finally, care tasks glimpsed for a week or two can seem less burdensome than when experienced daily on a protracted basis. Also, most care arrangements result from a slow succession of compromises as the older person's health deteriorates, rather than from clear choices. For example, a son may struggle for months to get his widowed father to accept a hired worker to clean his house, finally settling for his father's concession of permitting his bathroom and kitchen areas to be cleaned. His sister may then arrive in town for her annual visit and scold him for "letting Dad live like a pig" when she sees the cluttered house. Visiting family members often do not consider that they are witnessing the outcome of incremental adaptations rather than irresponsible care.

Resenting the "Favorite"

An especially painful obstacle to fairness in caregiving occurs when siblings believe that their parents have always favored one of them. In retaliation, they may try to load the majority of the care tasks on the "favorite": "Mom always gave you the best deal, so now you help her out." In another variation, a sibling who had always envied the love and attention going toward this favored person may take on too much of the care, hoping to win similar notice from the parents at last. Bitterness may arise if the parents fail to grant the long-awaited recognition: "I do so much for Dad, day after day, yet he still lives for Jeff's phone calls from Colorado."

Jealousy can also arise if older parents choose their "favorite" to serve as a money manager or to be assigned power of attorney. It can seem to the siblings that this proves once and for all that their parents have greater trust or love for this person than for them. Try as they might, the parents may be unable to convince their other adult children that these money-management tasks were assigned on the basis of factors other than favoritism. They may also try in vain to reassure the others that their designating a money manager does not mean that this person will receive more than a rightful share of the estate.

Worrying about the Inheritance

How extensively to drain the parents' life savings for care expenses is a common area of contention. For example, a daughter may regard hourly payments to her mother's in-home helper as a waste of the future inheritance, preferring that she and her brother each take on half the care tasks themselves. Her brother may prefer to protect his time, claiming that their mother's money should be spent on her care. As their mother's condition worsens, the daughter may insist on keeping their mother in her own home to prevent the house from being sold to pay for nursing home expenses. Her brother may oppose her: "I'd rather our whole inheritance be blown on the nursing home than having to check on Mom every day, run all her errands, make sure she's taking her medicines, and worry about her all the time."

A sibling may decide to handle duties like these singlehandedly, both to protect an inheritance and to express dedication to a parent. In doing so, this person is likely to feel she deserves a larger share of the inheritance than siblings who are not helping: "I'm doing most of the work, so I should get most of the money." Unless her mother alters her will to reflect her greater time contribution, the daughter may boil inside each time she spends a Saturday morning cleaning her mother's house while her siblings are home relaxing. (See "Who Gets What," pp. 111–112.)

BUILDING ON FAMILY STRENGTHS

Achieving communication, rather than resolution, may be the most productive goal for siblings trying to join together in taking care of their parents. Having everyone see things the same way and agree on all the details is usually impossible. Instead, understanding and acknowledging each other's point of view may go a long way towards smoothing out differences and building on the strengths each person brings to the situation.

Family leaders often have to learn how to give up control over the care situation and to accept a less than perfect job from the others in the family. By pointing out the tasks which can be reasonably delegated to siblings, professionals can sometimes hasten the process of letting go: "Your sister's not a nurse, but she can certainly learn how to change your mother's sterile dressing. Then you won't have to drive over there every morning." Many family leaders become accustomed to getting things done their own way and they need prodding in order to recognize how much extra work they have taken on for the sake of retaining control. Allowing their siblings to do the best they can and learn new skills leaves the family leader free to get adequate rest and time away from caregiving.

Out-of-town and local siblings can prevent disputes by acknowledging their divergent perspectives prior to encountering them. It is particularly important for out-of-town family members to refrain from criticizing the care until they have gathered more information and stood in their siblings' shoes; likewise, local siblings need to realize their advantage in having been able to adjust incrementally to what visitors must face all at once. Professionals can help by reminding local caregivers that their siblings' anger is most likely at the older person's deterioration rather than at them. Emphasizing that all of the care dilemmas do not have to be resolved during the concentrated time when the family is reunited may further reduce the pressure.

When necessary, a natural logic to dividing up care tasks can be invoked. Certain errands, such as bringing over and organizing medications, tend to be easiest for the family member who lives the closest. Those who live farther away often help most efficiently by taking on assignments that can be done in their own home, such as preparing frozen meals or making advocacy phone calls. Those with back injuries or other physical limitations may need to confine themselves to telephone check-up calls and serving as phone liaison with professionals involved in the older person's care. Others who have their hands full with young children may be able to fit tasks for the older person into their other errands, such as grocery shopping for two households at once. A handy person in the family may prefer to be responsible for the upkeep of the parent's home, just as an accountant in the family may find paying the parent's bills a comfortable form of contribution.

Family members tend to vary in what they regard as easy or burdensome. Some family members find it less intrusive on their lives to provide help in predictable blocks of time, such as two or three hours of yard work every Saturday, rather than sporadic forms of assistance. Those who dislike regular commitments may prefer to take on needs that crop up intermittently, such as visits to the doctor. An adult child who has had a close, warm relationship with a parent may be able to perform intimate tasks more easily than one who has been alienated from the parent. Tasks that do not require face-to-face contact may give an emotionally distant sibling a chance to contribute to the family without first having to work through accumulated turmoil from the past. Cultivating preferences and avoiding aversions usually produces better care for parents than trying to go against such feelings.

The degree of psychological burden or vigilance that accompanies a particular duty is a factor which should be given special prominence. Although certain tasks involve minimal time and effort, they may weigh on the mind of the person responsible for them. Someone who volunteers to "stay available" in case the older person falls may find that the requirement of telephone accessibility becomes more burdensome over time. The person never feels free. Others in the family should recognize this captivity as a significant contribution.

Recognition, thanks, and appreciation may make a big difference for the person in the family doing most of the work. Whether by choice or default, imbalances in the workload may continue, and it is vital that others in the family concede that this is so. A brother can say to his sister, "I mow Mom's lawn every Saturday, but you're pretty much doing everything else. Thank you for doing so much." Words like these often go unspoken in families, because people think they are unnecessary. In truth, they may give someone renewed energy for what lies ahead.

In many instances, words alone cannot diminish a sibling's anger at being "stuck" with all the work. A daughter may feel justified in paying herself out of her mother's checking account for hours spent cleaning, cooking, and running errands, reasoning that her efforts will not be fairly compensated later and that this is the only way she can keep from resenting her brothers. Others in the family may view these payments as stealing, especially if the checks are written secretly. A family meeting is often necessary to bring divergent feelings and opinions out into the open and to address injustices directly.

FAMILY MEETINGS

Holding a family meeting may help siblings divide up the care of their parents more fairly. Many families benefit from having a professional conduct the first meeting, but some are able to hold productive meetings on their own if made aware of a few precautions. In either case, asking family members to review the section, "Sources of Unfairness in Caregiving," before the meeting may help them recognize how each contributes to the unfairness. This section will portray the circumstances in which family meetings are most useful and offer a model for conducting them effectively.

Before the Meeting

Simply announcing the need for a family meeting and setting a date is often fruitless. Unless considerable effort is exerted, a meeting intended to relieve overloaded caregivers could consist solely of participants who are already contributing to the care. The very barriers that have kept the others uninvolved will tend to keep them away from a discussion meant to draw them in. For this reason, much of the effort involved in a successful family meeting is often invested prior to the meeting.

Phoning each of the siblings and listening to their concerns is an essential first step in planning a family meeting. The goal is to find out why certain members of the family have avoided doing their share and to determine the extent to which historic resentments are impeding cooperation. In some families, old conflicts are so bitter that bringing everyone together for a meeting would be more destructive than helpful. Explosions may erupt which would not have occurred in more scattered discussions, and fragile forms of cooperation may be harmed. When siblings cannot talk without being verbally abusive, it may be more constructive for professionals to help resolve disputes behind the scenes or simply convey information between family members.

In talking with the siblings, professionals may discover that some are uninvolved because of grief rather than resentment or lack of concern: "I just can't stand to see Dad in that condition. He's always been a rock in my life, someone I could depend on." Feeling that the person who is needing so much care has already been lost, they may avoid visiting or even asking the primary caregivers how they are doing. When a professional suggests that they may be able to help with the care without coming into direct contact with their parent, they may be glad to attend a family meeting.

Other siblings may claim that they did not realize that the primary caregiver needed their help: "Our older sister has always held everything together in the family. We never think about her getting tired or stressed out." They may respond to the call for a family meeting with gratitude, saying that they need concrete suggestions on how to support this sibling whose strength they take for granted and whose skills in this area seem so much better than theirs.

A common question during the planning process is whether or not to include the older person. The answer depends upon the purpose of the meeting and the private agendas likely to underlie the discussion.

If the primary caregivers need to express their weariness, they would not be able to do so in front of their parent. Among siblings still competing for a parent's affection, a parent's presence may provoke unrealistic contests over who can offer the most help, instead of more reasoned planning and negotiation. On the other hand, including the older person in a practical discussion of care dilemmas may help her recognize the family's physical and emotional limits and permit her to become involved in finding ways to reduce the strain.

When the older person is not to be included in the meeting, some family members may ask professionals to conceal the fact that it is taking place: "Let's not tell her about the meeting. She'll think we're ganging up on her." Although such concealment may seem convenient in the short run, professionals expecting to have further contact with the older person can spare themselves and family members later awkwardness by advising against keeping the meeting secret. Instead, a family meeting can be described to the older person straightforwardly: "We're holding a meeting next week to see how each person in the family can be of help to you. We'll let you know what we figure out." Worried about being a burden to their children, most older people have no desire to hear this kind of discussion, but appreciate being informed.

The timing and location of a family meeting is often pivotal, if these factors exclude some family members while making it easier for others to attend. Careful consideration in setting up these arrangements establishes an overall stance of fairness. For instance, if the meeting is held at the home of a family leader, the others may resent this reinforcement of the existing power dynamic. Holding the meeting at the home of a family member who has felt peripheral to the caregiving may have the effect of drawing this person into a more central role.

Conducting the Meeting

At the outset, the person conducting the meeting should remind everyone present that the purpose is to improve the current care situation rather than to resolve longstanding family issues. Handing out copies of the following model structure for family meetings, along with the "Family Plan for Task Delegation" on p. 77, may help the family stay focused on issues pertaining to the care situation.

The meeting begins with each person writing an individual wish list, describing the problems they are experiencing and their ideas for how these problems can be solved. The discussion leader should instruct family members to write their suggestions in clear, measurable terms. For instance, instead of writing, "I wish I could be relieved of doing Mom's housework once in a while," a daughter should write, "I wish I could take a week off from Mom's housework once a month." These lists immediately point the discussion toward improving the situation, rather than allowing the family to become mired in complaining about how bad things have been. The call for specific terms also avoids global statements which tend to feed conflicts, and thus gives the family a basis for constructive discussion.

A STRUCTURE FOR FAMILY MEETINGS

1. *Identify the problems*
   - Each family member makes an individual wish list of ways the situation could be improved.
   - Pass the personal lists around and identify areas of conflict and agreement.
   - Make a general list of problems and conflicts.

2. *Exchange solutions*
   - Family members trade favors and solutions back and forth until some semblance of fairness is found.

3. *Write out a time-limited plan for task delegation*
   - Record what each family member has offered to do and how often each task will be carried out.
   - Set a date for revising this plan after a brief trial period.

From Wendy Lustbader and Nancy R. Hooyman, *Taking Care of Aging Family Members* (New York: The Free Press, 1994). Copyright © 1994 by Wendy Lustbader and Nancy Hooyman; copyright © 1986 by The Free Press.

Next, the personal lists are passed around or read aloud. This process may result in some problems being resolved spontaneously. For example, a brother may say to his sister, "I didn't know you felt so bad every time I took Mom out to dinner. Why don't you come along with us on my tab, since you work so hard on her housework?" In many instances, recognition of extra effort, along with some sort of concrete compensation, relieves pent-up resentment.

	Who Helps	How Often	Notes on Trades
FAMILY PLAN FOR TASK DELEGATION **Suggestions for Deciding and Dividing Tasks**			
Grocery shopping			
Laundry			
Bill paying			
Check-up calls			
Yard work			
Trips to doctor			
Meal preparation			
House cleaning			
Medicine setups			
Random errands			

Signatures:

_____

_____

_____

The leader's primary role during a discussion of wish lists is to maintain the family's focus on identifying problems, rather than trying to solve them. A large piece of paper taped to a wall can serve as a way to keep track of the different points of view. Tasks which family members want reassigned should be posted, as well as the terms of any spontaneous agreements. Repeatedly, the leader may need to stop side conversations and draw attention back to the wish lists, an arduous responsibility in talkative families. Most importantly, the leader should make sure that each person gets a chance to explain their wish list.

In guiding the meeting into the next phase, the leader should first select the most solvable problems. Allowing the family to achieve a few simple successes permits skeptical family members to feel more confidence in the process and gives the family a sense of unity before tackling the more difficult problems. The strategy to be emphasized is that compromise is a give-and-take process; favors must be traded and consideration must be reciprocal. For example, a brother may ask his sister, "What can you give me in return if I take over Mom's housework once a month to give you a week off?" His sister may reply, "I'll stop complaining. I won't nag you to do anything else." Weary of the nagging, her brother may regard her offer as a satisfying trade.

The third phase, writing out the plan, can be carried out while the bartering winds down. For each listed task, the name of the family member who has volunteered to take responsibility for it should be recorded, along with a specific notation of how often this task will be accomplished. At the bottom of the page, each family member should sign their name as a statement of their commitment to this process of attaining fairness. Signatures confer added dignity and power to the written plan that may help ensure that participants remain true to their word. As soon as possible following the meeting, each family member should receive a copy of the plan.

In the relief of expressing themselves and resolving conflicts, some family members may offer to take on more tasks than are practical for them in their day-to-day lives. Warning participants of this tendency can help them be more realistic. Most families benefit from a trial period when the plan can be tested and unworkable commitments identified. Predicting that the initial plan is likely to need adjustment sets the family up for successful revisions later, rather than disappointed expectations. Choosing a specific day and time when a follow-up meeting will be held clearly establishes the trial period and allows the family to muster the patience and flexibility necessary for true experimentation.

Joining together to take care of an ill parent can give siblings an enduring feeling of strength and confidence. When siblings do not manage to achieve cooperation, caregiving can worsen old rivalries and produce fresh bitterness. Trying out some of the suggestions discussed in this chapter may provide a conflicted family with the means to resolve their differences, or at least may help them to do a better job taking care of someone to whom their lives are bound in common.

SUGGESTED RESOURCES

Articles

Brody, Elaine. "Parent Care as a Normative Family Stress," *The Gerontologist*, 25 (1985), 19–30.

> Provides a framework for understanding the dynamics of the child-parent caregiving relationship and implications for social policy.

Cicirelli, Victor. "A Comparison of Helping Behavior to Elderly Parents of Adult Children with Intact and Disrupted Marriages," *The Gerontologist*, 23 (1983), 619–625.

> Adult children with disrupted marriages (divorced, widowed, remarried) gave less help, perceived lower parental needs, had fewer filial obligations, and were more limited in helping, primarily due to job responsibilities, than those with intact marriages.

Cicirelli, Victor. "Siblings as Caregivers in Middle and Old Age," in Jeffrey Dwyer and Raymond Coward, ed., *Gender, Families and Elder Care*, (Newbury Park, CA: Sage), 1992, 84–101.

Book

Steinmetz, Suzanne. *Duty Bound: Elder Abuse and Family Care* (Newbury Park, CA: Sage), 1988.

> Presents findings from a survey of adult children regarding the causes and consequences of abuse and neglect of parents.

Recognizes the role that caregiver stress and burden play in precipitating such behavior.

Organizations

Children of Aging Parents. 1609 Woodbourne Road, Suite 203A, Levitown, PA 19057. (215) 945–6900.

This organization provides starter information for those first becoming caregivers, and a matching service for people starting a support group. They also offer workshops for the general public, printed materials, and a bimonthly newsletter.

Family Service America, Inc. 11700 West Lake Park Drive, Milwaukee, WI 53224. (414) 359–1040

FSA is a network of nonprofit counseling agencies serving families throughout the US and Canada. Their member agencies provide individual and family counseling for caregivers, as well as other services. Contact the national office for local referrals and information.

4

Special Considerations in Caregiving

Women perform most of the hands-on, personal care for older relatives. When men assist with caregiving, they tend to help with paying bills, home repairs, and giving rides to appointments and errands. Awareness of the different strengths and weaknesses that women and men bring to the caregiver role allows other family members and professionals to tailor their support to fit a family's needs. This chapter also considers the special needs and distinctive abilities of grandchildren, stepchildren, only children, and in-laws, as well as people in their sixties and seventies who are taking care of parents in their eighties and nineties. Recognizing which dilemmas are situational, rather than personal, helps determine what can be changed and what must be endured.

WOMEN AND MEN AS CAREGIVERS

Many women work all day at jobs outside the home and then come home to work all evening at housework and caregiving. In families with traditional sex roles, husbands and brothers come home from their jobs and feel entitled to put their feet up and rest after a hard day's work. Most women feel no such entitlement, even if they have worked the same number of hours outside the home. For them, to be a "good wife" or a "good daughter" means taking care of the men in the family as well as the children and elders. While the men eat and rest, they cook, clean, and take care of others' needs.

When an older relative becomes ill and extra tasks are added to this pattern, a woman may find herself overwhelmed. Simply stated, there may not be enough time in the day to accomplish all that is demanded of her. In desperation, she may appeal to her husband or brother for help: "Look, I can't do all the housework, run all the errands, go to work every day, and still take care of Mom. I can't tear myself into a hundred pieces." Instead of feeling sympathetic, men in traditional families may view the woman who says, "I can't," as deficient, ridiculing her for not measuring up to their standard of boundless womanhood. But the worst pain comes from women blaming themselves for not being able to do it all.

Women in the Work Force

It is estimated that at least 60 percent of all working-age women will be employed outside the home by the year 2000, yet women continue to provide the majority of the care to children and aging family members.[1] Women earn considerably less than men on the average and fill a higher proportion of low-status jobs, which often do not permit the flexibility of taking time off during the day to tend to a sick child or parent. Even when such flexibility is granted, pay is deducted for missed hours. Lower-status jobs may also mean close supervisory scrutiny of how sick time is used, forcing a woman to feign illness as a cover for helping a family member.

Women in higher-status positions may possess greater worktime flexibility, which allows adjustments for caregiving demands. Ironically, however, using this flexibility may place women at a disadvantage for promotions and other types of recognition, when juxtaposed to male colleagues who do not take time off for caregiving. Women will tend to drop a project at work to attend to family needs, while men more easily insist that they are too busy. Managers find that caregiving employees often have more instances of lateness, absenteeism, excessive telephone use, and unscheduled time off from work than employees without such responsibilities.[2]

Increasing numbers of women have been delaying childbirth until after they have established themselves in careers. This means that their parents may be needing their help just as they are immersed in coping with the demands of juggling a career and the care of young children. In contrast, their mothers and grandmothers frequently faced caring for their parents after their own children were grown. Although women with established careers may be able to command higher salaries and higher-status jobs, giving them more financial options and worktime flexibility, they may struggle just as intensely as ever with the inner conflicts entailed by all of this juggling.

Fortunately, some employers are making changes to accommodate the greater number of caregivers among their employees. Supportive policies such as permitting check-up calls, providing flexible hours, and allowing employees to use their sick time for child or elder care can greatly improve the lives of employed caregivers. For instance, making quick check-up calls to an ill partner or parent at home may actually increase a worker's productivity, if she is less distracted once she has been reassured that her loved one is safe. The right to use sick time for ill family members, regardless of their age, enables a worker to take planned sick leave for a relative's care following surgery, rather than having to feign her own illness and take time off without giving adequate notice.

Employed women who are also primary caregivers often end up feeling they are not doing any job well. They may try to resolve such conflicts by changing jobs or reducing their hours, but such efforts do not address their problems at the source. The reality is that caregiving and employment outside the home do not mix well, unless employers implement supportive policies, men assume their share of workload at home, and affordable options are available for substitute care during the workday and on weekends.

Women's Work and Men's Work: Letting Go of Traditional Roles

Traditional roles often imprison both men and women. For many women, hiring in-home workers or using community services feels like an admission of failure. Accepting help violates their image of themselves as strong and competent women. They may need emphatic encouragement to take care of themselves: "Let's face it. You're not sleeping at night, and you look terrible. You've got to take some time for yourself." Professionals should put a priority on helping such women recognize the line between doing their utmost and threatening their own health and well-being.

Hearing other women in similar situations testify to the impossibility of doing it all is one of the best ways for women to free themselves from unrealistic standards. For instance, attending a caregiver support group may enable a woman to stop condemning herself for saying "no" to excessive demands on her time and nurturance: "When I realized that all the other women in the group had someone helping them clean the house, I stopped kicking myself for not being a wonder woman."

Attempting to involve husbands and brothers in caregiving, rather than following the path of least resistance, is another professional imperative. When assisting families with organizing their division of care tasks, professionals can suggest to the men in the family that they try to learn skills which cross the lines of traditional sex roles: "George, maybe you could take over washing the sheets when your mother wets the bed, so your wife will have one less thing to do in the morning before she goes to work." At times, suggestions originating from someone outside the family are more easily accepted than those from siblings or partners.

Men who grew up with traditional roles tend to feel demeaned by what they see as women's work. Pushing a grocery cart or folding laundry may violate their sense of what it is to be a man. Attempting to talk a man out of these feelings by claiming that "times have changed" is more likely to inspire his wrath than alter his feelings. Such reactions tend to be emotionally complex, having been forged during childhood and reinforced in adulthood by like-minded peers.

When traditional men abruptly become caregivers or widowers, lack of familiarity with "women's work" often leaves them feeling inept and overwhelmed. Grocery shopping, mending, laundry, cooking, and cleaning require attention to a host of details which can be bewildering to beginners. After years of having these tasks performed for them by women, these men often find themselves lapsing into helpless passivity while housework piles up all around them. Having too much to learn at once, they throw up their hands and wait for a sister, daughter, or female neighbor to rescue them.

Traditional men also tend to experience conflict with their sisters when their parents need care. They are often accused of not doing their share of the daily menial tasks, such as changing soiled bedding, scrubbing the bathtub, or doing the laundry. If they contribute at all, they usually prefer to handle the bill paying or the driving, or to take their parent out to dinner. Expecting their sisters to take care of the situation comes naturally, since they have always relied on women in the family for these basic aspects of life. Yet their sisters may view parent care as a duty which should be shared equally, no matter how uncomfortable men feel with the "women's work" that dominates caregiving.

Expressing sympathy with a traditional man's feelings may be the

best starting point in these situations, even though this is usually difficult for an angry or frustrated sister to do. For instance, she can say to
her brother, "I know you feel humiliated pushing a grocery cart. To
you, grocery shopping just isn't what a man does." She can go on by
detailing all the tasks burdening her and then ask her brother to
choose those which feel the least demeaning to him. This is far more
effective than trying to tell a traditional man what to do, an approach
which tends to evoke resistance to being controlled by a woman.
Giving him the room to choose among a list of tasks allows him to save
face and exert some control. He may surprise his sister later by con-
fessing enjoyment in folding laundry or a willingness to learn how to
cook special meals for their mother.

Teaching a traditional man household tasks without demeaning
him requires respect for how profoundly lifelong sex roles can influence both perception and self-concept. For instance, a woman may
take for granted the ability to perceive dirt, thinking her brother is
being obstinate when he fails to clean under a dresser or in the corners
of a kitchen floor. It may not occur to her that he does not see what she
sees. Similarly, a man who is skilled with a table saw and an electric
drill may fumble at first with a vacuum cleaner and a washing ma-
chine, needing his sister to suppress any impulse toward mockery as
he learns to operate these unfamiliar machines.

Supporting Male Caregivers

For men socialized to suppress their feelings, giving care to an ill family member can be emotionally trying. For instance, the impulse to
weep arises naturally around a person who is suffering pain or humiliation from an illness. Stifling this impulse takes its toll. Unable to release sorrow or frustration through tears, some men explode in rages
which they barely understand. They then feel tortured by guilt for having yelled at an ill person who could not help what was happening or
having berated another family member who was only wanting to offer
assistance. Others get increasingly depressed as their sorrow accumulates and is permitted no outlet.

Having someone to talk to makes a great difference for any care
giver. Ideally, a confidante listens without making judgments and gives
the caregiver a place to express feelings which cannot be spoken elsewhere. In the generations currently serving as caregivers, women tend
to have close female friends to whom they regularly divulge their
struggles, while men are much less likely to have such intimate friends.

Many have their wife as their sole confidante, leaving them utterly isolated when they need someone else to complain to while serving as their partner's caregiver.

Recognizing that rage is often disguised sorrow and that depression is often stifled heartbreak can be immensely helpful to those trying to assist male caregivers. When a daughter notices a few tears in her father's eyes, she can say, "Dad, go ahead and cry if you feel like it. You've got so much to deal with right now." Hearing his feelings acknowledged out loud may help a man attain the release of weeping; at the very least, it will put a name to his emotions. Later, when no one is around to evoke the shame he learned in boyhood, he may be able to cry.

Making the most of time alone with an isolated male caregiver is another valuable response. An out-of-town sister visiting a brother who is serving as the primary caregiver for their mother should give him every chance to talk about his dilemmas and air his complaints. Instead of rushing to offer suggestions, family members who dedicate themselves to listening may be able to induce a brother or a father to express buried feelings. Nothing may change outwardly, but a male caregiver who is able to get sorrow off his chest may feel more energy and patience.

As members of a small minority, male caregivers deserve recognition for their efforts. Becoming more expressive emotionally and learning new roles are not easy attainments in the midst of already difficult situations and in the face of lifelong patterns. Although some men move easily into giving care to aging family members, most have to grapple with challenges for which their prior life experience has not equipped them.

ONLY CHILDREN

Adult only children experience caregiving differently than those with siblings to share responsibilities. Their feeling of being alone can be pervasive—of having no one to complain to, to express worries with, or even to resent for not doing more. They may have more difficulty coping with their aging parents' frailty and mortality, realizing that with their parents' deaths they will be totally alone, without immediate family. This awareness of being alone in the face of care tasks can result in futile attempts to be all things to their parents.

Those who became their parents' sole offspring because a brother or sister died may have a still greater sense of duty. In other instances, a sibling may have become unavailable to the parents due to mental incapacity, jail sentence, or longstanding alienation from the family. Left behind, the surviving or available adult child often bears the weight of having to compensate for the missing sibling. Filling in for this kind of absence can feel especially burdensome when the person feels guilt from having survived or having had a better life than the missing sibling.

Regardless of how one becomes an adult only child, relationships with parents tend to be intense without siblings as buffers. Often, the singularity of focus can function as a positive force, with no siblings to dilute the parents' appreciation and support. Caregiving may become an opportunity to express gratitude for this closeness. The paradox is that adult only children may feel bound by this very devotion to defer their own needs too extensively while taking care of their parents. For example, they may agree to their parents' moving near them at retirement, even when they prefer the privacy afforded by geographic distance. The very warmth of these relationships can make adult only children feel that they do not have a right to set limits when their parents need them in later life.

Conversely, adult only children who manage to maintain boundaries may feel they are not doing enough for their parents, especially if a sizable inheritance awaits them. The prospect of the inheritance may quietly dominate their contacts with their parents. Aware that they will be sole heirs, adult only children often feel that their sacrifices must be commensurate with the size of these resources. They may feel compelled to avoid putting their parents in a nursing home at all costs, perhaps by bringing their parents to their homes against their partners' wishes or pursuing other equally stressful options.

When adult only children have long-standing mates, their partners may be more involved in caregiving than those of adult children with siblings. In recognition of the intense relationship with the parents, these partners may make special efforts to be close to their in-laws. In the most fortunate instances, their in-law relationships may approximate those of biological children. The adult only children and their partners can then collaborate on care decisions much as siblings do, taking turns with time-consuming tasks and offering each other ongoing emotional support.

More frequently, partners of adult only children do not develop relationships of equivalent strength with the parents, but instead resent the closeness, time, and energy devoted to them. A husband may insist, "I married you, not your parents," disliking his wife's daily contact with her parents. He may feel intruded upon by lengthy visits and phone conversations, comparing these to the relatively infrequent visits and calls from his parents.

Grandchildren can also be drawn into the fray. Contacts with them are often similarly asymmetrical, with expectations that they will write, call, or visit this one set of grandparents more than the set who have other grandchildren. Grandchildren can find themselves in intensified roles that approximate those of only children, even if they have siblings with whom to share the additional expectations. They may feel equivalent affection for both sets of grandparents, but they may feel forced to extend themselves to this one set, perhaps hurting the other grandparents' feelings.

Efforts to compensate for the absence of other children and grandchildren in their parents' lives and to be fair in contacts with in-laws can produce overwhelming pressures on adult only children. Their free time may be filled with obligations to relatives, which leave them feeling that they cannot do enough for either side of the family. These conflicts are heightened if the parents move nearby at retirement or into the family's home after a medical crisis. Resentful of this encroachment on their lives, their partners may withdraw, making little effort to relate to the parents or to assist with extra work. As a result, adult only children may be left feeling more alone than ever.

Adult only children providing care at the expense of their own needs may benefit from professional encouragement to use community resources and to accept assistance from outside helpers. Professionals can also work with adult only children to help them identify realistic limits to their responsibilities and to maintain interests outside of caregiving. Referral for individual counseling may be the best way for them to resolve feelings about their parents' aging, inheritance pressures, and the absence of immediate family ties. Similarly, disputes with partners over how to handle the parents' needs may be best handled through referrals to couples counseling.

GRANDCHILDREN

Two generations removed, grandchildren often possess greater tolerance for their grandparents' idiosyncracies than do their parents. Grandparent relationships are generally not complicated by past authority conflicts, and warm childhood memories of the grandparents may contribute to bonds of affection. For these reasons, grandchildren often approach caregiving with an energy and optimism which greatly exceeds that which their parents are able to supply.

The ages of grandchildren at the time that grandparents need care is one of the key factors in these relationships. Even though young grandchildren are unable to assist directly with the care, their naturalness and spontaneity may bring pleasure to the grandparents and some relief to the parents. For instance, young children tend to be uninhibited by a grandparent's severe memory loss. The physical affection given readily by toddlers can fulfill a grandparent's need to be touched and accepted, especially when cognitive changes have caused others to withdraw from such contact. In addition, the simplicity of games enjoyed by young children may fall within a confused grandparent's range of abilities.

Grandparents and school-age grandchildren may not blend as easily, due to differences in mobility, activity level, and noise tolerance. Caregivers in the middle generation may find themselves torn between the needs of older and younger family members, especially when they compete for listening time and help with transportation. A woman returning home from her job may be greeted by her twelve-year-old daughter asking for a ride to a basketball game and her seventy-two-year-old mother asking for a ride to a club meeting. Using car pools, taxis, or occasionally paying someone else to drive is often preferable to making a forced choice between these types of conflicting needs.

Needs may also converge usefully for these generations. A grandparent who is alone all day may celebrate a grandchild's return home from school, with the child gaining the security and comfort of being welcomed home. Often, a grandchild's assistance with incidental needs in the afternoon can be instrumental for an older person who would otherwise have to wait until working parents returned home. Help with finding misplaced glasses, opening jar lids, or retrieving things from hard-to-reach places are examples of tasks which children can handle.

Some parents try to protect their children from caregiving, believing that children should be free to play or do homework after school. Structuring a grandchild's help into regular hours and offering extra allowance for this time both frees the child to plan other activities and acknowledges the importance of these duties: "You'll help Grandma from 3:00 to 4:00 every day, right after you get off the bus. Do whatever she needs, and then you're free. We'll raise your allowance, because Grandma will be relying on you." Allowing the grandchild to share this assignment with neighborhood friends or cousins can make it more pleasurable, as well as lend status to the grandchild's helping role.

Including grandchildren in care decisions which affect their lives is another valuable strategy. When they are involved from the start with difficult choices, rather than learning of decisions after the fact, they are less likely to resent changes which impinge on them, such as missed vacations or staying off the phone "in case Grandma needs to reach us." For instance, a teenager who will be asked to forgo having friends over and listening to loud music when his grandmother visits should be permitted to participate in planning the timing of her visits. Giving up a private room for a grandparent is a particularly sensitive issue which can be helped by including the grandchild in prior efforts to make other options work. (See "Living Together in the Caregiver's Home," pp. 269–285.)

Grandchildren left alone with an ill grandparent are often afraid the grandparent will die in their presence, yet fears about death may remain unspoken. Young grandchildren may be especially apprehensive when they see their grandparents asleep. Making clear statements on this topic can bring significant comfort: "When Grandma is asleep, it may look as if she's not breathing even though she is." Books written for children which discuss death can also help them talk about their fears. Rehearsing what to do "if something happens" may enable children to handle different types of emergencies effectively and increase their security when charged with the role of "watching over Grandma," even for brief after-school periods. In any case, children should never be left alone with a grandparent without a list of phone numbers of reliable adults who can be reached to talk with them when they are worried or afraid.

Giving grandchildren specific information about how to respond to their grandparents' needs, such as problems with memory or hearing loss, can greatly improve their competence as caregivers. Instead of feeling embarrassed when his grandfather asks the same question five times in front of his friends, an informed grandson can learn how to change the topic cheerfully and relieve his grandfather's anxiety through a reassuring tone of voice. A granddaughter disappointed by her grandmother's inability to hear about her day at school may need to be instructed about speaking slowly, enunciating her words, lowering her voice, using hand gestures, and sitting where her grandmother can see her lips.

Grown grandchildren may face the same strains as their parents in handling full-time employment and giving care to a grandparent.

Resentment can also arise when one adult grandchild is providing the bulk of the care while the other grandchildren do little for the grandparent: "I can't believe I have eleven cousins and no one else seems to have time for Grandma." It is common for a grandchild in this situation to feel wronged when the grandparent's will calls for an equal share for each grandchild instead of a greater portion for the one who gave of her time and affection so much more than the others.

The grandparent-grandchild bond can be a powerful and intensely satisfying one. The opportunity for a grandchild to contribute to a grandparent's life can be a rich learning experience as well as create cherished memories. Parents exhausted by working outside the home and giving care after their workday should not disregard the benefits of having their children participate in the daily care tasks. Such involvement can make grandchildren acutely aware of the dilemmas their parents face and make them less prone to criticize their parents if further contributions and compromises from everyone in the family become necessary.

IN-LAWS

Relationships with a partner's mother or father may be troubled from the start, but these feelings often intensify when an in-law begins to need care. Antagonism toward the care effort by a partner who does not regard the in-laws with affection can place a great strain on an adult son or daughter. Although some couples approach the care of both sets of parents with a spirit of partnership, others evolve an adversarial stance which interferes with a rational consideration of care options. Deciding where one's loyalties lie and how to mediate the strain may be much harder than the care itself.

Conflicts may worsen because partners differ on their attitudes toward traditional roles. For instance, a son raised in a traditional family may believe that care for his parents in their old age is his wife's duty, no matter what her feelings about his parents. She, on the other hand, may give priority to her personal goals, her immediate family, and her own parents. If her husband attempts to pressure her into providing care, she is likely to resent his allegiance to his parents' needs over hers. In turn, he may interpret her resentment as disrespect for his parents and for him.

Whether her husband's family contains other female relatives in the vicinity is often another key factor. A woman whose husband has two unmarried brothers is more likely to be targeted as the primary caregiver than one whose husband has sisters or sisters-in-law. In the absence of other female relatives, her in-laws may fully expect that she will take care of them, despite her employment pressures and other commitments. The daughter-in-law herself may have so absorbed traditional roles that she overlooks her husband and his brothers as potential helpers in the day-to-day aspects of tending to her in-laws' needs.

Competition between in-laws may also create tension, especially around holiday visits, time with grandchildren, and care efforts exerted for one side of the family more extensively than the other. For example, if a daughter enjoys contact with her in-laws more than with her own parents, she may need to hide her frequent calls and visits to her in-laws in order to prevent her parents from making hurtful comparisons. Anxieties about fairness may also arise when a couple wishes to invite one set of parents to live with them, yet fears the other will interpret this invitation as a sign of greater love. A couple may worry generally about setting precedents by including one partner's parents in their lives in ways they would not be willing to replicate later with the other's parents.

Unresolved parent-child issues can further complicate these situations. In a belated attempt to obtain her mother's respect and affection, a daughter may make considerable personal sacrifice for her mother's care. Her partner may feel frustrated watching her submit to demands which are not rewarded with either recognition or tenderness: "Why are you bothering? Can't you see that your mother's never going to change?" A partner's protective feelings may feel more like interference than support when early life issues have been engaged during caregiving, as commonly happens.

Divergent perspectives on what is actually occurring with each other's parents can feed such rifts between partners. A partner's claim to greater objectivity may trigger defensiveness: "She's *my* mother, not yours, so stay out of it." Splitting off into the territory of "mine" and "yours" is the last thing a couple needs during these times, but emotions tend to be stronger than reason when fundamental questions are at stake. It is often helpful to remember that one's partner may be replaying early life issues and that caregiving sometimes provides precious opportunities to work through longstanding problems with parents.

Ironically, close relationships between parents and adult children can also complicate caregiving. A mother and son may maintain such a deep intimacy that his wife feels like an outsider when mother and son are reunited during visits. Over the years, geographic distance may have enabled wife and mother to share each other's claims to his attention amicably. As the mother-in-law's care needs increase, however, the daughter-in-law may regard the prospect of her joining their household or immediate community as the ultimate intrusion on their married life. Accordingly, her husband may feel that her jealousy and guardedness are unwarranted, insisting that he is capable of balancing his loyalty to his mother and his wife.

Negotiating the simultaneous desires to please one's parent and one's partner can spur fears of being a failure at both relationships. Furthermore, the middle tends to be a lonely position. Fending off a partner's complaints about one's parent and a parent's grievances about one's partner leaves a person isolated within a wall of secrets. Breaking out of this isolation may mean bringing conflicts out into the open and risking damage in the hope for resolution.

A concept which may prove helpful is that strength in adulthood is best derived from one's partner rather than one's parent. For example, a son who spends most of his weekends and evenings at his mother's house, no matter how legitimate her need for his presence, is likely to have a bitter partner. Over time, his absence will wear out his partner's patience, and he may face the withering of this intimacy when he most craves it. A more productive strategy in this type of triangle is for the adult child to set respectful limits with the parent: "Mom, I can't come over here all the time without hurting my relationship. I want to be good to both of you, because I need both of you." Parents then face a recognizable truth with which to grapple, rather than a distortion which could only have diminished the person on whom they are depending.

With divorce and remarriage rates increasing, loyalty to former in-laws can add yet another dimension to in-law relationships. A woman leaving a thirty-year marriage may find that divorce does not lessen her affection for her in-laws. Grandchildren and years of shared experiences may tie them together. Should she remarry, her relationship with her new in-laws may seem superficial in its recency compared with the depth of this longer-term bond. Assisting her former in-laws may feel more natural than helping her current in-laws, leading to conflict with her present husband. Few models exist from previous generations for approaching dilemmas created by remarriage.

STEPFAMILIES

Relationships between stepparents and adult stepchildren can also pose distinctive problems. As an increasing number of older people remarry, more adult children acquire stepparents and stepsiblings later in life. Although there are success stories of joined families in later life, these new relationships can be perplexing and stressful. This section first explores concerns which can arise while a parent is courting prospective mates, and then examines the impact of later-life stepparent and stepsibling relationships on caregiving.

Family members with lives rich in companionship may be unable to comprehend the power loneliness has to engender changes in a parent's social behavior. Divorcing from a spouse of many years can result in a bereavement as intense as being widowed. For newly single older people, loneliness can command startling changes. For example, a previously reserved and conservative parent may join a club for older singles, lose twenty pounds, purchase a new wardrobe, change her hairstyle, and begin keeping late hours. These transformations may dismay family members, evoking a mixture of grief and shame, because they feel the parent they have always known is vanishing and this new person is not acting in a manner befitting their station in life.

The parent's choice of mate may provoke further uneasiness. Adult children may react with incredulity upon meeting their parent's new companion, wondering how their parent could possibly be attracted to this person. They may be unable to comprehend their parent's joyful obliviousness to obvious faults in the prospective partner. During courtship, adult children's efforts to point out these faults are likely to be met with defensiveness: "You just don't know what he's really like." Often, the parent already has made unconscious tradeoffs before introducing the mate to adult children, blocking out the person's disadvantages in order to enjoy the companionship.

Compared to men, women face difficult remarriage odds, primarily because women outlive men by an average of nine years. A man searching for a spouse in later life is likely to encounter a large number of women seeking partners, whereas an older woman is likely to face a scarcity of available men. She may lower her standards, taking on a mate with unattractive qualities, "just to have someone." Among the current generation of older women, many moved directly from their family of origin into marriage; thus, their need "to have someone" may be made more urgent by their prior upbringing to depend on a man, as well as their limited experience in living alone.

Financial considerations also frequently force older women to compromise in their choice of mates. A woman who is widowed or divorced in her fifties must wait several years until she receives Social Security. If she has spent her adult years as a homemaker, she may possess few skills to give her an advantage in the job market and may face age discrimination for the low-paying unskilled jobs usually held by younger adults. Under these constrained circumstances, marrying a man who has a reliable income becomes an act of survival more than a quest for companionship. To a woman faced with little or no income of her own, these pragmatic concerns can be far more important than personal freedom or the desire for a mate with a pleasing personality.

Just as women in later life tend to seek economic protection, older men generally want someone who will take care of them. A man who has never learned to cook or clean may value a woman's housekeeping skills more than her conversation or affection. Similarly, a man with a progressive disabling condition, primarily concerned about his future care needs, may hope to find a nurturant woman who will spare his grown children the demands of caring for him. Since it is socially acceptable for men to marry younger women, men's chances of finding women healthy enough to be caregivers are enhanced.

Adult children's unhappiness with the parent's choice may be further complicated by suspicions that the prospective partner is taking advantage of their parent's loneliness. A son may try to instill mistrust in the very affection which his father has found so rewarding: "Dad, she's marrying you for your money. I'm sure of it." Similarly, a daughter may urge her mother to reconsider: "Don't you see that he just wants a woman to wait on him hand and foot?" Whether or not such concerns have legitimacy, efforts to dissuade a parent from planning a new marriage are likely to meet with determined resistance.

Prior to advising a parent against remarriage, adult children should examine the underlying sources of their discomfort. For example, a future stepparent's physical frailties may be the chief focus of the family's wish to prevent the marriage. They may fear that the eventual care needs will become their burden, as well as a strain on their parent's health and financial resources. In some instances, they may worry that the future stepparent will squander their inheritance through undisciplined spending habits. Other concerns may hinge on financial disincentives, such as a woman forfeiting her deceased husband's pension upon remarriage.

Marriage contracts are a way to resolve both anxieties about an inheritance and a spouse's financial worries about losing income by marrying. For instance, a woman who forfeits a sizable alimony check can be guaranteed an equivalent monthly payment from the spouse's estate in the event of his death. If she also fears being asked to leave a house that one of her spouse's children will inherit, a living trust can be included which grants her the right to remain in the home after the spouse dies. Adult children concerned about financial exploitation by the stepparent can suggest a marriage contract that protects against this possibility, without needing to inject mistrust into their parent's happiness.

Another source of discomfort with a parent's companion may be the perception that the new partner will intrude upon time alone with the parent. For example, after her mother's death, a daughter may have enjoyed one-to-one contact with her father which she fears losing upon his remarriage. These possessive feelings are understandable, but they may translate into ongoing dislike of her father's new companion until the daughter identifies the basis for her reserve.

Similarly, when a parent seizes upon another partner shortly after the death of a lifelong spouse, adult children may feel resentment which has little to do with the new partner's personal attributes. They may fear that their parent is making a poor choice by using the partner as an antidote to grief. In such instances, family members can suggest that the marriage ceremony be delayed until at least a year after the bereavement, out of respect both for their feelings and for a decision of this magnitude.

After the marriage, if a stepparent comes to need care, further problems may arise. Giving care as an expression of devotion differs greatly from providing care out of obligation. As a result of too much geographic distance or having had too little time, adult children may not have developed a close relationship with a later-life stepparent. In some instances, personality clashes or unresolved resentments from the courtship period may have precluded all possibility of closeness.

Watching a parent become stressed and exhausted from caring for their stepparent can intensify existing resentments. Even if an amicable relationship has been achieved, adult children may feel angry at the stepparent whose needs are tiring the person they most want to protect. They may increase their assistance to relieve pressure on their parent, but find that their anger at the stepparent increases proportionately to the effort they exert. In situations where the care needs become extreme, they may reach the point of pleading with their parent to place the stepparent in a nursing home for the sake of self-protection.

Another aspect of the strain in these circumstances can be adult children's perception that their stepsiblings are not doing their share. Opportunities to know the stepsiblings as people and therefore to have empathy for their life situations may have been minimal prior to this stressful period. In divorce situations in which both parents have remarried, adult children may have to deal with two sets of stepsiblings as well as two stepparents. The complexities can increase exponentially if care needs emerge simultaneously from both sides.

In contrast to these difficult scenarios, some adult children develop affectionate ties with their later-life stepparents and are able to negotiate these challenges smoothly. Some of the experiences most likely to forge good relationships with stepsiblings occur when the family has to work together to provide care for the parents. During this time, adult children may witness self-sacrificing and dedicated acts by the stepparent and stepsiblings which give them a deeper appreciation for the strengths of the family into which their parent married.

THE OLD TAKING CARE OF THE VERY OLD

The fastest-growing population group in the United States is people over the age of eighty-five. The world of the oldest old is comprised largely of women. Taken together, these facts mean that increasing numbers of women in their fifties are worrying about mothers in their seventies who are still taking care of their mothers. In many instances, the caregivers in their seventies are facing physical problems of their own.

One advantage of the old taking care of the very old is the potential for understanding each other. When a seventy-two-year-old daughter takes care of a ninety-two-year-old mother, they may find that they are both dealing with similar issues, such as encountering hurtful stereotypes about older women everywhere they go and facing the lack of useful activities after retirement. They may both be widowed, as well as mourning the deaths of lifelong friends. The commonality of their daily experience may be greater than ever before in their lives, allowing them to draw closer together than was previously possible for them.

In the last third of the lifespan, chronological age holds less meaning as one's functional age becomes more significant. For example, a ninety-two-year-old mother with mild heart problems may be functionally younger than her seventy-two-year-old daughter with disabling arthritis. Possessing much more dexterity in her hands, the mother may need to help her daughter do her laundry and prepare meals. Any decline in her mother's health would present a double threat to the daughter, since she depends on her mother's assistance on a daily basis and is not in a position to become her mother's caregiver.

Even when a daughter in her sixties or seventies is in relatively good health, she may still have difficulty with lifting, bending, and climbing steps. If her mother's care requires helping her in and out of a wheelchair or running up and down steps throughout the day, the daughter may find that she does not have the physical flexibility or strength necessary to meet her mother's needs. Many women continue to provide heavy physical care to older relatives in spite of back injuries, muscle strain, and other maladies they incur by doing so.

Professionals may have to help women in this position recognize their physical limits and take steps to protect their own health. Encouraging the use of adaptive devices and ensuring that these women have received training in transfer techniques is essential. On a deeper level, prompting them to see how strongly their self-esteem as women is entwined with caregiving may help them to recognize when they are doing too much.

Grandchildren in midlife or nearing retirement age may find that they have their hands full with two or three generations of relatives needing their assistance at once. Eighty percent of people between the ages of forty-five and fifty-five have at least one living parent.[3] Contrary to expectations of an empty nest, these same individuals are increasingly finding that their adult children are returning home because of divorce, unemployment, or the high cost of housing. Some of these midlife grandchildren become primary caregivers to their own grandchildren whose parents are unable to provide adequate care, often because of substance abuse. Their older relatives may require their assistance just as they are trying to help the next generation recover financially and handle their offspring.

Human situations are so variable that no two instances of caring for aging relatives are truly alike. Men and their female relatives face challenges of breaking out of traditional sex-role expectations to achieve a more equitable sharing of tasks. Adult children without siblings may bear a particularly heavy and lonely burden. Grandchildren can be valuable resources to both their parents and grandparents, but may require extra training and support for their efforts. Conflict is often inherent in in-law and step-family relationships. The old caring for the oldest-old may be struggling with their own age-related issues. Yet there are strengths that can be applied to all relationships, such as open communication and the willingness to deal directly with conflicts.

NOTES

1. Marjorie H. Cantor, "Families and Caregiving in an Aging Society," *Generations*, Summer 1992, 69.

2. Older Women's League, "Failing America's Caregivers: A Status Report on Women Who Care," 1989, p. 9.

3. Robyn Stone, Gail Cafferata, and Judith Sangl. "Caregivers of the Frail Elderly: A National Profile," *The Gerontologist*, (27) 1987, 616–626.

SUGGESTED RESOURCES

Articles

Guberman, Nancy, Pierre Mahue, and Chantel Maille. "Women as Family Caregivers: Why Do They Care?" *The Gerontologist*, 32 (1992), 607–617.

The authors maintain that attempts to understand women's caregiving must take into account the sexual division of labor, its reinforcement through social policy, and how women internalize ideas regarding appropriate gender-role behavior.

Horowitz, Amy. "Sons and Daughters as Caregivers to Older Parents: Differences in Role Performance and Consequences," *The Gerontologist*, 25 (1985), 612–617.

This study found that sons tend to become caregivers only when a female sibling is not available and provide less overall assistance to their parents, especially hands-on services. Husbands were more likely to name their wives as caregivers to their parents than wives were to report that their husbands were caregivers to their parents.

Miller, Baila, and Lynda Cafasso. "Gender Differences in Caregiving: Fact or Artifact?" *The Gerontologist*, 32 (1992), 498–507.

The authors found no significant gender difference in total caregiver involvement in personal care or money management tasks. They suggest that future research focus on the meaning of the caregiving experience, rather than on documenting specific gender differences.

Stoller, Eleanor. "Males as Helpers: The Roles of Sons, Relatives and Friends," *The Gerontologist*, 30 (1990), 64–70.

> Women were more likely to provide regular help with routine household chores and personal care, while men tended to provide intermittent assistance with other tasks.

Books

Abel, Emily. *Circles of Care: Work and Identity in Women's Lives* (Albany, NY: Sate University of New York Press), 1990.

> Drawing upon a feminist perspective, this book examines gender differences in the meaning, motives, and consequences of the caregiver role. Includes the negative consequences in old age for women who have provided care to dependent family members throughout their lives.

Alexander, Jo, Debi Berrow, Lisa Domitrovich, Margarita Donnelly, and Cheryl McLean. *Women and Aging: An Anthology by Women* (Corvallis, OR: Calyx Books), 1986.

> This moving anthology of poems and short stories provides insights into problems, concerns, and images about women and aging.

Brody, Elaine. *Women in the Middle: Their Parent-Care Years* (New York: Springer), 1990.

> The author focuses on daughters and daughters-in-law, their multiple responsibilities, and their feelings of strain, which are greater than for sons. How caregiving affects mental and physical well-being, lifestyles, and family relationships are vividly portrayed.

Finch, Janet, and Dulcie Groves. *A Labor of Love: Women, Work and Caring* (London: Routledge and Kegan Paul), 1983.

> An insightful analysis of women's caregiving for dependent persons and how social policies fail to support their efforts. The analysis is based upon the tension between women's economic independence and their traditional role as caregivers.

L'Engle, Madeline. *The Summer of the Great-Grandmother* (New York: The Seabury Press), 1979.

A beautifully written, moving account of a daughter's caring for her mother and the daughter's approach to her mother's dying.

Norris, Jane, ed. *Daughters of the Elderly: Building Partnerships in Caregiving* (Bloomington, IN: Indiana University Press), 1988.

This collection of essays by professionals and family caregivers is both inspiring and informative.

Wharton, William. *Dad* (New York: Avon Books), 1981.

Through fiction, an intimate glimpse of a son caring for a father with dementia.

Organization

Brookdale Grandparent Caregiver Information Project. Center on Aging, University of California, 140 Warren Hall, Berkeley, CA 94720 (510) 643–6427.

This project is dedicated to determining nationwide the state of the art of supportive interventions to assist grandparents raising their grandchildren.

5

Making Difficult Decisions

Many of the dilemmas that older people and their families face have no clear solutions. Choosing one option means forfeiting others, and each choice may contain a bewildering assortment of benefits and losses. Confounding things further, each member of the family may have a separate slant on the situation, leading to differences of opinion which can be painfully divisive. This chapter grapples with four challenging dilemmas: long-distance caregiving, families in conflict about care decisions and managing a potential inheritance, facing end-of-life choices, and older parents who allow an adult son or daughter to abuse them. The process of struggling through difficult decisions can itself be a basis for spurring individual growth and finding family strengths.

LONG-DISTANCE CAREGIVING

Geography often separates children from parents in early adulthood and, to a large extent, arrests the evolution of their relationships. Although most older people who have adult children live near one of them, growing numbers of adult children live at a distance from their aging parents. Giving care to parents from a distance poses special tactical and emotional challenges. Deciding whether or not parents in this position should move to be closer to their adult children is a complex choice requiring considerable discussion and deliberation.

Professionals in the field of aging often feel especially worried about living at a distance from their older relatives. In their daily work, they see the difference it makes when family members are actively involved in older people's lives. They tend to carry an extra degree of guilt about their own parents and grandparents: "Here I am helping everyone else's grandmothers, while mine gets hardly any help from me." They hear themselves giving advice to others that they are unable to follow in their own lives: "How can I counsel other people to do what I'm not doing?" Professionals do not have the luxury of ignorance about the implications of their absence, often extrapolating painfully from current circumstances to what the future is likely to bring.

When Visiting Is Stressful

Making the most of privacy afforded by distance, some older people conceal their problems when talking by phone with out-of-town family members. They omit mentioning their physical decline for long periods of time, until a mishap such as a broken hip reveals their true level of frailty. Arriving in town for the crisis, family members may feel resentful when they discover how much had been hidden from them. Yet their relative may not have intended to deceive them as much as protect them: "My daughter's got her own worries. What could she have done about my dizziness and my falls from 2,000 miles away?"

While visiting, family members often feel pressured by the need to settle as many matters as they can during their stay, aware that follow-up on any actions they initiate will be through long-distance phone calls. Employed people using up precious vacation days for the visit tend to feel an extra urgency to try to solve everything at once. Family members may be further strained by a lack of familiarity with the older person's community and worries about their unattended commitments at home. For those visiting alone, the separation from family and friends may also heighten the tension of the situation.

Prior to visiting or immediately upon arrival, out-of-town family members may benefit from contacting a professional in their relative's community who can provide an appraisal of the local services. Increasingly, many communities have private geriatric care managers who can spare families the time involved in randomly calling agencies out of the telephone book. These managers are listed in the Yellow Pages under "Senior" or "Elder" services. Some may charge a flat fee for going out to the home, assessing the older person's situation, and recommending appropriate services. Others may charge on an hourly basis, according to the actual time spent. Still others offer ongoing monitoring and support for a monthly fee, once the older person has had an extensive initial assessment session. (See "Care Managers," pp. 237–239.)

Other sources of information are staff persons of organizations targeted to serve older people, such as senior centers, adult day care centers, and home health agencies. Most towns and cities also have a senior information and assistance hot line listed in the community services section of the telephone book. Associations such as the American Cancer Society, Alzheimer's Association, Arthritis Foundation, and Lung Association can be particularly helpful in recommending services for specific health problems.

The amount of lead time needed to set up care arrangements can be exasperating to visiting relatives. For example, the older person may be eligible for state-funded home services, but the delay before someone comes out to do the required assessment may be weeks. Another waiting period may occur before the service actually begins. In addition, the older person may resist having a stranger in her home and may want to have family present when a worker first arrives. Hiring someone through a newspaper advertisement may not be feasible because of the need to stay in town long enough to ensure that the person is trustworthy and handles the care responsibly. Private-pay services through agencies, which require only a day's notice, are expedient but too expensive for most families.

Another frustration for visiting family members is how little time they get to spend with their relative's doctor and other health-care professionals. They often encounter doctors, nurses, and social workers who are too pressured by their heavy caseloads to spend adequate time with them. These abbreviated discussions tend to frustrate everyone involved. A helpful strategy is for families to contact these professionals by letter or telephone in advance, notifying them of their impending visit, the questions they will be asking, and the kind of services they hope to arrange. In response to this courtesy, a physician may schedule a longer time for the appointment which will occur during the family member's visit. (See "Talking to Doctors," pp. 115–16.)

When family members first get word of a relative's hospitalization, calling ahead to the primary nurse or discharge planner immediately helps personalize the care. Describing specific problems which the older person had been facing at home aids hospital staff in establishing realistic discharge plans. Providing the names of friends and neighbors who have been actively assisting the older person saves hospital

SUGGESTIONS FOR LONG-DISTANCE CONTACT

Establish routines for calls	Calls are most satisfying if they occur regularly, on a specific day. This permits anticipation.
Obtain an extension phone for a couple	Extension saves time; both can participate in the conversation at once. Eliminates the need to repeat information.
Exchange phone numbers with the older person's neighbors	Phone contact on an occasional basis with supportive neighbors serves as a source of information and a means of expressing thanks.
Send brief, newsy letters frequently	Letters are especially helpful for those who tend to forget what is said on the phone. The older person can reread letters at will.
Provide the older person with preaddressed envelopes and return address labels	Many older people fear that their handwriting is not legible enough for the postal service. A stack of envelopes ready for mailing serves as an encouragement.
Send clippings, photographs, books, home videos, etc.	These are easier to send for family members who are not letter-writers. The older person still feels acknowledged and remembered.
Recording and sending cassette tapes back and forth	Tapes are especially useful for low-vision people. They save on the expense of lengthy long distance calls.

staff the time needed to identify such helpers. By informing staff of solutions which have been tried in the past without success, out-of-town family members help reduce duplicated efforts. Above all, a family's phone contact tends to hasten the planning process and ensure that necessary service referrals are made in a timely manner.

The preceding chart suggests ways that out-of-town family members can maintain supportive contact with their relative. Such efforts not only provide the older person with ongoing links with people seen infrequently, but may also help relieve pressure on local caregivers. (See "Out-of-Town vs. Local," pp. 69–70.) The out-of-town family can also become better acquainted with their relative's neighbors, friends, and other helpers, as described in Chapter Six, in order to establish regular communication and to offer them assistance and appreciation.

Should the Older Person Move to the Family's Community?

After the stress and expense of flying back and forth to repeated crises, out-of-town family members are often attracted to the idea of moving the older person to their community: "Mom, if you lived near us, we could really help you instead of just putting out fires." From the older person's perspective, the losses in such a move may seem much greater than the gains. The thought of leaving lifelong friends, moving out of a long-term home, and learning a new area implies an immensity of effort that some find overwhelming. The older person may also wonder if she will find a physician with as much warmth as her family doctor or if she can rebuild a supportive network of friends and neighbors.

Despite these doubts about moving, an older person may tell herself, "At my age, I should be near my kids." She may be afraid of delaying the move until "something happens" which will make her regret having waited. Many people believe that it is always better to move near family in later life, no matter how attached they are to their own community. Even though decades may have elapsed since they last had daily contact with their adult children, they assume that blood ties matter the most at the end of life.

One problem with an older person's move to an adult child's community is that it can abruptly overload their relationship. Having left friends and neighbors behind, the older person becomes entirely dependent on family members for social contact and practical assistance. Renewing family relationships requires a certain amount of stamina and patience under any circumstances, but doing so under the compulsion of care needs does not allow a gradual approach. For instance, a daughter may convince her mother to move to her community after an unsuccessful cataract operation. All at once, her mother's vision problems would force their relationship into a pattern of daily face-to-face contact, in contrast to their previous pattern of occasional long-distance phone calls. They would have no transitional time to reestablish their bond on a happier basis.

The daughter is likely to discover that she cannot possibly fill in for the friend with whom her mother talked on the telephone every morning for twenty years. The daughter may realize that she is making room in her life for someone she calls "Mom" but whom she does not know very well as a person. Even when their parents are still independent, adult children may react with anxiety to the idea of a move: "Will we get along if we see each other more often?" Relationships which have succeeded within the safety of distance may need considerable reworking when geographic boundaries are removed.

Deciding how often to see each other and how often to call becomes a sensitive process of negotiation. Both parents and adult children may experience uncomfortable feelings of intrusion as they gain unaccustomed access to each other's private lives. Finding a livable rhythm of contact under these conditions requires open discussions of feelings and preferences, an achievement which is easier for some families than for others.

To avoid situations of regret, family members should urge the older person to consider a trial period in the new community. It is usually not difficult to convince someone that the cost of maintaining two residences for a few months is worth it to preserve the possibility of moving back. Such trial periods are especially useful following a spouse's death or another event that may have hastened the decision to move. Many older people are not aware of the value of remaining in their own communities until after they move away.

FAMILIES IN CONFLICT

There tend to be as many truths in a family as there are family members. When a family faces decisions about the long-term care of an elderly relative or managing a potential inheritance, opinions may diverge widely. Instead of trying to find consensus, professionals and family members often have to accept multiple and conflicting viewpoints. This section illustrates ways to consider differing views while seeking workable compromises.

Keep-at-Home vs. Nursing Home

One of the most painful splits within families revolves around deciding when to resort to a nursing home. Often, one side of a family argues that the older person should be placed in a nursing home "for the sake of health and safety," and the other side claims that the older person should be maintained at home "no matter how much the family has to do." One sibling may become a spokesperson for the nursing home faction and another may represent the effort to keep the older person at home. Each would-be family leader may then try to enlist alliances with other siblings who support their position. Unless reconciled, such a rift can force the older person into the center of an uncomfortable battle as each side tries to undermine the other.

When an older person goes into the hospital, such simmering disagreements tend to reach a flashpoint. The leaders from each faction immediately try to recruit the support of the medical staff involved in the older person's care. The keep-at-home faction may seek reassurance that the increased care demands are manageable at home, requesting training in care techniques and referral to community resources. The nursing home faction may seek advice about local nursing homes and request help with the mechanics of the placement process, trying to use the momentum of their relative's separation from the routines of home.

At such junctures, hospital staff can decisively influence the course of events to the extent that they provide information to one of the factions or lend an authoritative stance to another. A nurse whose philosophical beliefs support the use of noninstitutional alternatives may be tempted to side with the keep-at-home faction. A discharge planner influenced by Medicare incentives for shorter hospital stays may be drawn toward the nursing home faction, especially if she learns that a bed is available at a nearby facility. A physician in a hurry may remark that the older person's condition is "too much to handle at home." Those family members who are eager to be released from home care duties may then use "the doctor's recommendation" to break the will of siblings who were not yet ready to stop trying.

Since each faction's information will be colored by their point of view, hospital staff trying to advise a divided family are likely to hear two entirely separate versions of the home situation. Hidden agendas within the rivalry of the two family leaders can so widen the gap between the two versions that staff may be unable to decide which account to believe. Hoping to arrive at one indisputable truth, professionals sometimes ally with one side of a family against another, thereby deepening the family's strife.

A better approach is to hear out all sides during disagreements about care arrangements and financial resources, promoting a family's ability to listen to each other's ideas and feelings. This approach is more time-consuming but is more likely to serve the best interest of the older person. There is usually merit in all sides of a dispute of this nature. For instance, a son arguing against nursing home placement "so Mom can stay in familiar surroundings" may also be trying to avoid having the house he hopes to inherit sold to pay for the nursing home. His sister's claim that their mother would be more comfortable in the nursing home may be correct in terms of skin care and other physical needs but wrong in terms of her mother's own desire to stay home and protect the inheritance.

Proposing a time-limited trial period at home, without excluding the option of later nursing home placement, is often the best strategy at these junctures. A trial period can be presented as a chance to gauge the effects of changes in the older person's condition on the family's caregiving capacity. The services of home care professionals can be enlisted for help obtaining the proper medical equipment or for teaching caregivers specific techniques for managing the care. As long as a date is set for when the home care situation will be reevaluated, the nursing home faction may be satisfied.

In testing her new needs against the reality of the home situation, the older person may be able to reconcile herself to the necessity of nursing home care. Family members who had been opposed to a nursing home may slowly become more accepting as they experience how complex their relative's care has become. In the example above, the older woman may realize how much worse her bed sores are getting without nurse's aides available at night to help her change positions in bed. Her son may see that his mother's discomfort from inadequate skin care is not worth trying to preserve the inheritance. (See "Setting Up a Trial Period at Home," pp. 316–317.)

Families can also choose to place their relative in a nursing home on a trial basis. In this way, they gain a period of relief from caregiving and can use the time both to rest and to assess their ability to go on providing home care. During such trial periods, the older person's home can be left intact and occasional visits home can be arranged. Using a nursing home for a few months often revives caregivers whose personal needs had been too long neglected. If they manage to use the time away from caregiving to catch up with themselves, they may be able to retrieve their relative from the nursing home with fresh vigor for providing care at home.

Who Gets What?

To siblings, the choices involved in "who gets what" of the family's possessions and resources have a tendency to symbolize who the parents love, respect, or trust the most among them. For this reason, inheritance issues often surpass all others in their power to disrupt sibling relationships. Older parents can become sickened by these tensions within the family, and caregiving arrangements can dissolve, leaving a legacy of injured relationships behind.

Conflicts may first arise when parents leave a private house for a smaller, easier-to-manage apartment. When an item such as an heirloom piano will not fit in the apartment, an older couple may be forced to consider who among their children would take the best care or make the greatest use of it. After finally offering the piano to one of their children, the couple may discover that they have hurt the others, who interpret the choice as a negative judgment against themselves or a positive judgment in favor of the selected sibling. Feeling slighted, these siblings may be less inclined to be helpful to their parents, or they may become hostile toward the sibling who received the gift.

When anticipating the need to distribute possessions, an older couple can defuse the potential for hurt by asking adult children to make a list of the items which mean the most to them, in the order of their importance. This strategy places the discussion out in the open and incorporates the adult children as participants in the choice process. The lists of their preferred items function as a survey of the emotional territory, providing the older couple with an advance view of the items which may be disputed. Preventive discussions can then be initiated by questions such as, "If you had to choose between the oriental rug and the piano, which would you take?" The essence of this strategy is for parents to remove themselves from the deciding role as much as possible, thereby stripping the choice process of its symbolic power.

Other strains arise when a sibling chosen by the parents as their money manager is mistrusted by the others, or when the siblings become suspicious that the parents are giving this person secret bonuses. The money manager can allay worries by opening up financial records to the siblings' view. Similar to companies issuing financial statements, a family financial manager who wishes to dispel anxiety can periodically send copies of bank statements and other documents to family members. Including a page which itemizes the ways income has been spent or reinvested reassures siblings that the money manager is not "borrowing" the money for personal uses or otherwise benefiting from the role.

Finally, professionals may be drawn into the fray concerning inheritances by becoming privy to family financial secrets. For instance, an older person who has become close to a visiting nurse may confide her inheritance plans, asking the nurse not to divulge these plans to certain members of the family. Although such confidences may be harmless as long as advice is not offered, the nurse may then feel awkward when facing those family members who have been excluded from secret information. A professional can say to an older person, "I'd rather not know about your plans to disinherit your son, because I am trying to play a neutral role in the family. This way, I can be helpful to everyone."

The worst situations are those in which professionals inadvertently stumble upon long-held financial secrets. While assisting with a Medicaid application, a hospital discharge planner may learn that a son secretly arranged with his mother years ago to put her savings in his name. If exposed during the already emotionally charged medical crisis, such secrets can trigger explosive conflicts between siblings. Professionals perform an important service for families by warning them not to establish such secrets in the first place. There is little that can be done later to repair the trust which shatters once such secrets are revealed.

END-OF-LIFE CHOICES

Dying has become more complicated than ever. Medical technology presents so many choices that older people and their families are becoming increasingly bewildered and conflicted as they try to figure out what to do. Many people yearn to have these decisions taken out of their hands by an abrupt death, such as a heart attack, which would allow them to bypass difficult decisions altogether. This section gives some ideas about how to handle end-of-life choices when they arise, as well as long before these decisions become urgent.

To Die at Home or in the Hospital?

People of all ages are haunted by images of dying in an intensive care unit. However, respecting a relative's wish to die at home is not always possible. For instance, holding back from calling an ambulance when a loved one goes into severe respiratory distress goes against instinctive impulses to take rescuing measures. When the dying process moves more slowly, sustaining a person's last weeks and days at home can be exhausting. Waking several times a night to administer pain medications or help someone to the bathroom is physically draining. Feeling helpless while watching a spouse or parent deteriorate adds emotional fatigue to this nightly weariness.

When their relative pleads, "Promise me I can die in my own bed," family members often do not realize that community services for carrying out such wishes are limited. Hospice programs to support the families of people who choose to die at home are not available in all communities, and Medicare restricts these services to the last six months of life. Even when someone's condition qualifies for Medicare-covered hospice services, home visits by hospice nurses and aides only supplement the family's efforts. The majority of round-the-clock care must still be carried out by family members and friends. Although hospice agencies increasingly make use of volunteers to provide time off for family caregivers, such relief is for short periods of time and constrained by the volunteer's schedule.

The bind is that when dying people and their families resort to a hospital at the end stage of illnesses, they forfeit much of their control over their medical options. For instance, a wife caring for her husband at home may decide, after considerable discussion with him, to stop administering antibiotics for his pneumonia in order to respect his desire to die naturally. If she becomes frightened and hospitalizes him at the last minute, she is likely to encounter resistance to their chosen strategy. Hospital staff may ignore her request to continue withholding antibiotics, claiming that doing so constitutes murder. She and her husband become, at that juncture, captives of the health care system and of the legal establishment which judges its actions.

Discussing Difficult Choices

Of all medical choices, "doing nothing" is usually the most difficult. When a hospitalized older person announces that he has had enough of life and prefers to be left alone, he is likely to continue to be probed by strange hands and urged to undergo humiliating and uncomfortable procedures. Expressing the desire to die rarely finds a receptive audience among those whose profession it is to promote life. Also, once the reality of the person's death is upon them, family members themselves may plead with their loved one to accept "everything that can be done."

The Patient Self-Determination Act, implemented in January of 1992, was intended to ensure that older people and their families are informed in advance of the implications of their medical choices and are provided with an opportunity to make their preferences known in writing. Since laws about end-of-life choices vary from state to state, specific documents for implementing these choices also differ. The following chart explains the types of documents that older people now face when they are admitted to a hospital or nursing home.

DOCUMENTS FOR IMPLEMENTING END-OF-LIFE CHOICES

Durable Power of Attorney for Health Care

A person designates another ("Agent" or "Proxy") to make health care decisions in the event the person becomes incapacitated or unable to communicate.

Living Will

A person signs this document to express a wish not to have their life prolonged when terminally ill.

Advance Directive

A person states which treatments would be unacceptable with any illness, not only when terminally ill.

From Wendy Lustbader and Nancy R. Hooyman, *Taking Care of Aging Family Members* (New York: The Free Press, 1994). Copyright © 1994 by Wendy Lustbader and Nancy Hooyman; copyright © 1986 by The Free Press.

Ideally, completing these documents serves as an opportunity for an older person, her physician, and her family to discuss end-of-life choices. Yet many people resist any discussion of death and shun those who try to break through their resistance. When a document such as a Living Will is placed before them, they insist on putting it away until "later." The law requires that such documents be made available but does not require an older person to complete them. Family members may be left fretting behind closed doors about the medical choices which are looming and which the older person refuses to face.

Family members encountering such resistance or who find raising the topic too painful should ask a medical professional to conduct a discussion of these issues. When an older person avoids discussing her preferences for emergency medical intervention or the use of life-sustaining technology, it may be helpful to ask, "Are you afraid of dying or are you afraid of death?" This question generally opens the discussion wide enough for people to give voice to their fears. Some will readily admit that their dread is focused on the suffering that may precede death rather than on death itself: "I don't mind dying, but I can't stand the thought of that ambulance ride and what they'll do to me in the hospital."

It is sometimes helpful when family members explain that declining "last ditch" measures would be easier if they had a signed document on hand: "Mom, I have to be sure that I understand what you want so I can carry out your wishes. Otherwise, it would be too hard for me to make those decisions." Putting the situation in terms of making things easier for family members during a painful time may prompt an older person to go ahead and get the documents completed.

Talking to Doctors

The time allotted to family conferences in hospitals tends to be filled with necessary explanations of the risks and mortality rates of proposed treatments. A doctor responsible for many other acutely ill people may not have the time to address a family's grief and fear, nor to handle their many practical questions about the aftermath of surgery and the nature of the home care that will be required. Called upon to give informed consent for life-prolonging surgeries and procedures, family members may feel hurried by the doctor's urgency and confused by all the medical terms thrown at them at once. They may conclude the conference with a helpless abdication of choice: "Whatever you think is best, doctor."

This abdication results in many surgeries and procedures which would have been omitted if doctors had both more time and more skill in presenting medical choices in ordinary language. Unless the likely consequences of each option are depicted in sufficient and realistic detail, older people and their families are usually unable to imagine what life will be like following the hospital stay. For example, hearing that their mother's leg amputation may mean difficult wound care and a long nursing home stay may enable family members to respect her wish to forgo the surgery. In contrast, if a rushed physician cites only the survival statistics after performing rather than omitting the amputation, family members may be left with the emotional impetus to prolong their parent's life and their ignorance of what it means to do so.

To slow down the discussion, the older person or a family member may have to say, "Doctor, I am so upset and scared that I didn't understand a word you said." The doctor is then alerted to the fact that communication has not been achieved and that the person being asked to sign the consent form cannot be construed as "informed." Stating outright which terms or phrases make no sense then helps the doctor begin to translate medical jargon into everyday speech. Many people hold back from asking questions because they do not want to appear ignorant or they do not want to keep the doctor from attending to other patients. Nurses and social workers may need to coach families prior to medical conferences, assuring them that it is normal to have a hard time comprehending medical language and that they have a right to understand before they make life-and-death decisions.

Another helpful approach is for older people and their families to make a list of their questions prior to talking to the doctor. Since memory tends to falter under stress, many people find that they cannot remember what they wanted to ask when they are finally face-to-face with the doctor. As soon as the doctor leaves the hospital room, the questions come surging back. Making a list along with the older person also gives family members a comfortable way of voicing their concerns without alarming their relative: "Mom, let's jot down some of those questions we had about blood transfusions, like how do they know that the blood is safe, just so it doesn't nag at us." This may liberate the older person from her own reticence about questioning the doctor.

The majority of the money spent on medical care in a person's lifetime tends to be paid out for services received during the last few months of life. On a societal level, this reality translates into major expenditures of funds for limited results. On a personal level, many people find that the medical technology which allows them extra time does not provide them pleasure or meaning. Family members often need professional support as they attempt to find ethically and emotionally acceptable responses to their relative's preferences. In many instances, helping the older person obtain a good death is the most loving response that family members can offer and professionals can facilitate.

PARENTS WHO ACCEPT ABUSE FROM ADULT CHILDREN

In a family, there may be one sibling who does not do as well in life as the others, due to drug or alcohol addiction, mental illness, or personality factors which have interfered with forming relationships and earning a living. If this person becomes the parents' caregiver in their old age, a host of problems may arise in the family. This section probes what can be done when parents find themselves exploited or neglected by a troubled adult child, either because they are maintaining a long-standing pattern or because they are protecting their grandchildren.

Destructive Entwinement

Situations in which older parents allow themselves to be abused by their grown children are probably the most difficult instances of self-neglect to unravel. For example, a seventy-five-year-old mother may take no action after her fifty-two-year-old drug-addicted son steals from her, destroys her property, or hits her. She may then feel degraded and ashamed by her very failure to take care of herself, and may believe she is entirely powerless to protect herself from further harm.

Substance abuse tends to be a primary ingredient in situations in which parents accept harm from adult children. Long into later life, some parents continue old patterns of sacrificing their financial resources for the sake of an addicted son or daughter. Their adult child may plead for rescue from bill collectors and landlords, for assistance with business ventures which never come to fruition, or for other seemingly legitimate enterprises which turn out to be a means of siphoning off money for drugs or alcohol. The older parents may keep telling themselves that "this time" their son or daughter will succeed, or that this is the "last time" they will be fooled, only to go on repeating a pattern of futile rescue.

Years may pass as this pattern repeats, with the older parents becoming ever more weary and frightened. Their resources may become significantly depleted, and they may wonder with increasing urgency how this dependent son or daughter will manage after they die. They may turn to their other adult children with the hope that their protective role will be taken over by one of them, finding instead that their other children's sympathy had been used up long ago. Resentment and anger may have taken the place of any remaining compassion.

In these situations, the siblings frequently want nothing to do with this member of the family. They may bitterly cite the many times this sister or brother caused their parents distress. They may lament all their useless attempts to persuade their parents to stop throwing away money on this sibling's behalf and to stop accepting emotional or physical battering. Claiming they have been cheated of their future inheritance, they may harbor rage toward their parents for what they perceive as their display of favoritism toward this "spoiled" member of the family.

Recognizing the toll their actions have taken on their other adult children may come as a blow to older parents. If this awareness occurs just as they are needing their other children's assistance as caregivers, the blow may be especially painful. Their children may try to force them to set belated limits on the errant sibling's abuse as a condition of their providing care: "Mom, we won't take care of you unless you get the locks changed and stop letting Johnny into your house. We're sick of how he exploits you." These adult children may feel it is pointless to provide care so long as their parents continue to accept abuse.

These worst predicaments tend to arise when older parents permit a substance-abusing adult child to reside in their dwelling and live off their income. An all-too-common scenario is a son or daughter spending large portions of the parents' Social Security income on alcohol or drugs. Once their funds are depleted, the parents may fail to fill necessary prescriptions, purchase foods in accordance with their dietary restrictions, or keep medical appointments vital to their health and safety. Household bills may go unpaid for long periods of time, resulting in disrupted telephone service or in threatening collections or eviction letters.

Living at the mercy of an addicted son or daughter often means more than financial strain. With inhibitions blurred by drugs or alcohol, the adult child may lash out at an older parent verbally and physically. There are cases in which older parents regularly accept beatings from their adult children. Too humiliated to seek help, older parents may then avoid medical appointments in order to conceal bruises which have become their badges of shame. Their failure to protect themselves from harm may then spiral into serious medical problems and a resulting loss in function that renders them physically dependent on the very person who had been harming them.

When professionals try to assist such families, they often encounter intense resistance. Years of well-intentioned "helping" is at stake. The parents may feel as unwilling as ever to set limits, believing this to be tantamount to abandoning their troubled son or daughter. They may strive to preserve a role they continue to see as protective, rejecting professionals or family members who try to get them to see the situation differently. Some will go to their deaths rather than risk examining their own contribution to these damaging patterns, or permitting their adult child to face the consequences of substance abuse or a destructive lifestyle.

Blaming other people or outside circumstances for their son or daughter's problems is a common defense employed by these beleaguered parents. As they hand over money to their adult child that would be better spent on their own care needs, they may insist that no one else understands their loved one as well as they do: "Johnny has just had a hard time getting going in his life, and now no one will give him a chance to prove himself." When self-neglect is supported by such extensive and impenetrable self-deception, the best that professionals or family members can do is to leave behind suggestions that may yield results later.

These concepts can be presented as questions: "Since you're not going to live forever, have you considered stopping your help now so you can be there for your son when he gets his life together?" The goal here is to help parents begin to separate financial rescue from emotional support. The idea that they can stop the financial dependency while continuing to "be there" emotionally may never have occurred to them before. Another is: "Can you see that each time you pay his bills, you're saving him from the consequences of his addiction? You're helping to keep him addicted, because he doesn't have to pay the price for what he's doing." These ideas should be offered to weary parents in a neutral, respectful tone, along with acknowledgment of their love for their son or daughter. This allows parents to hear the ideas and give them some later thought, as these concepts contain the seeds of positive change. The key is to avoid negative judgments which will only arouse the parent's self-defense and will interfere with their thinking over these ideas on their own.

In some instances, the parents may come to recognize the destructive effects of maintaining the adult son or daughter's dependency, but they feel helpless about their tendency to crumble in the face of angry threats or pleas for rescue. Such parents may need one further concept to inspire change: "Have you thought about the legacy of resentment you are leaving your other children? Maybe if you stopped giving away their share of the inheritance, your other children might be willing to help your daughter after you're gone." The idea of leaving a legacy of better feelings between the siblings may serve as a motivation where nothing else does. Some parents who are unable to say "no" to an exploitive adult child may then allow one of their other children or a neutral third party, such as a bank, to take control over their finances.

Assisting older parents with making these arrangements for money management is often an effective intervention, so long as the parents are prepared for the adjustment period that will ensue as soon as the dependent adult child loses access to the money supply. For instance, giving the son or daughter ample notice may ease the transition, as well as implementing a gradual withdrawal of financial support: "This month you'll get $300, next month $200, and then $100 a month for six months. After that, you're on your own." Warning the parents that there may be a period of acting out and testing the limits may help them endure while their son or daughter slowly attains a more constructive manner of living. Assisting the adult child with referrals to drug and alcohol treatment, mental health counseling, and subsidized housing may further bolster the parents' determination to put an end to the exploitation.

Understanding the power of parental guilt should be the basis for any intervention. Parents in these predicaments tend to be burdened by remorse about errors made earlier in their lives which they fear may account for their son or daughter's lack of happiness in life. Parents who physically or sexually abused their children or who neglected them due to their own problems with substance abuse may be especially fearful of talking about the past. A professional or family member who hopes to assist older parents with such difficult memories must be prepared to do a great deal of listening. When pent-up feelings and fears are released, the process of sorting them out and making sense of what happened is both time-consuming and complex. If sufficient time is not available, it is preferable to make referrals to other sources of help.

Protecting Grandchildren, Neglecting Themselves

As drug and alcohol abuse have become more prevalent in recent decades, increasing numbers of grandparents are sacrificing their own needs for the sake of grandchildren whose parents are addicted. The grandparent may go so far as to move into the household of substance-abusing parents in order to ensure that the grandchildren have food on the table and emotional support in their daily lives. Another common scenario is for the family to move into the grandparent's residence, having been evicted from their own. In either instance, the grandparent's income may be taken over to serve the addictions, leaving the grandparent unable to meet his or her basic nutritional or health care needs. A battle may ensue in which the grandparent manages to retain control of just enough money to care for the grandchildren while neglecting personal needs, such as medications and special diets.

In other tragic variations, some grandparents manage to maintain a separate residence and separate finances, but they provide more child care than is good for their health or for the safety of their grandchildren. For instance, a woman with severe arthritis in her hands and knees may take a two-year-old grandchild into her home during the day. Fearing that she might drop the child or be unable to pursue him fast enough to keep him out of harm's way, she may nevertheless prefer her risky care to that which the child's drug-addicted mother provides when the older grandchildren are at school. The fact that her joints become swollen and painful under the stress of these exertions may be yet another sacrifice that she bears for the child's sake.

Such dilemmas induce heartbreaking binds for grandparents. Aware that their self-neglect may shorten their lives or erode their ability to take care of themselves, they may persist because they see no other options. Many grandparents in these situations say that they live from day to day, trying not to think too far ahead in their quest to provide basic protection to their grandchildren. It is enough to get through each day with the grandchildren adequately fed, clothed, and sheltered, and to stand by as a bodyguard to prevent physical or sexual abuse. Giving up a potentially longer life or longer period of independent functioning in the future may seem justified when measured against the urgent needs of the present.

When professionals and family members face a grandparent in this situation, an intense need to try to rescue both the grandchild and the grandparent may be kindled. Reporting the grandchild's parents to the state's child protection agency may be one option; another may be to report the elder's situation to the state's adult protection agency. Workers from both agencies may be hampered by the realities of case overloads and insufficient resources to offer in terms of child care or elder care assistance. Additionally, state regulations may be such that the grandparent's protective efforts may be just successful enough to prevent the state from having grounds to remove the child from the parents' home. Similarly, the state's capacity to protect frail elders who are mentally competent hinges upon their cooperation. In these instances, grandparents generally refuse to be rescued, especially if such rescue entails their pressing charges against their own son or daughter as an abuser of children or the elderly. Most choose instead to go on from day to day and to do their best to protect their grandchild on their own.

The most useful interventions in these predicaments center around what the grandparent chiefly desires: a better life for the grandchild. In this regard, a professional or family member may be able to assist the grandparent with making the best possible use of existing resources. For instance, if the grandparent's Social Security check is being used primarily for alcohol and drugs instead of food, the grandparent may accept help setting up a direct-deposit bank account to which the addicted parents do not have access. Finding a community volunteer who would be willing to accompany the grandparent to the bank and grocery store at the beginning of each month may be an effective intervention. In this way, the house may be supplied with good food at least part of the month. The elder's prescriptions can then be filled a month or two ahead, and any remaining money can then be subjected to the usual household priorities. These changes can be introduced slowly, with the majority of the elder's monthly income gradually going toward groceries and medications.

Helping a grandparent gather the inner strength to assert herself in this manner may require many discussions in which the long-range benefits are emphasized: "This way, you'll live a lot longer and your granddaughter will have a grandmother to protect her a lot longer." Pointing out that setting an example of self-care is as important as any other lesson taught to a grandchild may further motivate the elder to bear the initial strains that will result from her resuming even partial control of her finances. Access to education about substance abuse may be helpful in this regard, such as through attendance at Al-Anon meetings. The presence of the community volunteer each month can be supplemented by visits from a case manager, with the idea that extra witnesses to what goes on in the household may reduce the misuse of funds.

In some communities, self-help groups have formed expressly for the purpose of strengthening and supporting grandparents in this position. Connecting an isolated grandparent with such an organization, even if the closest is accessible only by mail, may serve as a vital source of strength. Hearing how common this situation has become, some grandparents may then be able to transcend their shame about their particular circumstances and reach out for help to members of their religious congregation or other groups in their community. Some may learn thereby that they have the capacity and the courage to gain custody of their grandchild, because members of their community will stand by them and other forms of assistance will be made available to them.

Uncertainty is inherent within many of the dilemmas that family members confront while caring for aging relatives. As much as families crave the "right" answer, they often have to accept imperfect compromises and bear with successive trials and errors. Longstanding problems feed into current tensions, making it difficult to know which way to turn. This is particularly true with end-of-life decisions and instances of abuse and neglect. Eventually, through a combination of experience, knowledge, consultation with professionals, and the vagaries of life itself, older people and their families find some resolution of these painful issues.

SUGGESTED RESOURCES

Articles

Lee, Melinda, and Karen Berry. "Abuse of Durable Power of Attorney for Health Care: Case Report," *Journal of the American Geriatric Society*, 39 (1991), 806–809.

> This case report highlights typical problems with the Durable Power of Attorney for Health Care, including improper execution, proxy decisions that are contrary to the wishes or best interests of the patient, and conflicts of interest between the patient and the proxy. Practical and procedural recommendations for resolving such problems are presented.

Puma, Helena. "Advanced Directives on Admission: Clinical Implications and Analysis of the Patient Self-Determination Act," *Journal of the American Medical Association*, 266 (1991), 402–405.

> The author reviews the potential benefits of the Act and clinical, legal, and ethical barriers to successful implementation. Recommendations to maximize the Act's effectiveness are presented.

Books

Macklin, R. *Mortal Choices: Bioethics in Today's World* (New York: Pantheon), 1987.

A thorough and sensitive review of common ethical dilemmas in medicine, including gaining informed consent, determining competency, and forgoing life-sustaining therapy.

Minkler, Meredith, and Kathleeen Roe. *Grandmothers as Caregivers: Raising Children of the Crack Cocaine Epidemic* (Newbury Park, CA: Sage), 1993.

Drawing upon in-depth interviews, the authors portray the experience of grandparents in the African American community who are caring for children whose parents are casualties of the crack cocaine epidemic. They conclude with implications for social policy.

Quinn, Mary Joy, and Susan Tomita. *Elder Abuse and Neglect: Assessment and Intervention* (New York: Springer), 1986.

Comprehensive review of the nature of elder abuse, types of abuse, causes, and guidelines for detection and intervention. Includes case examples from the authors' clinical experience and detailed protocols.

Organizations

Choice in Dying (formerly Society for the Right to Die). 250 West 57th Street, New York, NY 10107. (212) 246–6973

This nonprofit group protects the rights of all Americans to a natural and dignified death. Their publications provide information about the right to refuse medical treatment and they offer forms such as "Durable Power of Attorney for Health Care" and "Advance Directive: Living Will and Health Care Proxy" tailored to each state's laws.

American Association for Retired Persons (AARP). 601 E. Street, N.W., Washington, DC 20049. (202) 434–2277

AARP has many useful publications. Call or write for a list of all their publications. These are only a sample of those relevant to this chapter.

"Domestic Mistreatment of the Elderly: Towards Prevention," D12810.

"Miles Away and Still Caring: A Guide for Long Distance Caregivers," D12748.

6

Neighbors, Friends, and Other Helpers

Neighbors, friends, and other helpers are vital to older people striving to live independently. Based on decency, friendship, or a perception of mutual need, the help rendered in these relationships is often more acceptable to older people than formal agency services. Professionals and families can strengthen these helpers' efforts by sharing information, affirming their crucial role, helping them set limits, and linking them with others. This chapter suggests ways to identify and support such helping networks and presents approaches for creating fresh networks. It concludes with a discussion of ways that neighbors and other helpers sometimes take advantage of vulnerable older people, with suggestions for preventing such abuse and distinguishing between supportive and exploitative helpers.

IDENTIFYING AND SUPPORTING NETWORKS

Asking older people directly to identify their helping networks often yields little information. The human instinct to avoid acknowledging dependency, combined with pride in their friendships, may prevent older people from recognizing their extensive reliance on others for their daily survival. This section suggest ways to identify and support these helpers without harming someone's pride.

Helpers in Employment Roles

Some individuals offer special assistance to older people while fulfilling their prescribed employment roles. In many instances, the difference between what they are supposed to do as part of their job and the "extras" they provide out of kindness becomes blurred into one spontaneous act of caring. Many older people do not recognize special assistance when it occurs as such a subtle extension of an employment role. In small towns or urban neighborhoods with stable businesses, customers' relationships with proprietors and staff tend to resemble friendships more than functional contacts. The chart below depicts examples of helpers in employment roles and the ways they assist older people. It can be used as a guide by professionals or family members to begin to assess an older person's informal support network.

Locating such helpers is time-consuming for professionals and family members, but worth the effort in terms of the information and support gained. These helpers are akin to field anthropologists observing people in their natural context. A grocery clerk may notice that an older person wanders the aisles, repeatedly looking for the same items. A bus driver may find that an older person fails to get off at the stop nearest home unless reminded. Family members who see their relative within the known and mastered environment of a lifelong home may be unaware of problems the person experiences in the outside world. For this reason, families often find it valuable to introduce themselves to clerks and owners of local businesses as a way to check on the older person's functioning out of the home.

Another strategy is for family members to accompany their relative through a typical day, learning thereby what help occurs, by whom, and how often. For example, a son going with his father to a frequented restaurant will be able to glimpse which customers and staff greet his father by name. The son may also see how a waitress cajoles his father out of ordering foods which violate his restricted diet. Similarly, a daughter who witnesses her mother's conversations at a beauty salon may sense that a hairdresser's caring responses to her mother are based on an intimate knowledge of the family circumstances.

During this process of network exploration, family members may also discover that an older person has more social contacts and a more attractive public personality than they thought possible. A man who is relatively silent and contained around his wife may be boisterous among his cronies in the neighborhood tavern. His charm and

HELPERS IN EMPLOYMENT ROLES

Nurses and receptionists at doctors' offices: help with insurance forms, arranging transportation to and from appointments, liaison with other helpers

Bus drivers: give help getting on and off the bus, reminders to get off at the right stop, directions to specific destinations, assistance with packages

Apartment managers: assist in facilitating helping networks in the building, checkup calls, simple errands

Grocery store clerks: help reaching for items on shelves, carrying packages, reminding about needed items and special diets, cashing checks

Postal carriers: note daily checkup; read important items to low-vision people; bring mail to the door

Bartenders: assist by social introductions, lengthy listening, referral to other sources of help, relaying messages

Deliverers of fuel oil, meals, and oxygen: aid by periodic checkups; friendly visiting; referrals to other sources of help; encouragement toward self-care

Cab drivers: help getting up and down steps, locating destinations, carrying packages

Pharmacists: offer leeway on bill payment, repetition of instructions to older people with memory loss, education about side effects of medications

Hairdressers and barbers: are resource for social introductions, lengthy listening, opportunities to be touched, referrals to other sources of help

Restaurant staff: assist by special food preparation, nutritional reminders and encouragements, social introductions, special discounts, credit until the next month

Home health aides and chore workers: help by daily telephone calls; stopping by after work for checkup visit; bringing needed items on weekends or evenings

congeniality in that setting may surprise his son, who accompanies him there for the first time while learning about his father's helping network. The son may discover that the bartender knows a host of people who would help his father during a time of need, out of affection formed during years of pool games.

Meeting these helpers and gathering information from them also gives them recognition. Their help may assume added importance when family members point out its value within the overall helping effort: "Without your making sure she gets the right groceries, we'd have a much harder time keeping her in her own home." When they sense collaboration from the older person's family, helpers are often further motivated to personalize their aid. For example, when their questions about the older person's health status are answered by the family, they may feel more trusted and included. Family members can affirm the helpers' interest and support by offering their home phone numbers and inviting the helpers to share further questions and concerns.

Another appreciated gesture is to let each helper know what the others in the informal network are doing. Such people tend to be pleased to hear about others in the community who are concerned with the older person's welfare. Linking helpers in this way eliminates overlapping efforts as each becomes more aware of the others' assistance. Cooperative problem-solving can occur when family members or professionals convey information between helpers. For instance, if a bus driver learns that a teenage grocery clerk is willing to walk an older person home during an afternoon break, he could cue the person to stop at the store as he drops her off, thus solving her problem of getting lost between the bus stop and her house. A postal carrier may be willing to check with the apartment manager when he notices mail accumulating in the box. The potential for such linkages between helpers is limited only by the helpers' imagination and willingness to become involved.

By providing motivation against becoming homebound, helpers in employment roles can deter depression in older people. A woman may maintain her weekly visits to her beauty salon more for her beautician's listening and touching than for attractive hair. As she enacts her weekly ritual, the trip gives her the exercise of walking to the bus stop, the social contact of talking with others on the bus, the mental stimulation of varied sights and conversations, and the mood elevation inherent in a change of scene. Looking forward to this outing one day each week can make the rest of the week's monotony easier to bear. Without the draw of her beautician's warmth and friendliness, the pull to stay in the safety of home might have won out and depression might have resulted.

Such friendliness increases in value with the intensity of the older person's isolation. A waitress who automatically places an older man's order as soon as he enters the restaurant acknowledges his existence and provides a feeling of belonging. A clinic receptionist who converses at length with older patients inspires compliance with follow-up appointments and personalizes the health care experience in a way that busy doctors and nurses cannot. A bus driver who greets an older woman by name or notices when she resumes riding the bus after a long illness may give her sufficient reason to get herself dressed and out to the bus stop. The motivation of anticipated warmth can help an older person overcome hazards such as slippery steps, uneven pavement, steep hills, and busy traffic.

Families can acknowledge helpers in employment roles by giving them gifts or sending letters of appreciation to their work supervisors. Inviting them to speak up when the older person's needs begin to exceed their time constraints is another form of acknowledgment. Some may need encouragement to set limits on their help, as in the case of a clerk who allows an older person to build up excessive debts to a pharmacy. Periodic checking with an older person's helping network functions both as a support to ongoing efforts and as a way to identify problems before they erode the helpers' good will.

Neighbors as Helpers

As the most accessible natural helpers, neighbors provide more frequent assistance to older people than other types of helpers. Those in employment roles have defined work hours and private lives outside the context in which help occurs, but neighbors are within reach on a potentially unlimited basis. Not surprisingly, one of neighbors' chief problems in helping older people is finding ways to limit their involvement. Many who could offer specific help remain aloof out of their fear of being overwhelmed by an avalanche of needs if they make themselves available at all.

When they do become involved, neighbors are often the keystone of the support needed to keep older people in their homes. A relationship that begins with stopping over for coffee can become the provision of indispensable services. A neighbor who first notices that her older friend has difficulty reading medication labels may respond by giving her the morning dosage. Recognizing next that her friend cannot prepare hot meals without help, the neighbor may begin preparing break-fast during their morning conversation. As the helping gradually mul-tiplies in response to the needs, a neighbor could eventually find herself assisting the older person with getting dressed in the morning and then returning to help with bedtime tasks.

Problems arise when a neighbor such as this realizes how confined or burdened she has become as a result of her kindness. Contemplat-ing a vacation, she may find no other neighbors willing to take over while she is gone. The older person may discourage her from contact-ing her family members, fearing that nursing home placement would be discussed. Neighbors in such predicaments often hear from the older person: "Go ahead on your trip. I can manage." Knowing too well how precarious the older person's survival would be in their absence, they may defer vacations indefinitely. The prohibition against contact-ing family members then leaves them in a bind between loyalty to the older person and their own needs for privacy and leisure.

Family members and professionals who assist older people may re-main unaware of such neighborly captivity for long periods of time. An older person's hospitalization often precipitates discovery of this type of situation. For instance, the neighbor may disappear on an extended vacation during the hospitalization. If their relative returns home while the neighbor is still away, family members then confront the full extent of the needs previously handled by the neighbor. Similarly, a hospital discharge planner may contact a neighbor while checking on the older person's support system, only to hear accounts of frustration and weariness: "Please don't send her home; I can't do it any more." Discharge planners often encounter such pleas from neighbors who have been the silent, behind-the-scene support for an older person's re-maining at home.

In order to prevent such untimely discoveries, professionals and family members must maintain an ongoing awareness of neighbors' ef-forts. For example, a daughter can determine who is most involved in her mother's life by asking her mother to describe the people she knows well in her apartment building. Asking to be introduced to these neighbors during her visits enables the daughter to convey her appre-ciation and awareness of how vital they are to her mother's well-being. Through these contacts, she can affirm that neighbors will not be left alone with future care tasks if the older person's condition worsens. This assurance may inspire them to be more innovative in the help they offer, rather than protective of their personal turf.

Another way to support neighbors' helping is for family members to incorporate neighbors' errands into those they do for their relative. Ringing a neighbor's doorbell to see if there is a need for extra groceries conveys a cooperative attitude. It also implicitly rewards the neighbor for taking an interest in the older person's welfare. These contacts with family members may fill older neighbors' practical and emotional needs unmet by their own families. The time added to errands by this extra kindness is not substantial and tends to be well worth the good will it creates.

When family members sense that a neighbor is becoming weary of helping, an effective way to broach the subject is to ask, "How can we make it easier for you to help?" Hiring someone to do the tasks the neighbor least likes to do may be a possibility. Another strategy is for family members to offer to pay neighbors for their time. Those who feel they should be compensated will accept it; those who do not want to be paid usually appreciate the chance to decline payment. Listening to neighbors' accounts of their efforts over the phone may be the best way to avert weariness, particularly in the case of out-of-town family members who cannot offer neighbors help with errands and other immediate tasks. If the acts of helping seem to be the neighbor's sole meaningful activity, family members can enhance the neighbor's satisfaction by taking the time to listen to these stories.

Daily check-ups is one of the most useful functions neighbors can perform without a substantial commitment of time. A neighbor in the house across the street can check to see that the blinds are opened by a certain time each morning. If they are not, she can use a house key to check on the older person's safety. In apartment buildings, a next-door neighbor can make sure that the daily newspaper is taken in by a certain time and alert the manager if it is not. The knowledge that someone will check on them removes an older person's dread of lying helpless for days because a sudden incapacitation prevents their reaching the telephone.

BUILDING NETWORKS

Most older people, no matter how isolated they feel, have some type of network which professionals and family members can activate. Even if neighbors have only a nodding acquaintance with a woman next door to them, they nevertheless will tend to be aware of her routines and deviations from habit. Concerned people to whom older residents can turn exist in most neighborhoods, but these individuals may be uncertain as to how they can help or wary of offering unless asked.

Some older people do alienate those who would help them. By complaining excessively or expecting too much without reciprocating, they erode others' good will. Some withdraw from neighbors' gestures of kindness out of pride and a desire to protect their privacy and appearance of independence. In these instances, professionals and family members are faced not only with creating a helping network, but with working through the older person's resistance to accepting help.

Building networks requires that families and professionals devote the time necessary for visiting the older person's locale to talk informally with neighbors and area business personnel. An outreach worker, for example, may visit with others in the lobby of a senior high-rise building. By questioning and listening, the worker can learn which neighbors have the reputation of helping. In many cases, these neighbors may have wondered about the person's need for help, but not known specifically what to offer. The outreach worker can suggest ideas, without violating the person's privacy: "The man next door to you might appreciate your picking up a loaf of bread or quart of milk for him once in a while." Once neighbors begin knocking on the man's door, offering to run simple errands, they may help spontaneously with other needs and develop an ongoing routine of looking in on him.

Professionals may feel awkward when they ask neighbors for information about someone in their building, while knowing that confidentiality constraints prevent them from answering neighbors' questions about the person. Professionals should make these boundaries clear through statements such as, "I appreciate any information you can give me, but I can't answer your questions without permission from your neighbor." Once these boundaries are established, neighbors will understand that their speculations about the person's private affairs can neither be confirmed nor denied by the visiting professional, but that their observations are still helpful and important.

In contrast to professionals, family members have much more freedom to exchange information about their relative's situation with neighbors and others who may be of help. They can put out the word in the apartment building, for instance, that driving restrictions have left their relative in need of rides to the pharmacy and the nearby senior center. They can answer specific questions about the nature of their relative's health problems, especially if doing so generates further commiseration from neighbors and a greater understanding of what help is needed. They can put up a sign in the lobby offering mutually beneficial exchanges, such as rides to the grocery store for anyone interested in doing their relative's laundry once a week.

Not all professionals are comfortable or skilled in working with informal helpers. To be effective, professionals must be committed to the concept that these helpers can be a vital resource, a perspective sometimes contrary to their advanced training. In addition, professionals and informal helpers may differ in how they define adequacy of care and the need for professional intervention. For example, neighbors may believe that an older man living alone should be placed in a nursing home, having grown tired of taking out the rotting garbage they find in his house when they drop off his groceries. They may become angry at the professional who insists on honoring the man's right to self-determination rather than trying to convince him to leave the home he cherishes. Working with weary neighbors and attempting to reduce their sense of burden is a response that expresses respect both for the central role these helpers play and for the dilemmas they face when someone's needs exceed what they are willing to handle.

WHEN FRIENDSHIP VERGES ON EXPLOITATION

Although neighbors and helpers in employment roles are a major support to older people and their families, abuse can arise in such relationships. For instance, when vulnerable older people offer gifts or cash to gain extra help, the line between legitimate payment and abuse can become blurred. A homebound woman who gives a neighbor cash to retrieve her mail or pick up her groceries may eventually be persuaded by the neighbor to pay more for these services than is warranted. The more dependent she becomes, the more the neighbor may take advantage of her vulnerability in extracting further payments. Loneliness and need can deprive people of their ability to approach others selectively and to protect themselves assertively.

Sensory and memory deficits can also interfere with older people's ability to protect themselves. In fact, hearing, vision, or memory loss combined with loneliness are red flags for checking to see if anyone in the older person's environment is taking advantage of the situation. Families and professionals should translate an alertness to this possibility into a scrutiny of the older person's natural helpers.

Detecting Abuse

A useful starting point is to determine how long an older person has known the people who help her. A neighbor who became friendly only after the person needed help paying bills and cashing checks compares poorly with someone who extended friendliness prior to the onset of the person's vulnerability. In general, longstanding friendships with a history of reciprocity are more trustworthy than newer friendships with little history of mutual helping.

Acceptable motivations for helping tend to be visible. People with kindness as part of their nature usually demonstrate this inclination in their overall conduct with others. Those with religious reasons may readily explain how their acts of helping fit into their beliefs. Those who help with the hope of investing in their own future or the promise of someday being helped in return tend to be obvious in their attitude of storing away good will. When such clear motivations are not apparent, suspicions of abuse are generally worth exploring.

Family members and professionals who suspect abuse should make themselves known as widely as possible within the older person's support system. Those who might have information about abuse need to be assured that their disclosures will be handled tactfully and constructively. For example, a neighbor possessing incriminating information about another neighbor may fear retaliation if her role in exposing the abuse is not kept confidential. Another potential informant may worry that the older person's feelings will be hurt if the illusion of friendship created by the abuser abruptly collapses. Acknowledging and demonstrating sensitivity to these issues can help bystanders feel better about becoming involved in what they may perceive as a "touchy" situation.

Watchful helpers in employment roles are likely to confide that they suspect abuse after family members and professionals make themselves known as advocates of the older person. A store clerk may notice that ever since a neighbor began shopping for an older person, expensive items have been purchased on her behalf that do not fit her customary selections. If this woman's case manager introduced herself at the store and left her business card, the clerk might be willing to phone in his suspicions and report any further questionable occurrences. Similarly, a bank teller might be willing to report each time she sees an older customer hand over sizeable sums of cash to a young companion, if a daughter alerts the teller in advance about suspicions of financial exploitation.

Some of the most commonly occurring forms of abuse are those perpetrated by in-home workers. Neighbors who are able to make unannounced visits to the home can be especially helpful as observers in these instances. A neighbor who drops in unexpectedly may catch a paid homemaker watching television instead of cleaning, or walking out with a bag of "gifts" from the older person. An apartment manager with an office near the lobby may notice that an aide leaves the building sooner than the conclusion of her scheduled hours, or that a live-in companion leaves the older person alone most of the day. Because victimized older people are often reluctant to report such abuse, neighbors and other helpers who are willing to report it for them can function as valuable safeguards. (See "Fearing Victimization," pp. 244–246.)

Intervening in Situations of Abuse

In most instances, abusers do not like to prey upon an older person who has a variety of unpredictable visitors and therefore potential witnesses. Family members may want to emphasize their visibility by attending social events in their relative's building or taking walks with their relative at times when they are most likely to be observed. Establishing routines of contact with neighbors, under the guise of running errands or dropping off groceries, can serve as a pipeline of information as well as a sign of involvement that might discourage abusers.

Professionals and family members can also set up additional services which increase the number of visitors to the home. For instance, a church or synagogue in the neighborhood may have a "friendly visitor" program in which a volunteer may be assigned to visit the older person on a regular basis. Signing the person up for home-delivered meals adds another knock at the door on a weekly basis. Generally, the more people who have access to and are concerned for an older person, the less chance there is for abuse to continue or intensify.

When the abuse is by someone posing as a friend, the consequences of breaking the illusion of friendship should be carefully considered before any action is taken. The benefits which the older person gains from the relationship should be weighed against the harm inflicted. For example, if a neighbor who helps with bill paying, steals thirty dollars every time she cashes the older person's Social Security check, family members and professionals may decide against confrontation. The hurt that would follow from forcing the older person to recognize a helper's friendliness as insincere may not be worth protecting her from this small financial drain. Although it is demeaning for anyone to admit to being duped, it is especially humiliating for someone who already feels powerless in response to necessary dependence on others.

Rather than direct confrontation, strategies that reduce the abuser's power may be effective without hurting the older person's pride. Finding someone else to help with bill paying or household tasks can remove an abuser's pretext for opening the checkbook or entering the residence's private areas. An extra measure of protection is to make the abuser aware of the discovery of the abuse when introducing an alternative helper. This indicates to the abuser that gracefully bowing out is the only viable option.

In situations of advanced memory loss, stronger measures of protection may be necessary. Someone who is unable to recall daily events cannot protect herself from inappropriate actions, such as a neighbor insisting on cashing a check for her after a family member has already done so that day. In such situations, threats of legal action against the neighbor may be necessary to halt the abuse, with concerns for the older person's feelings about the neighbor becoming less important. Since older people with this degree of cognitive impairment are in constant danger of abuse, a guardian may be needed to oversee the finances.

Some of the most fortunate people are those who manage to live in the same neighborhood for decades and who amass good relationships with their neighbors. During a time of need, helpful neighbors can sometimes make the difference between someone staying in their own home and their having to find an alternative living situation. Knowing the owners of local businesses and maintaining friendly contacts with service people further supplements this protective web. Family members often find that their pressures as caregivers are greatly reduced when they can count on neighbors, friends, and other helpers to give their relative a hand with incidental or unpredictable needs.

SUGGESTED RESOURCES

Articles

Buckwalter, Kathleen, Marianne Smith, Peter Zevenbergen, and Daniel Russel. "Mental Health Services of the Rural Elderly Outreach Program," *The Gerontologist*, 31 (1991), 408–412.

> Presents an innovative elderly outreach program for the rural elderly that integrates a variety of health, mental health and human service agencies in the planning and delivery of services.

Korte, Charles and Vasudha Gupta. "A Program of Friendly Visitors as Network Builders," *The Gerontologist*, 31 (1991), 404–407.

> Describes a new conception of the friendly visitor role. The program trains volunteers to function as network builders who become directly involved in an isolated elderly person's social network.

Pynoos, Jon, Barbara Hade-Kaplan, and Dorothy Fleisher. "Intergenerational Neighborhood Networks: A Basis for Aiding the Frail Elderly," *The Gerontologist*, 24 (1984), 233–237.

> Portrays a neighborhood intergenerational project built on residents' capacity to help each other. The elderly participants served as donors as well as service recipients and were found to develop new friends, participate in more social activities, and enjoy increased life satisfaction.

Book

Barbara Myerhoff, *Number Our Days* (New York: Simon and Schuster), 1978.

> As an anthropologist, the author lived with and observed elderly Jews in Venice, California, to discover how they assigned meaning to their own and other people's lives. She movingly portrays how their culture and support networks gave them the strength to face and overcome enormous problems.

Organizations

Gatekeeper Program. Spokane Community Mental Health Center Elderly Services, South 107 Division, Spokane, WA 99202. (509) 838–4651.

> This program utilizes nontraditional referral sources who come into contact with high-risk elderly individuals. They offer a training video, training manual, and other material relative to the concept of active case finding and in-home delivery system.

National Parish Nurse Resource Center. 1800 Dempster Street, Park Ridge, IL 60068. (708) 696–8773.

The center provides information about the philosophy and activities of nurses in congregations across the country. Parish nurses are registered nurses who volunteer or work for a modest stipend to aid older members of their congregations. They do not provide hands-on nursing, such as wound care, but serve as health educators and referral persons.

Senior Companion Program. c/o ACTION, 1100 Vermont Avenue, N.W., 11th floor, Washington, DC 20525. (202) 634–9108.

Matches volunteers over age sixty with frail elderly who need care and assistance. Volunteers receive reimbursement for travel expenses. Local programs are listed in the phone book or can be located through the national headquarters.

Shepherd's Centers of America. 6700 Troost, Suite 616, Kansas City, MO 64131. (816) 523–1080.

This national nonprofit group is comprised of a network of ninety-six centers. Older adults volunteer to provide services such as meals on wheels, transportation, and telephone reassurance.

7

Coping with Memory Loss

M emory loss is one of the most dreaded conditions associated with old age, yet many people do not realize that it is rare to lose the kind of memory which matters the most. There are two types of memory, short- and long-term, located in physically separate areas of the brain. Short-term memory consists of daily events such as where a car was parked in a parking lot, whether noontime medications were taken, or which items need to be purchased at the grocery store. Long-term memory consists of long-standing knowledge, such as where one was born, the number of siblings in one's family, or the type of work one performed prior to retirement. It is possible to have problems with short-term memory without losing long-term memory. This chapter first examines normal memory loss and ways to cope with it, and then looks at more severe kinds of memory loss.

NORMAL MEMORY LOSS

Many people over the age of seventy-five experience problems with short-term memory. In fact, short-term memory loss is so common with increasing age that it is termed "senescent memory loss" in medical texts, a normal condition rather than a pathological disorder. Only a small percentage of these individuals will go on to experience the progressive loss of long-term memory which is the locus of everyone's dread.

Assessing Memory Without Causing Shame and Anxiety

People of all ages have trouble with burnt pots, lost keys, remembering to take pills, locating their car in massive parking lots, and forgetting grocery items. Short-term memory is like a basket that is filled hour by hour. If someone is distracted, stressed, or overly busy, the basket can seem to have a hole in the bottom where information leaks out. Concentrating, relaxing, and slowing down can often bring an immediate improvement in someone's capacity to retain short-term information. In old age, this "basket" for storing daily material begins to show signs of wear, resulting in the need to find other ways to hold onto information.

Putting someone on the spot with memory questions tends to arouse anxiety, which then interferes directly with the retrieval of memory-dependent information. Many older people experience a slower retrieval process generally, and this slowness only worsens when they know they are being tested. For instance, it is humiliating to struggle to recite one's birthdate in front of a younger person who is awaiting an answer. Often, as soon as the questioner goes away and performance pressure is lifted, someone who had been struggling to retrieve a name or a date will suddenly come up with the information.

During their visits, well-intentioned family members sometimes practice checking their relative's memory, imitating heath-care professionals by asking their relative to name the current month, year, and day of the week. Although the older person may conceal her uneasiness, these questions tend to cause intense shame if the person has trouble answering them. Similarly, a physician asking these questions at every medical visit may lead to an older person's refusal to return to that physician.

A more subtle and caring way for family members to check a relative's memory status is to refer back to the content of recent conversations to see how much has been retained. If the older person consistently needs a review, then it is better to provide a review on a regular basis rather than test each time for its necessity: "Mom, you know how Billy fell off his bike last week and scraped his knee. Well, now he's got an infection." If an older person starts to tell a story already told the day before, it is more respectful to say plainly, "Yes, you did tell me that," rather than to endure a repetition and then indirectly convey impatience.

Similarly, professionals should place the ethical mandate to "do no harm" above their need for quick methods for testing older people's memory. Mental status exams consisting of a series of "silly" questions such as, "What month is it?" can only degrade older people who have difficulty answering. It is preferable to incorporate memory-dependent questions into the conversational flow, such as by asking what year someone was born while talking about their hometown. Letting someone immediately off the hook when the answer is not forthcoming helps reduce embarrassment: "It doesn't matter. We can get your birthdate later. Tell me more about your hometown." Explaining how common it is to experience slow retrieval with names and dates and describing the difference between short- and long-term memory may also help make it safe for someone to confess problems with memory, rather than trying to hide from a professional's scrutiny.

Creative Compensations for Short-Term Memory Loss

Older people often devise diverse and creative strategies to compensate for memory loss. For example, those who always forget to mark off the days on their calendar may begin wearing a watch which displays the date and day of the week. Some older people keep their daily newspaper on the kitchen table for a prominent reminder of the date. If their medications are not linked to mealtimes, some people set watches or stove timers to alert them when it is time for the next dosage. Such creativity knows no limits, as long as an older person is able to see memory loss as a condition requiring adaptation rather than a sign of the beginning of the end.

Families should avoid reacting to these coping efforts as a cause for alarm. The person may finally be putting his need to adapt ahead of his need to conceal. Such efforts should be acknowledged in an encouraging manner: "Dad, that's great to tape reminder notes to your refrigerator. I think I'll copy your method." When family members come up with their own ideas of how memory problems can be solved, they should offer these suggestions in a way that does not hurt their relative's pride or arouse fear that memory lapses are being probed: "Mom, wearing a front door key around your neck could save you long searches in that bottomless purse of yours." The following list of problems and solutions is meant to stimulate inventive strategies for helping an older person cope with the loss of short-term memory.

COPING WITH SHORT-TERM MEMORY LOSS

Problem	Possible Solution
Losing purse, wallet, or keys within the home	Install a hook near the door for hanging a purse or keys, or put a large bowl near the door for depositing a wallet and keys upon entry.
Losing the car in parking lots	When parking in huge lots, make a written note of a nearby landmark instead of trying to rely on short-term memory. Tie a plastic flower to the top of the antenna or some other marker that can be sighted from afar.
Adding some ingredients twice while cooking; forgetting to add others	Lay out the ingredients all at once when starting to cook and then put each item away after using the required portion.
Mixing up medication times and dosages	Obtain a medication box with compartments for each day of the week and each dosage time.
Forgetting to get tasks done or to show up at appointments; forgetting what was said during phone calls.	Obtain a pocket-size memo book on which to make notes of each day's tasks and appointments, calls made, and the gist of what was said or learned from each call. This notetaking gradually becomes a habit.

MEMORY LOSS BEYOND THE NORM

Signs of memory loss beyond normal forgetfulness tend to occur in the areas of long-term memory and of basic orientation to time and place, such as failing to recognize an immediate family member or becoming confused about the current season or the town where one resides. Other signs are difficulties with problem solving, such as becoming unable to complete sequential tasks. The first step when such problems are noticed is to rule out the treatable causes of memory loss through a medical examination.

Types of Severe Memory Loss

People experiencing memory problems are often afraid to go see a doctor. They fear having their memory checked, yet this is precisely what their family members want the physician to do. It may be helpful to emphasize the physical focus of the exam and to downplay the issue of checking memory, since the physician will have to rule out the many reversible causes of memory loss before drawing any conclusions. Talking about physical problems reduces the person's sense of threat and may allow for a trusting relationship with the physician to develop. A complete medical workup requires more than one visit, and there are many occasions during this process when the physician can check the person's memory through casual, respectful conversation.

Alzheimer's disease is often misheard by people as "Old Timer's Disease," which makes it sound far more common than it is. Studies vary, but most estimate that Alzheimer's occurs in a small percentage of people over the age of sixty-five. There is no single test which proves that someone has, or does not have, the disease. To make a diagnosis, physicians must go through the process of ruling out all the treatable causes of memory loss (see following chart). If no other cause of memory loss is found, Alzheimer's is diagnosed as the cause. A definitive diagnosis can be made only after death, by examination of the brain during an autopsy.

There are several conditions besides Alzheimer's disease which can lead to severe memory loss. Multi-infarct dementia, or a series of small strokes, may produce abrupt downturns in the person's memory capacity, followed by long periods of stability in which memory does not seem to worsen. This condition can sometimes be helped by medications which bring the person's blood pressure under better control. In other instances, the condition progresses in this step-down fashion and cannot be remedied. A CAT scan of the brain may reveal areas of damage, but often the strokes are so small that they do not show up. Distinguishing between Alzheimer's and multi-infarct dementia is often possible only by observing a gradual vs. a step-down progression.

Heavy alcohol intake over a lifetime can also lead to significant memory loss. Liver damage from alcohol can become so severe that the liver loses its capacity to filter toxic substances from the blood. These toxins reach the brain and interfere with memory and cognition. Liver damage can be determined through medical tests and may serve as undeniable proof that someone has not been immune to the detrimental effects of alcohol. There are some individuals who will stop drinking when confronted with both this evidence and the pronouncement that liver damage can produce memory loss. Since liver function may improve somewhat with the cessation of alcohol intake, this information may serve as additional motivation for an older person to enter alcohol treatment.

There are several other kinds of dementia which can be diagnosed through a neurologic evaluation, many of which are treatable. Excessive pressure on the brain from spinal fluid is an example of a cause which can usually be treated. Although rare, vitamin B-12 deficiency has been linked to memory loss. The list of treatable causes of memory loss can be used as a checklist for common conditions that may need medical attention and for which family members and professionals should be on the alert.

Responding to Personality Changes

Changes in a relative's personality tend to be more painful for many family members than coping with the memory loss itself. These changes may include loss of interest in others' lives, mood swings inconsistent with past personality patterns, increasing negativism and suspiciousness, and episodes of depression as the person struggles with his awareness of cognitive losses.

Loss of memory for recent events, conversations, and even the story line of a television program can be deeply disturbing as someone gradually becomes aware of this lost capacity. Hearing the refrain, "Dad, you told us that already," over and over again may stifle an older person's willingness to embark on a conversation, lest he be accused of repetition. He may become leery of asking any questions about a loved one's job or health status, fearing that he might have been given the answer several times already. He may hold back from asking others to

TREATABLE CAUSES OF MEMORY LOSS

Poor nutrition: Body chemistry can become imbalanced from the "tea and toast" syndrome, eating meals lacking the full range of necessary nutrients.

Dehydration: Many people do not drink enough fluids, or they consume primarily caffeine beverages which flush fluids out of the body.

Fluctuating blood sugar: People who develop diabetes late in life may go for years without realizing they should ask their physician to check their blood sugar.

Thyroid deficiency: Possible deficiency can be checked by a physician and remedied with medication.

Infection: Urinary tract or bladder infections are most common, but any infection can cause memory loss.

Medication combinations: Taking multiple pills every day can result in mix-ups or medication interactions.

Medication toxicity: Occasionally, too much medication accumulates in the blood. For example, digoxin (Lanoxin) is a heart medication which can become toxic.

Depression: Some people lose interest in others and become confused when they get depressed. Antidepressant medication may help significantly.

Sensory losses: Loss of hearing or sight may interfere with orientation to time and place.

Lung disease: Decreased lung capacity may mean insufficient oxygen for the brain. Memory loss may completely resolve when the person goes on oxygen.

Cancer: Tumors in the brain, liver, or other organs can lead to memory loss. Prompt diagnosis may mean that the tumor can be removed or reduced through treatment.

Toxic house: Furnaces sometimes malfunction and leave carbon monoxide in the air, producing confusion and sleepiness. Fixing the furnace may restore alertness.

explain the plot of a film they are seeing together, afraid of revealing the extent of his memory problems. Retreating into silent watchfulness may seem the safest course, even though this may appear to family members as a loss of concern about their lives and a loss of interest in activities that were previously valued.

Moodiness often accompanies this retreat into watchfulness. Frustration is rampant for someone unable to remember daily or hourly occurrences, and incessant frustration tends to produce short temper. Blaming others for misplaced wallets and car keys, or barking at those who issue too many anxious reminders are reactions which may bruise family members' feelings. Yelling at those who try to help when a car is lost in a parking lot or an important appointment is missed may be examples of misplaced rage. The pent-up anger belongs to the memory loss but is dumped onto loved ones.

Confabulation and Suspiciousness

Reactions to memory loss which resemble paranoia are particularly disturbing to families. A woman may move her treasured diamond necklace from its customary location and then forget both that she moved it and where she put it. Groping for an explanation for its disappearance, she may blame her daughter who often helps clean her home and therefore has access to her jewelry: "Mary, why did you take my diamond necklace?" If Mary insists that she did not take the necklace, her mother may only get more angry and accusatory.

In this instance, mistrusting her daughter is less painful to the older woman than facing her memory loss. The admission, "I can't remember where I put my valuable necklace," may be unacceptable because it would undermine her confidence in her ability to manage her own life. Belief in one's abiding mental capacity is a conviction which tends to be more vital than any other, including belief in a family member's trustworthiness. The false accusation protects the older woman from the distressing awareness that she is, in fact, losing her mind.

Confabulation is the process of inventing false information to fill in a gap in memory. The motivating force behind confabulation is the need to explain memory failure in a way which places blame outside the self. Trying to defeat a confabulation by using rational argument or presenting someone with undeniable proof that their ideas are false tends to evoke anger and more strenuous insistence as to their correctness. For instance, an older man may tell his family that his local bus route has been discontinued, rather than admit that he can no longer find the bus stop near his home. If his daughter were to hand him a printed schedule proving that his route was still functioning, he would probably be more outraged than mollified. His daughter might accuse him of being stubborn or lying, unless she knew that such false information arises from confabulation, a desperate form of self-preservation.

In contrast to true paranoia, which tends to affect several areas of life at once, the delusions expressed by older people with memory loss are usually confined to an aspect of life directly affected by their memory loss. A woman who regularly misplaces her keys and her purse when she comes home may assert that "little men" are coming through her window and hiding these items when she turns her back. Her seemingly paranoid delusion is best understood as confabulation, because her belief about her miniature intruders serves the single function of explaining lost objects. As with any confabulation, attempts to dissuade someone that the "little men" are not real is likely to meet with adamant protest as to their reality.

The best way to handle confabulation is by understanding the purpose it serves. Rather than becoming upset by their relative's false statements or accusations, family members should be encouraged to see the self-protective function at the basis of these invented ideas. Working with, or around, the confabulation usually leads to a better outcome than trying to disassemble it.

Depression and Isolation

When it succeeds, confabulation serves to shield the older person from awareness of memory loss and therefore also from the sorrow that would have accompanied awareness. Depression often develops when someone is unable to deny his recognition of progressive memory loss through these and other protective measures. The person may begin making statements such as "What's the use of being alive if I can't remember anything?" More than any physical limitation, the loss of mental ability can seem to remove someone's foundation for continuing to live. In these instances, families should seek professional assistance, since supportive counseling and structured activities may alleviate the depression. When family members find that their own sense of discouragement becomes heightened by their relative's depression, attending support groups with other family caregivers can be especially helpful.

People with progressive memory loss often fall into a cycle of depression and isolation. Unable to keep up with others in conversations and with activities dependent on memory, the older person may refuse social invitations and recreational outings. The loss of stimulation caused by staying home day after day then leads to increased disorientation, since clues to time of day and the sequence of days in the week are lost through the omission of outings. The isolation and loss of stimulation may, in turn, feed the depression.

Devising activities to counteract this cycle is sometimes effective. People who can no longer follow the content of a sermon may nevertheless enjoy the rituals of a religious service. People in the middle stages of Alzheimer's disease often retain their skill at conversational banter, able to exchange pleasantries and superficial remarks at social gatherings. Similarly, activities such as musical events, long walks, window shopping, and drives in the car do not depend on memory to be enjoyed.

Becoming accustomed to a relationship limited by memory loss requires practice and emotional agility. Family members may find that talking to a relative who cannot remember what they say feels useless. In addition, their relative's inability to express interest in their lives may quell their desire to listen. In such instances, reading to their relative, singing songs, playing music, or engaging in simple projects can fill in awkward silences and provide a soothing way to spend time together. Physical contact, such as giving the older person a backrub, can also take the place of conversations. Listening to often-repeated stories may be less frustrating if viewed as part of the visit's routine, rather than a hindrance. If the older person responds best to visual cues, looking at magazines and photographs together may become a mutual pleasure.

ADVANCED MEMORY LOSS

The later stages of progressive memory loss often include the breakdown of social inhibitions, failure to recognize family members, repetitive questions, episodes of pacing and restlessness, minimal attention span, and extreme mood swings. Keeping someone at home under these circumstances becomes an hour-by-hour challenge which can exhaust the patience and coping capacities of the most determined caregivers. The following questions are among those most frequently asked by families.

QUESTIONS AND ANSWERS FOR RESPONDING TO ADVANCED MEMORY LOSS

1. What can be done about questions that the older person keeps asking over and over again?

Answering the same question repeatedly can be extremely frustrating to families. When her mother asks every five minutes "What happened to my car?" a daughter may explain that the car was sold and money from the sale was deposited in the bank. This response may satisfy her mother only for the brief time that she retains the answer in her memory. Instead, the daughter could try to respond to the emotional tone behind the question, rather than to its content. After reassuring her mother with a touch on her shoulder that everything about the car has been taken care of, the daughter could distract her by switching the conversation to another topic. Similarly, if an older person repeatedly asks "Where are you going?" or "When will you be back?" reassurance on an emotional level, combined with a hug, may be more effective than facts in soothing feelings of fear or loneliness.

2. What are some ways to calm down an agitated and confused person?

The nonverbal sensing ability in older people with severe memory loss is frequently as keen as that possessed by young children. For example, a worried daughter may try to verbally reassure her father that he is safe with a substitute caregiver while she goes out shopping. Instead of listening to her words, her father is likely to read the worry in her tone of voice, body posture, and facial expression. If the daughter were to offer the same information in a calm voice, relaxed posture, and serene facial expression, her father's agitation might be greatly reduced. Learning to speak to feelings takes practice, but it can be much more effective than relying on words alone. Caregivers may need to separate themselves from the agitated person for a few minutes to compose themselves and master their own feelings before trying to calm their relative.

3. Are there any effective techniques for getting someone to bathe who puts up a struggle each time?

Refusal to bathe is a common problem in the later stages of progressive memory loss. Some confused people become terrified of showers

yet will still accept a bath if guided into the tub rather than asked be-
forehand. Others will pull back as soon as they see a tub full of water.
Telling a lively story while removing the older person's clothes may keep
her focus away from the reason for disrobing. If the story is sufficiently
animated, complete with broad gestures and exaggerated tones, the moment of getting into the tub may similarly go unnoticed and therefore
unprotested. This technique may work one morning and fail the next. In
many instances, older people with severe memory loss will get into the
tub for a hired caregiver but not for a family member, remaining obedi-
ent and cooperative only as long as this stranger assists them.

**4. What should be done when the older person speaks as if de-
ceased people are still alive or refers to events that never happened?**

It is usually not fruitful to try to force accurate information on someone whose thoughts are focused in another time and who is consequently uninterested in "reality" as known by family members. If, in
the middle of an otherwise rambling speech, an older person asks directly whether a deceased loved one is still alive, then it is important to
give accurate information. Families need to listen closely to distinguish this kind of reality testing from the speech which moves back
and forth in time without concern for current information.

**5. Is there a constructive way to respond when the older person
does not recognize family members?**

In the later stages of dementia, family members may find that they
need to introduce themselves at the beginning of each encounter, saying, for example, "I'm Mary, your daughter." To be mistaken for someone else or regarded as a stranger can be particularly painful to
members of the immediate family. Viewing nonrecognition as part of
the disease process is the only way to contain the recurrent hurt from
such experiences. Family members may need to remind each other of
this fact each time it happens.

**6. How can answers to important questions be obtained from a
confused person?**

When some people with dementia are in pain, general questions such
as, "Where are you hurting?" tend to elicit further confusion. In contrast, asking a series of specific questions that require only a shake of

the head may yield more information. The most productive method may be to ask, "Does your head hurt? Does your neck hurt?" while touching each area of the body until the pained area elicits a nod. The request, "Show me where it hurts," may work for some who do not need this successive cuing. Family members should take note of the particular questions and phrases which are especially effective with their relative and convey these to substitute caregivers or professionals who communicate with the older person.

7. Why does the older person become so much more irritable and anxious during the evening hours?

When the sun goes down, people with severe memory loss often become more confused and agitated. This problem is so common that it has been termed "sundowning." Solutions tend to vary from person to person, and sometimes from night to night for the same person. One response is to turn up the lights and play music, thereby increasing the amount of stimulation in the environment. Some people need to be taken for a brisk walk outside in order to release their anxiety through exercise. Others become calmer after a hot bath, a back rub, and a glass of warm milk. In situations where the person gets up at night and paces, sleep medications are sometimes effective.

8. How can a confused person be kept safely contained within the home when wandering is a problem?

A latch can be placed at the top end of doors, out of sight, where the older person will not remember to look for it. Installing a deadbolt is often enough, if the person is unaccustomed to doing more than turning a doorknob. Affixing a bell to the outside door to alert others when the door is opened may be helpful. For older people living alone, fire danger makes it unsafe to make door locks too complex for them to handle. The only safe strategy is have them wear an ID bracelet with name, address, and phone number.

9. What can be done in the situation where a person has severe hearing loss as well as memory loss?

The combination of hearing deficits with memory loss can be a particularly difficult mix, especially when a constantly misplaced hearing aid results. Many older people with moderate-to-severe memory loss remove their hearing aid when ringing or some other annoyance occurs.

When they need to put it back on, they cannot remember where they placed it. This practice can be especially frustrating to family members who phone to check on their relative's welfare and find that their relative does not hear the phone ring or cannot hear what is being said. A phone can be installed with a volume control which amplifies the speaker's voice enough to be heard without a hearing aid. Blinking lights on amps which are triggered when the phone rings may be vital for hearing-impaired people who need phone cues to overcome memory problems.

10. Are there ways to help someone retain the ability to put on their clothes correctly?

Some people can continue to dress themselves as long as their clothes are laid out for them in the sequence they will be put on. Others need someone to stand by, cuing each item one by one. Touching their bare foot while handing over a sock may be more helpful than saying, "Now, put on your socks." Reducing the number of surrounding distractions while the person is dressing also tends to be helpful, because many people can complete the familiar sequence of getting on their clothes as long so they are not interrupted in the process.

11. What are some strategies for helping someone who regularly mixes up medication times and dosages?

Setting up a series of envelopes or a medication box for each morning, noon, and evening dosage is helpful when the person is still somewhat oriented to time of day and day of the week. If not, cuing the person by phone for each dosage may be effective: "Dad, take those pills in the envelope on the kitchen table. I'll hold on while you get a glass of water." In some instances, it may be necessary to ask the person's physician to prescribe only one morning dosage, even when this schedule is not optimal, to insure that the person gets the right medicines. Often, neighbors are willing to stop by to make sure someone takes their morning medicines, as this favor only takes a few minutes and may make the difference for someone's ability to remain at home.

12. Are there ways to insure safety when the person insists on preparing hot meals?

Keeping an egg timer on the stove where the person sees it and remembers to use it may help prevent burnt pots. For some people, it is safer to disconnect the stove and obtain a countertop oven which is set to turn off automatically after a certain period of time. For making hot water, using a coffee maker may be safer than turning on an electric burner which can be forgotten. Phoning the person at mealtimes and giving verbal, step-by-step instructions is also a helpful strategy, but tiring for family members who are working full time. Leaving nonperishable food items where the person is likely to see them may help deter the person from attempts to prepare hot meals.

13. What can be done when someone drives dangerously and keeps getting lost when out on the road alone, yet insists on continuing to drive?

Some people will give up the car keys when a physician tells them it is time to stop driving. Others cannot remember that the doctor told them not to drive and will not listen to family members' pleas. Having a letter from the doctor which can be displayed repeatedly may help achieve cooperation. It is much less hurtful when the doctor's letter emphasizes physical problems, rather than memory loss, as the reason. In some instances, particularly with older men, allowing the person to retain the car keys in his pocket is sufficient. Some men like to go out and start the car occasionally, or wash and polish it, but will accept the prohibition against driving. Disabling the car by removing an essential wire or providing an old set of car keys that do not fit the ignition may be necessary in situations where a doctor's letter is ineffective. (See "Giving Up the Car Keys, pp. 251–257)

14. Are there methods to prevent a person from misplacing and forgetting to pay household bills, or paying the same bills over and over again?

Obtain a large, colorful shoe box that can be left on the kitchen table, with "Bills" marked on all sides. Repeatedly remind the person to place mail in the box so that it can be sorted when helpers visit. After considerable repetition, some people are able to develop this helpful habit. When registering the person for medical services, using a family member's address for the billing may reduce the number of confusing, computer-generated duplicate bills arriving at the older person's home. Marking old bills *"Paid"* may also help prevent double payments. (See "The Management of an Older Person's Financial Affairs," pp. 222–225.

Making the Nursing Home Decision

There comes a point in advanced memory loss when it matters less who is taking care of the person than that the care is rendered with kindness and compassion. When a nursing home has a unit specializing in the care of dementia patients or has aides experienced in this type of care, the person's quality of life may not diminish in the move from home to a nursing home. In some instances, the person's life improves because the staff only has to sustain their energy and patience for eight-hour shifts, as compared to the round-the clock efforts of family caregivers. The difficulty for families often lies in recognizing when it is time to seek nursing home placement.

Sleep deprivation is one of the major reasons that caregivers of people with advanced memory loss begin considering placing their relative in a nursing home. Their relative may confuse day and night, putting on all the lights in the home or pacing noisily in the middle of the night. Attempting to solve this problem through sleep medications does not always work, and hiring overnight help is expensive. When their sleep is interrupted on a regular basis, caregivers often become short-tempered, disoriented, and vulnerable to illness.

Another catalyst of nursing home placement is episodes of violent behavior. People with dementia may physically assault their caregivers in moments of extreme rage and confusion. Caregivers in such situations should seek a physician's help with trying various sedating medications and should experiment with behavioral techniques, but these interventions are not always successful. When caregivers are in danger of serious harm, a nursing home may be the only safe solution.

Dangerous situations beyond caregivers' control arise often in the later stages of progressive memory loss. For example, smokers with severe confusion may imperil the lives of caregivers and neighbors. Some manage to obtain cigarettes despite all efforts to prevent their doing so, and leave cigarettes burning near combustible material. In other instances, confused people manage to get out of the home and wander, leaving caregivers with frayed nerves and doubts about their capacity to go on.

Day after day, supervising someone with advanced memory loss can deplete even huge reserves of patience. Caregivers may gradually become prisoners at home, because their relative is too unpredictable and uncontrollable in public places. Visitors to the home may become scarce as friends and neighbors avoid contact with the person with dementia. Many caregivers reach the point where their isolation and exhaustion are extreme, but they need a professional to say the words, "It's time to find a nursing home." Hearing this sentence finally releases them.

As family members confront the need to place their relative in a nursing home, locating a facility which would be convenient to someone in the family often becomes the most important consideration. People in nursing homes who are visited frequently tend to receive the best care. The purpose of placement is not to end the caregiving, but to relocate it to another setting where it continues in a more bearable form. (See Chapter 15.)

Older people should be reassured that it is possible to lose some of one's short-term memory without losing memory of one's major life experiences. A variety of techniques can help older people cope with short-term memory loss. For the small minority of people who do lose their long-term memory, professionals should muster a full range of services to assist them and support their families.

SUGGESTED RESOURCES

Books

Cohen, Donna, and Carl Eisdorfer. *The Loss of Self: A Family Resource for the Care of Alzheimer's Disease and Related Disorders* (New York: W. W. Norton), 1986.

> The authors offer comprehensive recommendations about diagnosis, locating resources, handling behavior problems, and when and how to seek a nursing home.

Gwyther, Lisa. *Care of Alzheimer's Patients: A Manual for Nursing Home Staff*, (Chicago: Alzheimer's Disease and Related Disorders Association), 1986.

> Although this manual was written for nursing home care of Alzheimer's patients, its recommendations can also be useful to in-home caregivers, particularly the sections on managing behavior problems and communication strategies.

Mace, Nancy, and Peter Rabins. *The 36 Hour Day: A Family Guide to Caring for Persons With Alzheimer's Disease, Related Dementing Illness, and Memory Loss in Later Life.* (Baltimore: Johns Hopkins University Press), 1991.

> One of the best books for families who are taking care of a relative with dementia. Covers the importance of a thorough medical evaluation, typical problems in daily care, and family dynamics.

Organizations

Alzheimer's Disease and Related Disorders Association. 919 N. Michigan Avenue, Suite 1000, Chicago, IL 60611. (312) 335–8700.

> Serves as a clearinghouse for all aspects of Alzheimer's disease, including medical, psychological, research, legal, political, fund raising, and family support.

Alzheimer's Disease Education and Referral Center (ADEAR). P.O. Box 8250, Silver Spring, MD 20907 (301) 495–3311.

> Established by the National Institute on Aging, the center distributes information to health professionals, patients and their families, and the general public on Alzheimer's disease, current research activities, and available services. Publishes an Alzheimer's disease information packet.

American Association for Retired Persons (AARP). 601 E. Street, N.W., Washington, DC 20049. (202) 434–2277

> AARP has many useful publications. Call or write for a list of all their publications. These are only a few relevant to this chapter.
>
> "Coping and Caring: Living With Alzheimer's Disease." D12441
>
> "Reminiscence: Reaching Back, Moving Forward." D13186.

National Institute of Neurological Disorders and Stroke. P.O. Box 5801, Bethesda, MD 20824. (301) 496–5751.

> This institute offers information and publications on disorders such as dementia, stroke, brain tumors, and Parkinson's disease.

8

Coping with Physical Limitations

Deteriorating physically is one of the most challenging and infuriating aspects of old age. This chapter explores practical ways to compensate for problems with dexterity, mobility, vision, hearing, sexual functioning, and incontinence. Many of the suggested adaptations support independence and well-being, and do not require great expenditures of money or energy. Physical alterations of the home and types of medical equipment are considered, along with strategies family members can employ to help prevent accidents and injuries.

COMMON PHYSICAL PROBLEMS

Problems with dexterity and mobility can drastically detract from someone's quality of life, as can a decline in hearing, vision, or sexual functioning. Incontinence itself can become a kind of imprisonment. This sections surveys these common problems with the goal of offering practical hints for coping and ways to support a stance of creative adaptation.

Adapting to Arthritic Changes

People with dexterity and mobility problems often view each day as a succession of difficult hurdles, from getting out of bed and fastening clothing to opening mail and handling utensils for meals. Resting periodically may permit the person to control the pain or maintain safety, but this adds an infuriating slowness to the pace of daily life. Family members are often caught between wanting to take over some of the tasks to hurry things along and wanting to avoid diminishing their relative's independence by giving too much help.

The prime danger for people with arthritis is reducing their physical activity in response to pain. The saying "move it or lose it," summarizes the essence of the problem. Movement stimulates the secretion of lubrication in the joints and increases blood flow to joint areas. Movement tones the muscles which hold joints in place and which shield joints from excessive stress. When someone tries to avoid pain by sitting still as much as possible, the losses in lubricating fluid and muscular protection make movement still more painful. Eventually, the muscles surrounding immobilized areas lose their flexibility and affected joints freeze into rigid positions called contractures.

Obtaining practical aids and adapting the home can make daily life more manageable. Occupational therapists can suggest adaptive devices and safety modifications, particularly in the bathroom and kitchen. For instance, someone with painful hand joints would benefit from plastic extensions on cup handles, making them easier to grip. Built-up handles on utensils, faucets, lamp switches, stove controls, and door knobs would be similarly helpful. Someone with shoulder stiffness can be taught the use of a grasping device for reaching overhead items and for picking things up off the floor. A wall dispenser for liquid soap and shampoo may help someone who is unable to grasp slippery bars of soap and containers of shampoo.

People with arthritis also benefit from professional guidance in learning how to distinguish between pain which can be safely tolerated and pain which indicates that the optimal level of activity has been exceeded. Physical therapists can recommend appropriate types of activity and teach older people how to find the correct balance between exercise and rest. In addition, they can teach family members to perform passive exercises with their relative's arthritic joints, such as bending the person's knee up and down with gentle repetitions as he lies on a bed. Therapists also teach warm-up techniques for preparing muscles and joints for movement that relieve early-morning stiffness and serve as a prelude to exercise sequences.

The following chart lists practical aides for people with arthritis. To obtain items that are unavailable in local stores, families can phone for the catalogs of medical supply companies or consult with the rehabilitation departments of local hospitals and home care agencies. The local chapter of the Arthritis Foundation can also be contacted for information about adaptive devices and for obtaining their useful publications detailing self-help strategies for people with arthritis.

PRACTICAL AIDS FOR COPING WITH ARTHRITIS

Eating, preparing meals	Jar opener
	Electric can opener
	Food processor
	Portable cup and utensil handles
Handling common objects	Page turners
	Playing card holders
	Key extenders
	Cash and coin aides
Dressing, grooming	Zipper pulls
	Shoe horns with long extensions
	Brushes with long handles
	Velcro fasteners sewed into clothing
	Enlarged-handle tooth brushes

From Wendy Lustbader and Nancy R. Hooyman, *Taking Care of Aging Family Members* (New York: The Free Press, 1994). Copyright © 1994 by Wendy Lustbader and Nancy Hooyman; copyright © 1986 by The Free Press.

Adapting to Vision Loss

Normal age-related changes in eyesight can cause problems in daily life. Although able to see distant objects, most older people have difficulty shifting their vision to near ones. Depth perception may also be impaired, thereby increasing the risk of accidents from missing a step or a half-inch threshold. The aging eye also needs more time to adapt to levels of brightness and darkness. Sensitivity to glare may increase, as well as confusion about colors of similar intensity. Night vision may be greatly reduced.

More severe vision loss may be caused by glaucoma, cataracts, and macular degeneration. Glaucoma, a buildup of fluid causing high pressure within the eye, can generally be treated, but not cured, with medication drops or surgery. Older people and their families should be alert to the warning signs of glaucoma: loss of side vision, severe headaches, nausea, blurred vision, tearing, dull eye pain, and halos around light objects. An eyeball pressure test can detect glaucoma before vision is damaged and should be performed every two years.

Cataracts, a clouding of the lens, is the most common disability of the aging eye. Corrective lenses or an implanted lens can generally replace the damaged lens. Macular degeneration, the primary cause of blindness among older people, damages central vision. A simple test is to cover one eye and look with the other at the words on a page and then at a straight-line object; if blurring or waviness is noticed, an ophthalmologist should be consulted.

Severe vision loss can affect many areas of life. The person may feel uncomfortable entering into unfamiliar social situations when she cannot see other people's faces. Without the sight of facial expressions and features, it is difficult to gauge a new acquaintance's sincerity or to decide whether someone can be trusted. Sighted people often do not realize that smiling is also a responsive, visual act. The person with vision loss may seem cold or unresponsive, when in reality the person has been deprived of the warmth conveyed through the sight of someone else's smile.

Grooming is affected by vision loss. The inability to check whether a blouse has been put on inside out or if a dress is stained may leave someone feeling uncertain about leaving the house. Women accustomed to putting on makeup or doing their hair in a particular way may lose all desire to venture out. A trusted neighbor willing to drop by to perform inspections may help a great deal in increasing someone's confidence about their appearance.

Loss of the ability to read printed texts may be a source of continual grief to a previously avid reader. Adjusting to recorded books takes time, and the person may go on missing the printed page. Obtaining a tape recorder for sending cassette tapes in lieu of letters may reduce the frustration of written correspondence. Out-of-town family members and friends can send their address labels for the older person to place on envelopes. Having someone available on a reliable basis for reading mail and newspapers aloud also helps lessen frustration.

During visits to the home, family members can copy out the older person's favorite recipes in large print with a black marking pen and make lists of frequently used phone numbers. Visitors should avoid standing in front of bright lights or windows, because they will only make it harder for the older person to see their faces if silhouetted. Pulling up a chair and sitting close together may permit the older person to see the visitor's face, a step which may feel awkward at first but may greatly enhance the visit.

Paying attention to adequate lighting is a key strategy for supporting older people with vision loss. The following chart depicts ways that household lighting can be adjusted to promote safety and describes visual aides that can help sustain independence with daily tasks. In many communities, the services of an occupational therapist can be requested through agencies for the visually impaired. The therapist can suggest further adaptations and can teach an older person how to negotiate busy streets on foot.

ADAPTIVE STRATEGIES TO COMPENSATE FOR VISION LOSS

Lighting	Night lights placed throughout the house
	Multiple light sources, evenly distributed
	Horizontal blinds to control light and glare
	More intense light over work areas and stairs
Safety	Edge of steps marked with nonskid colored tape
	Throw rugs removed, clutter reduced
	Objects kept in the same place
Daily tasks	Color codes on medication bottles
	Raised number templates for telephones
	Stove and washer controls marked with colored dots
	Talking clocks which announce the time
	Adapted clothing, such as Velcro or large buttons
	Magnifiers for close-up activities
	Drinking glasses with painted rims

From Wendy Lustbader and Nancy R. Hooyman, *Taking Care of Aging Family Members* (New York: The Free Press, 1994). Copyright © 1994 by Wendy Lustbader and Nancy Hooyman; copyright © 1986 by The Free Press.

Adapting to Hearing Loss

A harmful consequence of hearing loss in later life for many people is social isolation. Needing to ask others to repeat what they said or finding that they miss essential pieces of conversations, older people with impaired hearing often feel that they are a burden to have around. Once this belief becomes established, a chain reaction of increasing isolation may ensue. They may eventually stay away from social situations altogether to avoid feelings of impatience and awkwardness.

Diminished contact with others often leads to a loss of the kinds of stimulation which maintain mental alertness and orientation to daily events. Older people with hearing loss may find that they have less to say to others, even when someone takes the time to initiate and carry out a conversation with them. This seeming "dullness" may cause family members to conclude mistakenly that mental deterioration has occurred along with hearing loss, resulting in further isolation as fewer people attempt conversations beyond a simplistic or routine level.

Unfortunately, some of the helpful strategies that friends and relatives attempt may be rejected by older people. Efforts to give a hearing-impaired person the best seating, or to post someone alongside him to speak directly into his "good ear" may be turned down by someone who fears being "too much trouble to have around." Many older people feel ashamed of their need for this consideration, unaware that up to 75 percent of people age sixty-five and older have mild to moderate loss of hearing.[1]

A problem which may embarrass family and friends during social gatherings is a hearing-impaired person's tendency to talk over others who have begun speaking. In such instances, the interrupted speaker typically stops talking and the person with hearing loss continues, unaware of having cut someone off. The visible embarrassment of others in the group may occur too late to alert the older person and prevent him from feeling foolish or rude. Even when people are aware that the hearing-impaired person cannot help talking over others, they may feel annoyed, thinking, "He should look around before he speaks to make sure he's not interrupting." A simple coping strategy is a signal system, where someone sitting beside the older person nudges his foot when he inadvertently interrupts someone.

A further problem is the tendency for people with hearing loss to speak more loudly than is necessary. Particularly in a close setting, such as a restaurant, the loudness may embarrass family and friends who notice others' stares or who are sensitive to the broadcasting of private business. In addition, side conversations may be difficult to keep going, if the person's loudness overwhelms quieter voices or is too distracting. Again, when this happens, someone sitting next to the person can discreetly cue him to speak less loudly. Establishing such cues is better than tolerating the situation and then withholding future invitations out of anticipated embarrassment.

Family members may eventually stop trying to include an older person with hearing loss in family gatherings. Their relative's lack of verbal participation may be mistaken for an absence of interest in other people's lives, especially if their relative has successfully hidden his progressive hearing loss. In other instances, the person may sit at the periphery of conversations, nodding and smiling no matter what is being said. Maintaining this falsely cheerful exterior may be the person's effort to conceal how isolated and embarrassed he feels during the inaudible discussion going on around him. Some family members may misinterpret the nodding and smiling as "senility," not realizing that the person's out-of-sync responses arise from a hearing impairment rather than disorientation.

The inability to hear what is being said in social situations can further lead to suspicious beliefs about unheard conversations: "They're talking about me over there. I just know they are." Presuming that the older person cannot hear them, family members often do talk about their relative while in the same room with him. They do not realize that the content of a conversation is easily conveyed through body language, gestures, and occasional glances toward the person being discussed. The older person is then faced with the choice of feigning unawareness or tolerating possible dishonesty when he asks what people were talking about. Even the most considerate family members and professionals may make this error, unaware of how readily the essence of a conversation can be visually discerned and how naturally suspicious feelings arise in these situations.

To avoid these problems, a standard practice at family gatherings or social occasions can be to position someone beside the older person to give periodic summaries of what is being discussed. The helper needs only to give the gist of what is being said, such as: "Mom is telling John about Billy's car accident. Dad's telling the same old jokes you've heard a million times." This role can be rotated among family members, as it requires patience and attentiveness. When stories are too complex to be summarized, the expectation can be established that specific details will be provided later. With practice, family members can become skilled at this role and may be rewarded by their relative's more animated facial expression and renewed participation in others' lives.

The phenomenon of selective hearing may be particularly annoying to family members: "He hears what he wants to hear." They may notice that their relative manages to understand conversations they are trying to conceal and then misses information they are trying to convey. Since reading lips and discerning body language require attentive effort, it follows that conversations become more audible the more the person with hearing loss wants to hear them. The ability to close off contact with others at will is also a powerful way to express anger, frustration, and the need for control. Family members' irritation often reflects the reality that their relative is effectively taking control in these instances. Viewing selective hearing as an exercise of control is more helpful than reacting to it as a deliberate attempt to make life more difficult for family members. In addition, restoring other areas of control in the older person's daily life is a strategy which may reduce selective hearing as a means of taking control.

One of the most challenging problems faced by families is the older person's denial that a significant loss of hearing has occurred. The person may complain that people are not speaking loudly enough or are mumbling their words. He may refuse to wear a hearing aid, regarding it as something "for deaf old people." Attempting to appease insistent family members, he may wear a hearing aid for a brief time and then claim that ringing sounds or distortions make it "impossible" for him to tolerate the device which he did not need in the first place. In some instances, it may be helpful to obtain an alternative device consisting of headphones and a microphone. The hearing-impaired person wears the headphones while others speak into the microphone. During card games, for example, the microphone can be placed in the center of the table to pick up the voices of all the players. This device does not carry the stigma of old age and therefore may be more acceptable than a hearing aid to someone who has tried to deny his hearing loss.

Telling their relative, "I really miss being able to talk to you," may be a family member's most effective encouragement. This message can be conveyed through a written note recalling the kinds of conversations that no longer are possible. A willingness on the part of both family members and their older relative to experiment with adaptive strategies is crucial for maintaining the motivation to keep talking to one another. Adaptive strategies for common hearing changes are provided in the following chart.

ADAPTIVE STRATEGIES TO COMPENSATE FOR HEARING LOSS

In the home	Install flashing lights on doorbell and telephone
	Add telephone amplification devices and volume control
By the speaker	Gain the person's attention before speaking
	Enunciate words clearly and slowly
	Keep facial expressions and lips visible
	Use low tones
	Speak slightly louder, but avoid shouting
	Use short, simple sentences
By the older person	Reduce background noise during conversations
	Ask people to write vital information

From Wendy Lustbader and Nancy R. Hooyman, *Taking Care of Aging Family Members* (New York: The Free Press, 1994). Copyright © 1994 by Wendy Lustbader and Nancy Hooyman; copyright © 1986 by The Free Press.

Adapting to Sexual Changes

Age-related sexual changes are often mistaken for signs that sexual activity should cease. On the contrary, these changes mean that older people may need information about adaptations and encouragement to experiment with solutions. Since there is a societal bias which ignores older, frail, or disabled people's sexual needs, health professionals should bring up the topic in a way that frees such individuals to voice their concerns. A doctor can say: "Sexual responses change as we age just like any other part of us." An older woman might respond, "Now that you mention it, I was wondering why intercourse has been so painful."

Due to a decrease in estrogen, women often experience a thinning of the vaginal walls and reduced moistness or lubrication, changes which can make intercourse uncomfortable. The time needed to respond to sexual stimulation may increase, and the intensity of response may lessen. For some, urinary tract infections occur more frequently because thinner vaginal walls offer less protection to the bladder and urethra.

Fortunately, there are ways women can adapt to these changes. Water-soluble lubricants, such as KY jelly and vaginal creams, can be purchased over the counter in most drug stores. Long, leisurely foreplay helps increase natural lubrication and allows time for a slower response. Consistent sexual activity, including masturbation, maintains vaginal lubricating ability and vaginal muscle tone, reducing discomfort during intercourse. These problems can also be treated and often reversed with estrogen replacement therapy. Drinking more fluids and urinating before and after intercourse may prevent urinary tract infections. Changes in sexual positioning can also help, such as aiming the penis down toward the rectum rather than toward the upper part of the vagina near the bladder and urethra.

Men often find as they age that the time needed to obtain an erection increases, and the erection may be less firm than when they were younger. Ejaculation may decrease in force and volume. Achieving a second erection may take longer or may not be possible. Men on blood pressure medicines and those with diabetes, circulation problems, or prostate disorders may find that they lose the ability to have an erection. The urgency to ejaculate may be reduced and the ability to delay ejaculation may increase. For some, orgasm may not occur during intercourse.

Allowing time for a slower physical response helps some men considerably. When the erection is not hard enough, placing the penis into the vagina by hand may increase hardness. Hormone levels may be higher in the morning, making this an optimal time for sexual activity. Medications with impotence as a side effect may occasionally be exchanged for those less likely to affect sexual function, if physicians are informed of this concern. Avoiding alcohol use prior to sexual activity can be helpful, since alcohol often increases desire, but decreases ability.

Fear of failure may also contribute to impotence. As they grow older, men often do not adjust their expectations of erectile performance. They misinterpret slowed responses as failures, and then try too hard on subsequent occasions. Such excessive effort only makes failure more likely, setting up a cycle of anxiety and defeat. Some men abandon sexual activity entirely, due to a false belief that their impotence is irresolvable. Many become depressed as a result, equating loss of sexual potency with personal inadequacy.

Some older men begin avoiding all affectionate contact, unwilling to risk revealing what they regard as weakness. They stop snuggling in bed, afraid this will be mistaken as their initiating sexual activity. Their partners then may feel unloved and rejected. For instance, a woman in this position may confide to her physician, "My husband's not interested in me anymore," hoping that the doctor will "have a talk with him" and bridge their silence on this topic. Worry that his partner is "getting what she needs elsewhere" may begin to consume the man who believes he is sexually inadequate, to the point where his suspiciousness keeps his wife homebound.

Health professionals can make a significant contribution to couples' sexual adjustment by urging them to focus on forms of intimacy other than direct genital stimulation. Long, leisurely foreplay reduces performance anxiety by removing the focus from erection and intercourse. Lying together in bed and giving each other massages can be substituted for genital sexuality. Finding varied forms of sexual expression and ways to express affection is particularly important when illness interferes with a couple's capacities. Experimenting with different positions, using protective devices such as pillows and knee pads, and giving each other physical contact through touching and caressing may enable a couple to restore this dimension to their lives.

Adapting to Incontinence

Incontinence is simply defined as loss of bladder or bowel control. It is estimated that up to twenty million Americans are incontinent. Of these, the majority are elderly and 85 percent are women. Most do not receive help from from their doctors, either because they are too ashamed to ask for help or their physicians are not aware of the successful treatments which have been developed in recent years.[2]

Many older people isolate themselves through worry and humiliation, going to great lengths to hide their problem from friends and family members. Some wash underclothes and sheets by hand to hide stains from those who assist them with the laundry. Some suffer sleep deprivation from waking themselves up during the night for frequent trips to the bathroom. Many avoid all social gatherings out of fear of leaving odors or stains on couches and chairs. They may decline car or van rides out of dread of an accident on the upholstery. Some give up grocery shopping because of the absence of convenient restrooms in the stores or worry about getting caught in a long line at the check-out counter. For a person living in an apartment building, even the elevator ride to the lobby mailboxes may have to be carefully timed and may include the dread of being detained in a conversation with a friendly neighbor.

Couples often maintain a taboo against discussing incontinence, despite their mutual awareness of the problem. A partner may be repelled by the stench on clothing and upholstery, yet say nothing in order to avoid humiliating the other. Some couples begin to sleep separately without ever discussing the reason. If the partner's smell sensitivity is keen, all affectionate contact may cease, adding yet another negative consequence to an already distressing situation. A partner who refuses to perpetuate the silence and instead confides in family members may feel guilty for violating the person's trust.

An older person's denial of incontinence is a tricky dilemma for both family members and professionals. For instance, many older people experience what is termed "dribble incontinence" in which small quantities of urine leak out during the day. Acclimated to the smell, or having lost a degree of smell sensitivity due to aging, some block out their awareness of the problem and thus avoid facing its implications. Visitors may be offered a dampened easy chair, finding themselves in an awkward position once they sit down. Yet confronting someone's denial head-on may provoke hostility, humiliation, or hurt feelings.

As a way to introduce the topic, family members or professionals can mention that many older people experience incontinence. An older person residing in a senior high-rise, for instance, may become more willing to discuss the problem after hearing a statement such as, "In this building alone, it's likely that at least half the people have difficulty controlling their bladders." Since few talk openly, most older people have no way of knowing that many others in their vicinity share their humiliation. Referring to the increased television and magazine advertizing about protective products may also help someone realize that incontinence is a common problem.

Once the topic is out in the open, the most important response is to make sure that the older person also tells her physician. Medical attention may alleviate or reduce these difficulties. Even when incontinence cannot be eliminated, its discomfort and inconvenience can usually be eased. Treatable instances of incontinence include those caused by bladder or urinary tract infections, which may be cured after a course of antibiotics. Sometimes prescription drugs cause urgent and frequent urination, and the physician may be able to adjust the dosage or prescribe a different medication. Women who are placed on estrogen sometimes find that their incontinence resolves. Men who experience incontinence following prostate surgery or as a result of prostate problems may be able to regain continence through medical treatment.

Medications for treating incontinence are worth a try under a physician's supervision. Bladder muscle relaxants are particularly useful with what is called "urge incontinence." Many people do not get enough warning prior to the urge to urinate and experience leakage on the way to the bathroom. Examples of these medications are Ditropan (oxybutinin hydrochloride) and Levsin (hyoscyamine sulfate). Medications which improve the tone of the bladder outlet muscle are occasionally effective, such as Rondec (carbinoxamine maleate) and Entex (phenylpropanolamine).[3]

Treatment techniques have improved in recent years. Many women regain bladder control through Kegel exercises, practice with starting and stopping the flow of urine. Weighted cones that fit in the vagina can be used for a few minutes each day to increase the effectiveness of these exercises. Biofeedback devices can also be employed to help women visualize their muscle activity and strengthen the muscles around the urethra. Another promising treatment is bladder retraining. In one study, more than three quarters of the women who participated reported improvement of 50 percent or more. The retraining program requires a strict urination schedule along with using relaxation techniques.[4] If the older person's physician is unfamiliar with these treatments, referral to a specialist should be sought.

In some instances, simple surgeries solve or reduce incontinence problems, such as repairing a prolapsed uterus. Through childbirth and the aging process, the ligaments supporting the reproductive organs become weaker and put pressure on the bladder. In some cases, the uterus may drop down and protrude from the vagina. Once this is repaired, many women find that their bladder control resumes.

Another important strategy is to restrict food and beverages which irritate the bladder or contribute to bladder leakage. It is not known in all instances how certain items affect the bladder, but older people should experiment with the list presented below. Urine control may improve markedly with the elimination of just a few of these items.

Many older people are reluctant to use protective pads with any resemblance to diapers. In recent years, an increasing number of products have been designed which fit the body comfortably and which are not detectable under clothing. These disposable pads can be attached to specially designed adult undergarments, allowing the person wearing them to feel dignified. These products are available in most drug stores and through medical supply catalogs.

FOODS AND BEVERAGES THAT MAY CONTRIBUTE TO BLADDER LEAKAGE

Coffee and tea (even decaffeinated)

Soft drinks with caffeine

Medicines with caffeine

Citrus juice and fruits

Alcoholic beverages

Highly spiced foods

Sugar, honey, or corn syrup

Milk and milk products

Tomatoes and tomato products

Adapted from *The HIP Report*, Help for Incontinent People, P.O. Box 544, Union, SC 29379.

Older people and family members are often confused about various types of catheters and their effectiveness for urinary incontinence. In-dwelling catheters, in which tubing carries the urine from the urethra to a catchment bag, require skilled nursing supervision, tend to be uncomfortable to wear, interfere with sexual activity, and often increase the older person's vulnerability to urinary tract infections. Despite these problems, an in-dwelling catheter may be preferable to the effort required to change and wash bedding several times a day. For men, externally worn condom catheters are available which have fewer disadvantages. Catchment bags designed to be worn on the man's leg are undetectable under loose pants and can be emptied easily. Unfortunately, externally worn catheters have not yet been developed for women.

Even when incontinence cannot be cured, its discomfort and inconvenience can usually be eased. As family members and their older relatives become more open about discussing incontinence, other solutions can become a collective effort. For example, the older person can be given a seat closest to the bathroom at family gatherings, and care can be exerted to keep the bathroom unoccupied as much as possible. On car trips, frequent stops can be planned on the itinerary, omitting the need for the person to keep asking for them. Washable upholstery covers can be placed on the person's favorite chairs, both at home and at family members' homes. An attitude of acceptance and support by family can, in itself, significantly reduce the older person's anxiety about the problem.

MODIFYING THE HOME

An attitude of adaptation to difficulties, rather than surrender, sets the stage for creative problem solving. When family members and professionals assert this stance, vulnerable adults feel safer about revealing their problems and seeking help to solve them. It is also important for all concerned to allow for trial and error as solutions are attempted and adjustments made. The following checklists for preventing falls and fires can be used by older people and their families to survey their homes and set a tone of working together to promote safety and physical freedom.

Modifying the home both supports the older person's independence and reduces the burden on caregivers. Families may feel overwhelmed when they first consider making these changes or obtaining medical equipment. Learning new care techniques and altering the ways they handle familiar situations may initially seem more burdensome than helpful. This section shows how specific adaptations can be well worth the effort.

Questions and Answers about Mobility Problems

1. What are some ways to make it easier for an older person to get out of a chair, couch, or toilet without assistance?

Wooden blocks placed under the feet of a chair or couch can often raise it high enough for an older person to stand independently. Even an able-bodied person may have difficulty getting up from a couch in which his knees are tilted higher than his waist. The blocks can be made on home shop equipment or obtained through the rehabilitation departments of hospitals and home care agencies. Professionals can advise how high to raise a particular piece of furniture and how to score the block's surface to prevent slippage.

Learning how to position the body for maximum leverage is also important. For instance, a person who moves himself forward to the seat's edge and then places his feet close in, under his center of gravity, will be able to stand more easily than if he extends his feet away from

FIRE SAFETY CHECKLIST

Light bulbs should be the proper voltage to avoid blowing fuses and causing fires.

Exits to the residence should not be blocked.

Ashtrays should not contain paper items and should be kept far away from the bed.

The insulation around wires should be kept intact.

Space heaters should be placed far away from bedspreads, drapes, and other flammable materials; they should be located out of areas where the older person walks.

Rugs should not cover electric wires.

Newspapers should not be stacked near the stove or near baseboard heaters.

Fireplaces and chimneys should be cleaned regularly.

Smoke alarms should be installed in the bedroom and kitchen.

The older person should establish the habit of using an egg timer when placing food on the stove.

Heat controls on the stove should be easy to read.

Clothing with loose sleeves (bathrobes, for instance) should not be worn while cooking.

Emergency phone numbers should be displayed on the phone itself.

From Wendy Lustbader and Nancy R. Hooyman, *Taking Care of Aging Family Members* (New York: The Free Press, 1994). Copyright © 1994 by Wendy Lustbader and Nancy Hooyman; copyright © 1986 by The Free Press.

where his body most needs support. Family members can help by reminding their relative to practice this technique until it becomes habitual.

A *raised toilet seat*, attached over an existing seat, can significantly ease an older person's getting up and down on his own. Some come with grab bars on either side of the seat which increase the safety of this maneuver.

PRECAUTIONS FOR PREVENTING FALLS

Nonskid mats or abrasive strips should line the bathtub and the floor beside the tub.

The shower or tub should have at least one grab bar within easy reach.

Sturdy rails should be available by all steps.

Adequate lighting should illuminate steps and hallways. Light switches should be located both at the top and bottom of stairs.

Light switches should be located by the doorway of each room.

Electric cords should be out of pathways.

A switch or lamp should be reachable from the bed.

Rugs should be smooth, with folds and wrinkles regularly removed.

Throw rugs should be eliminated unless they are secure around the edges and have slip-resistant rubber backing.

Areas of clutter should be cleared.

A long-handled sponge mop should be handy in the kitchen for mopping up spills.

Carpeting on steps should be in good condition and smoothly tacked down; steps should be sturdy and of equal height and width.

From Wendy Lustbader and Nancy R. Hooyman, *Taking Care of Aging Family Members* (New York: The Free Press, 1994). Copyright © 1994 by Wendy Lustbader and Nancy Hooyman; copyright © 1986 by The Free Press.

2. How can tubs and showers be adapted for someone to get safely in and out?

A *bath bench* is a small waterproof chair, placed inside the bathtub, onto which the person slides from the tub's rim. When the bench is the same height as the rim, getting in and out of the tub can be dramatically simplified. Instruction from a physical or occupational therapist and experimentation with benches of different heights and sizes may be necessary. Once on the bench, some people are unable to lower themselves to the bottom of the tub, but they can shower while seated on the bench with a hand-held spray device. *Grab bars* attached to the wall beside the tub are advisable for maximum safety in all instances.

3. What kinds of equipment enable people with disabilities to get in and out of bed?

A *triangle*, hanging from a bar attached to the bed's headboard, can be used by the older person to pull himself to a sitting position and to exercise arm and stomach muscles. If the older person's bed lacks a headboard or if the device cannot be securely attached, it may be necessary to obtain a hospital bed. However,a grab bar attached to the wall beside an older person's bed, along with a course of exercises for strengthening his stomach muscles, may enable him to sit up on his own without a hospital bed.

A *transfer board* is a polished wooden or plastic slab onto which an older person can slide when moving from his bed into a wheelchair. The chair wheels need to be securely locked and the board's surface may need powder to ease the slide, but an older person with sufficient muscle strength can usually learn to accomplish this transfer method independently. Often, the bed's height has to be adjusted to match that of the wheelchair, and a mattress with firm edges has to be obtained. Training in transfer techniques by rehabilitation therapists can be requested from home health care agencies if the person's physician approves. The older person may be able to use similar techniques for transferring himself onto a commode, toilet seat, or kitchen chair.

4. What if a caregiver is unable to lift the older person out of bed, in and out of chairs, or off the floor in the event of falls?

A *Hoyer lift* is a hydraulic device with a cloth sling. The caregiver positions the sling under the older person's body by having him roll to one side and then the other. The sling's ends are then attached to the device and a hydraulic arm is pumped until the older person is suspended in the sling. Becoming accustomed to the sensation of being suspended in this way generally requires a few practice sessions, but the advantages of being moved in and out of bed frequently are generally sufficient motivation for the ill person. Families can receive rental information and instruction in the use of this device from most home health care agencies or medical supply companies.

5. What can be done when steps separate crucial areas of the older person's home?

The transformation of a living room into a bedroom can make life easier for caregivers, especially partners who may have difficulty climbing steps to a second-floor sickroom. Placing the older person's bedroom on the same level as the kitchen eliminates going up and down steps to carry meals or tend to intermittent needs. With a more central location, the bedbound person may feel less secluded. Moving the bed near a large picture window may also improve the person's mood. A standing screen or a curtain run along tracks installed in the ceiling can create visual privacy when necessary. Another benefit may be lower energy costs from heating only one level of the house.

When the house's only bathroom is on the second floor and the kitchen is on the first, the strategy of moving the older person's bed downstairs becomes more complicated. A *commode*, or portable toilet, can be used, but carrying the catchbasin upstairs to empty into the toilet can be an onerous strain on caregivers. An older person living alone may have to deal with unpleasant odors until a family member or hired helper arrives to empty the commode. Nevertheless, commodes are an effective method of coping with toilet needs when accessibility is a problem. They are available from medical equipment suppliers at a wide range of prices and styles.

Installing a bathroom on the level needed is often worth the cost, especially if nursing home placement for an extended period of time is otherwise likely to result. Contractors are usually willing to give free estimates and recommendations regarding the feasibility of preferred locations. For example, a laundry room adjacent to the kitchen may already contain the necessary plumbing, if the homeowner is willing to forfeit space in that area. Some localities have loan programs for older people needing to make such adaptations and will send out housing rehabilitation advisers. Families can contact the senior hotline or housing authority in the older person's community to determine a program's availability and eligibility requirements.

6. What can be done to improve the safety of outdoor steps?

Installing sturdy railings alongside the older person's front steps can often prevent her from becoming homebound. The psychological security of having something to hold on to may induce her to go out, as well as make her safer when she does. If steps are particularly steep or uneven, rebuilding them or constructing a wooden ramp over them is often worth the cost.

The greatest disadvantage of ramps is the amount of space they require. Constructing a safe, gentle slope for the ramp may require more space than first estimated. Some older people have yards large enough for a long ramp, but dislike making their disability prominent to neighbors or resist having plywood intrude on their beloved garden. When cost is an obstacle, home repair programs in some communities provide free labor for such projects, if the older person pays for the materials.

Another option is for a physical therapist to teach the older person to maneuver safely on stairs, if this is feasible. In many instances, older people with walkers and canes do not know how to use these ambulation aids properly on steps. Some may need muscle strengthening exercises to increase their safety. Combining these efforts with railings of the proper height and shape can enable some homebound people to regain independent access to the outside world.

Obtaining Medical Equipment

Medicare provides for the rental or purchase of home care equipment, as long as a physician certifies its medical necessity. The purchase prices of items such as hospital beds and wheelchairs are almost always far above the amount Medicare reimburses; as a result, equipment purchased from providers not accepting Medicare assignment may leave the older person responsible for a considerable portion of the cost. Specially adapted wheelchairs, for example, can leave purchasers with as much as 60 percent of the cost after Medicare makes its payment, depending on how large the gap is between the allowable charge and the provider's actual charge. For equipment without special adaptations, providers can usually cite the amount that can be expected from Medicare, but may have to be pressed to do so. Those who qualify can also use Medicaid, or state medical assistance, for the purchase of equipment, but prior approval from the state's health services system must be obtained. (See pp. 201–214 for further explanations of Medicare and Medicaid.)

Purchasing or borrowing used medical equipment is an option which can save money, often without sacrificing safety. Nonprofit home health care agencies, medical clinics, senior centers, and Easter Seal, Multiple Scleroris, and Cancer Societies are examples of agencies which may maintain loan closets of used medical equipment. Some may sell reconditioned equipment. Even if equipment loans are only short-term, older people and their families can then gauge its utility before making purchases. Loans can also extend the time family members have for shopping around to different medical suppliers for the best prices or to advertise for used equipment to be purchased from private parties. For example, posting signs in the lobbies of senior apartment buildings or senior centers may yield wheelchairs, walkers, and bath benches which people are willing to trade, sell, or give away. For the sake of safety, used equipment should be examined for loose attachments and other defects, as well as scrubbed thoroughly with antiseptic cleaners.

One way for families to become familiar with the range of available equipment is to request catalogs from major suppliers, such as Abbey Medical, Sears, Care Medical, and others listed in the yellow pages under "Home Health Care" or "Hospital Equipment." Obtaining these catalogs also allows families to compare cost and quality without the pressures of salespeople and the inconvenience of visiting each supplier. Some of the most important questions to ask while phoning suppliers relate to how they handle Medicare billing, such as "Do you bill Medicare directly? Do we have to lay out a cash payment while we wait for Medicare reimbursement? How gradually do you permit payment for the uncovered portions of purchase prices?" In making phone calls to local suppliers, the phone contact sheet may be useful for organizing the information obtained. (See p. 233.)

Losing the ability to butter a piece of bread, read medication labels, hear conversations on the telephone, or walk safely down a flight of steps can be infuriating. Becoming dependent on others for help often means losing control over one's life. For these reasons, experimenting with adaptive devices and home modifications may simultaneously enhance someone's comfort and dignity as well as make life easier for caregivers.

NOTES

1. Lynne Olsho, Stephen Harkins, and Martin Lenhardt, "Aging and the Auditory System," in J. Birren and K. Schaie, Eds., *Handbook of the Psychology of Aging* (New York: Van Nostrand Reinhold, 1985), 332–377.

2. *The HIP Report*, Help For Incontinent People, P.O. Box 544, Union, SC 29379, volume 9, number 3, 1991.

3. From consultation with the office of Dr. Tamara Bavendam, Director of Female Urology, Department of Urology, University of Washington Medical Center, Seattle, WA 98195.

4. J. Andrew Fantl, "Bladder Training and the Management of Lower Urinary Tract Dysfunction in Women: A Review," *Journal of the American Geriatrics Society*, vol. 38, no. 3, 1990, pp. 329–332.

SUGGESTED RESOURCES

Books

Himber, Charlotte. *How to Survive Hearing Loss* (Washington, D.C.: Gallaudet University Press), 1989.

> The author shares her personal experience with hearing loss in later life, and presents the results of her intensive research of the hearing process, hearing loss, rehabilitation, and support groups.

Neal, Helen. *Low Vision: What You Can Do To Preserve—And Even Enhance—Your Usable Sight* (New York: Simon and Schuster), 1987.

> The author discusses the causes of low vision (the "gray area" between normal vision and blindness), the services and aids available, coping strategies, and future directions in eye care. Includes a useful appendix of resources, products, and support groups.

Organizations

Agency For Health Care Policy and Research. P.O. Box 8547, Silver Spring, MD 20907. (800) 358–9295.

> This clearinghouse has several helpful pamphlets they will mail at no cost. Dial the toll-free number or write for any of the following:
>
> "Pain Control After Surgery"
>
> "Cataracts in Adults"
>
> "Managing Urinary Incontinence: A Patient's Guide"
>
> "Pressure Ulcers"
>
> "Sickle Cell Disease"
>
> "Depression"

Alliance for Aging Research. 2021 K Street, N.W., Suite 305, Washington, D.C. 20006. (202) 293–2856

The Alliance serves as a clearinghouse for information on research about aging and conducts a variety of educational programs. They publish an easy-to-read brochure, "Incontinence: Everything You Wanted to Know But Were Afraid to Ask."

American Association for Retired Persons (AARP). 601 E. Street, N.W., Fulfillment Department, Washington, DC 20049. (202) 434–2277

AARP has many useful publications. Call or write for a list. One relevant to physical adaptations is "The Gadget Book: Ingenious Devices for Easier Living."

American Foundation for the Blind. 15 West 16th Street, New York, NY 10011. (212) 620–2000 or (800) 232–5463.

The foundation offers free publications on visual impairments, visual aids, and ways for the family and patient to cope with failing eyesight. They also make referrals to local chapters or community services for visually impaired persons.

American Printing House for the Blind. P.O. Box 6085, Louisville, KY 40206. (800) 223–1839.

Offers a catalog of writing aids, tape recorders, and educational materials, as well as "Catalog of Large Type Books."

Arthritis Foundation. P.O. Box 19000, Atlanta, Georgia 30326. (404) 872–7100 or (800) 283–7800.

The foundation conducts research into the prevention and treatment of arthritis and provides services and education. They publish many helpful pamphlets, including "The Self-Help Manual for Patients With Arthritis" which lists equipment and devices.

Better Hearing Institute. P.O. Box 1840, Washington, D.C. 20013. (703) 642–0850.

Helpline provides information about hearing aids, tinnitus, nerve deafness, special devices, and other problems related to hearing loss.

Help for Incontinent People (HIP). P.O. Box 544, Union, SC 29379. (800) 252–3337 or (803) 579–7900.

This is a self-help and patient advocacy group that offers encouragement, information, and resource listings for incontinent people. It also publishes a quarterly newsletter that provides practical advice, as well as the following helpful pamphlets:

"Bladder Retraining"

"Resource Guide of Continence Products and Services"

Independence Factory. P.O. Box 597, Middletown, OH 45042.

Nonprofit organization that sells practical aids (zipper pulls, enlarged handle toothbrushes, etc.) for those with hand and limb limitations.

National Society to Prevent Blindness. 79 Madison Avenue, New York, NY 10016. (212) 980–2020.

Publishes several pamphlets on specific diseases affecting eyes, including "The Aging Eye: Facts on Eye Care for Older Persons."

Self-Help for Hard of Hearing People (Shhh). 7800 Wisconsin Avenue, Bethesda, MD 20892. (301) 657–2248 or TTY (301) 657–2299.

Shhh is a national self-help organization for those who are hard of hearing. Shhh can help with information on coping with hearing loss and new hearing aids and technology. They publish a bimonthly journal.

9

Depression in Reaction to Illness and Disability

Depression is common among people coping with illness and progressive disability. Customary ways of getting through hardship tend to be disrupted by physical problems, leaving people in new situations without the use of their old strengths. The combination of fresh losses with fewer ways to surmount them accounts to a large extent for the prevalence of depression among ill or disabled older people. This chapter first considers the causes of depression, looking especially at what happens when an older person becomes homebound due to medical problems. Suicidal feelings are then explored, along with self-neglect as a form of slow suicide. The last section offers interventions for relieving depression that can be carried out by family members or professionals.

CAUSES OF DEPRESSION

Knowing what is causing depression and putting a name to it is often, in itself, a powerful source of solace. The list below portrays many of the losses associated with becoming ill, disabled, or homebound. Merging together, these losses can oppress even the most resilient spirit.

181

LOSSES ASSOCIATED WITH BECOMING ILL, DISABLED, OR HOMEBOUND

Loss of contact with friends and acquaintances; added dependence on relatives or caregivers for social contact

Loss of purpose; fewer ways to engage in useful activity or contribute to other people's lives

Loss of independence in self-care; decreased privacy and control in the activities of daily living

Loss of mobility; fewer opportunities for exercise and for obtaining a refreshing change of scene

Loss of sensory pleasures; diminished taste, smell, sight, hearing, or touch

Loss of patience; a short temper from chronic pain or a tendency to dump frustrations on loved ones

Loss of out-of-home activities; fewer pleasant distractions or healthy stresses to stimulate interests

Loss of self-esteem; fewer social roles or chances to affirm one's skills, knowledge, or creativity

Loss of meaning; fewer ways to construct a life that seems worth living

From Wendy Lustbader and Nancy R. Hooyman, *Taking Care of Aging Family Members* (New York: The Free Press, 1994). Copyright © 1994 by Wendy Lustbader and Nancy Hooyman; copyright © 1986 by The Free Press.

Feeling Lonely, Trivial, and Dull

In many senses, the sickroom or house becomes a world to the person confined within its limits. Details previously dwarfed by larger events assume a new importance. No longer confronting the novelty of outside experiences and a variety of social contacts, the homebound person may find that aspects of her illness are the only changing features of her immediate world. When someone calls, she may have little to say beyond reporting on meals, sleep, bowel movements, and the nuances of pain. "I'm sick of my sick self" is a common complaint under these circumstances, yet it is difficult to reach for other topics when physical rhythms and needs loom so large.

A sense of blandness gradually arises in someone who no longer has fresh experiences. The sameness and safety of home, unless occasionally interrupted, can leave an older person with too little stimulation. Healthy levels of stress inherent in venturing out into the streets are forfeited when a person faces a known environment day after day: "If I have to look at these four walls another minute, I'll go crazy." Activities such as preparing meals and watching television do not demand the degree of mental engagement required by unpredictable situations, such as negotiating busy crosswalks or handling transactions in stores. A homebound person may gradually adapt to the absence of challenge by paying less attention to what happens around her, including the needs of other people and events in the outside world.

When someone becomes homebound, the number of people who populate the person's life drops dramatically. Contacts with random strangers and conversations with store clerks, bus drivers, and acquaintances are lost. The older person's friends and relatives then become the recipients of a concentrated social need that was previously diluted by these other contacts. This new dependence on their visits and phone calls places pressure on family members, who previously felt free to come over or call less frequently. As the homebound person tries to satisfy her loneliness at each opportunity, visits and phone calls may be prolonged beyond family members' endurance.

The person's preoccupation with bodily needs may further exasperate family members who must listen repeatedly to her descriptions of physical concerns. They may come to dread visits and phone calls as intensely as the older person desires them. As busy people leading full lives, they may find it difficult to understand their relative's narrowed scope of attention. If her former range of interests was much wider, they may feel grief each time they encounter this focus on trivial matters. Efforts to interest their relative in other aspects of life, such as political events and concerns pertaining to the family, may be met with remarks which only draw the conversation back to her immediate reality.

Loss of Control

The basic human need to exert control is often frustrated by disability. For instance, a man feeling powerless as a result of a stroke may insist that his son return items to precise locations in his room. He may state exactly how he wants his laundry folded and specify when he is to be helped getting dressed. His son may feel irritated by this insistence on needless detail and strict timing, noting that the tasks take twice as long to complete when done according to his father's specifications. Attempts to hurry his father or dissuade him from his demands may be met with anger seemingly disproportionate to the situation.

Exploding at helpers who fail to perform a task correctly can take both the ill person and his family members by surprise. Such bursts of anger may be uncharacteristic at the same time that they come forth with irresistible force. The ill person may feel intense regret for yelling at the very people he needs the most, yet go on feeling angry at things that have not been done the way he would have done them if he were not disabled. Each incomplete task or period of waiting for help can seem to goad him as a reminder of his helplessness, while family members wait in vain for gratitude for all the things they did manage to do correctly. His repeatedly finding fault with efforts made in good faith may anger his caregivers and make them feel even less willing to comply with his demands. A depressing cycle may evolve between them of rage and regret, helplessness and resistance.

Feeling Useless

Using time purposefully is another basic need impeded when an older person becomes ill and homebound. Past sources of meaning, such as volunteer work or club memberships, are often lost when out-of-home activities become too costly or difficult. Vision, hearing, or dexterity problems may interfere with in-home activities, such as reading, writing letters, doing needlework, or listening to educational programs. Exclusion from even ordinary activities, such as doing the laundry or making dinner, may multiply feelings of uselessness.

With good intentions, family members often compound the problem by rushing to make life easier for their disabled relative. They may unwittingly remove all tasks and challenges from their relative's daily life, leaving an existence devoid of productive effort. Even if putting on his shirt takes a stroke patient fifteen minutes, this small exertion may be all he has left of feeling effective: "At least no one has to help me get dressed." Family members may turn down an older person's offers to help around the house, wanting to spare the person extra effort, while the person then feels that he has nothing to contribute to the household.

In other situations, family members may try to insist that the older person accomplish certain tasks on her own, only to be met with self-defeating beliefs such as, "Forget it. I can't do anything anymore."

Once such beliefs become established, people begin to view their daily lives through this lens and to notice only those occurrences which support these beliefs. For example, a woman with arthritis may drop a dish while helping to load the dishwasher and may view this accident as proof of her uselessness. She may then despair the next time she has trouble buttoning her blouse, refusing to get dressed on her own from that day forward. She may eventually shun all activities which emphasize her loss of dexterity, preferring surrender to fighting through her frustrations.

Touch Deprivation

The need to be touched is as fundamental as any other physical need. Adults of all ages enjoy being held as much as children do, but this need is much less acknowledged in adulthood. People often free themselves to satisfy this need within the sphere of sexual relationships, but accept the absence of physical contact in other types of relationships. Initiating a hug from a friend or relative is especially difficult for older people unaccustomed to expressing affection in this way or fearful that such gestures will be met with rejection. Touch deprivation can be a significant loss for unpartnered older people, who may go for years without being held or embraced.

Ways to be touched during everyday life become increasingly scarce when opportunities for intimacy decline. Weekly visits to her hairdresser may be a precious ritual for an older woman who lacks anyone else in her life to touch her. The sensation of strong hands lathering the soap on her head and positioning her shoulders while combing out her hair may be deeply soothing. In the same way, an older man may cherish the way his clinic nurse lets her hand linger on his wrist after taking his pulse. Illness and mobility problems tend to interfere with even these fleeting opportunities for physical contact.

The need to be touched is often most acute when it is least available, a paradox that can intensify feelings of loss and depression. For example, adult children frequently urge their parents to set up separate beds or bedrooms when one of them has an incapacitating illness. In these instances, the healthier parent's need for uninterrupted rest is presumed to take precedence over their sleeping together. More than at any other period of their marriage, however, the ill spouse may need to be cuddled during the night. People derive considerable comfort from being held, especially after disfiguring surgeries such as mastectomies, colostomies, and amputations.

RESPONDING TO A RELATIVE'S SUICIDE WISHES

Toward the end of life, death often becomes attractive as a release from suffering. In many instances, the balance between an older person's will to live and her longing to be released from life is so tenuous that an apparently small loss can tip the balance toward her wanting to die. A major difficulty for family members and professionals lies in distinguishing between appropriate acceptance of death and situations which call for active intervention.

Some older people indicate their readiness for death through anticipatory actions. Such preparations may include completing or updating a will, giving away treasured items, writing letters to distant friends and relatives, informing family members where vital documents are located, and initiating conversations about the significance of their life and relationships. These actions, when gradual, may be practical responses to an awareness of the approaching ending. When carried out all at once or accompanied by an extended depression, they may evoke family members' alarm that a suicide plan is in the early stages of enactment.

Suicide Threats

Families confronted with outright suicide threats or who suspect that their relative is contemplating suicide usually feel overwhelmed when trying to decide what to do. Failing to take preventive action feels irresponsible, yet instigating an involuntary commitment to a psychiatric ward may seem too dramatic and intrusive. The stress and humiliation involved in the legal process of commitment often makes families feel that they would be inflicting yet another form of suffering on an already pained person. Furthermore, those who feel sympathetic with their relative's desire to die may fear that the older person will misinterpret their inaction or their expression of sympathy as a wish to be free of care responsibilities.

When a relative with a debilitating disease requests assistance with committing suicide, family members tend to face still more intense internal conflict. Their compassion toward the person's suffering may be as deep as their repugnance toward the idea of helping someone end her own life. People with degenerative diseases sometimes make pacts with themselves or with loved ones to end their lives when they reach a certain stage of physical or mental incapacity: "When it gets to the point where I can't feed myself, that's it for me." When the self-assigned timetable for enduring runs out, the disabled person may not be able to commit suicide on her own. If family members then refuse to obtain pills or supply a lethal weapon, their relative may accuse them of cruelty or indifference: "If you really loved me, you'd help me die."

Removing a person's means of committing suicide is an immediate way to buy time for the consideration of other options. Items not readily replaceable by a homebound person, such as a loaded gun or accumulations of prescribed medications, can be moved to a neighbor's or family member's home. This intervention is usually difficult to enact because it requires that the older person be confronted directly about her suicidal feelings. For instance, a daughter may fear her father's anger if she removes his hunting rifles without his permission. She may need professional encouragement to remove his rifles as a dramatic statement of caring: "Dad, I love you and I don't want you to die, so I'm storing these guns at my house for a while."

Calling an involuntary treatment team can also be presented as an act of caring: "Believe me, Mom. If we didn't love you so much, we wouldn't bother going through all this." A mental health professional's arrival at the home signals to the older person that her feelings are being taken seriously and that family members are not yet ready to accept her dying. The professional can then assess the person's potential for implementing her plan. Many people fantasize about ending their lives but are actually frightened or repelled by the methods available to them. Others express anger toward family members through their threats of harming themselves but have no intention of taking their lives. Permitting a professional to make these distinctions often clears up family members' confusion about how to respond to future suicidal statements.

Assessing Suicide Potential

In most states, mental health professionals cannot come to the older person's home unless he has directly threatened suicide and possesses the means of carrying it out. The kinds of statements troubling to family members are often more subtle, such as, "I wish I could just stay asleep," or "I wish God would take me." If their relative is receiving home care from a visiting nurse, family members can request that the agency send a social worker to evaluate the person's feelings of despair and to help him address his reasons for wanting to die. Also, adult protection workers from the state social services office can often be dispatched to assist family members who are worried about a relative's potential for self-harm.

The following questions can be used by professionals to assess an older person's suicidal feelings:

1. Why do you want to die? Why now? Did something just happen, a "last straw?"
2. Who would care if you died? Who would be hurt by your dying? Whose life would be easier?
3. How would you end your life? Do you have (a gun, a stash of pills, etc.)? Do you feel capable of harming yourself?

The last question is the most important. Determining whether someone possesses a means of committing suicide and feels capable of following through dictates a professional's next response. If the means and capability are there, along with the intent, the only tenable course of action is to respond protectively: "I can't leave you now unless we take away (the gun, the pills) or you agree to go into the hospital." It is helpful to remember that someone would not have revealed their suicide plan unless they were hoping to be saved. Those who do not want to be prevented from taking their own life generally do not tell anyone who is in a position to stop them. To tell a professional is to ask to be rescued, no matter how strenuously someone denies this intention. With this maxim in mind, a professional can take protective action without worrying about ethical ambiguity.

Research has shown that most suicide attempts occur impulsively, when someone is in an especially bad mood. Depression creates tunnel vision in which nothing but bleak alternatives can be seen. A caring response or decisive intervention during this peak of depression is crucial, since people saved from suicide tend to express gratitude later when they are able to see a broader picture of their possibilities. Informing a suicidal person of this tendency toward tunnel vision may help considerably in obtaining their consent for help: "Right now, you can't see any other way. That's what depression does. Give us time to help with your depression and you'll start to see that you do have other choices."

Occasionally, the sheer act of airing suicidal feelings diminishes their hold on someone's mood. The opportunity to vent disgust with life, anger at relatives perceived to be neglectful, and weariness from chronic medical problems can facilitate a change of attitude which brings relief, even though external circumstances remain the same. Feelings sometimes emerge in these interviews which professionals can translate into suggestions for family members, such as, "When you're telling your friends on the phone about hard days taking care of your mother, make sure she's not overhearing you in the next room." Conveying messages between the older person and family members is often a prime component of a professional's intervention, especially around sensitive topics.

SELF-NEGLECT AS SLOW SUICIDE

Many family members face the dilemmas involved in caring for a relative who is committing slow suicide through such means as eating the wrong foods, smoking through oxygen tubing, or continuing to drink alcohol despite the harm it is causing them. Depression may be at the heart of their relative's self-neglect. This section offers ideas on how to respond productively to situations which may have no clear or immediate solutions.

Violating Medical Restrictions

When someone refuses to follow medical recommendations, it is sometimes helpful to confront the person's self-neglect head on: "You're eating cookies even though your blood sugar is sky-high. You're killing yourself by inches." Speaking the truth of someone's actions out loud may startle the person into discussing what has been denied or rationalized. Underneath anger about dietary restrictions may lie rage at the perceived deprivations of a lifetime. Until such anger is released, discussions may circle around, going nowhere. Letting someone express this rage for what it is may clear the way for more constructive discussions about self-care.

Some older people go against medical advice as a rebellious act, a way to assert personal freedom within constraining circumstances. Life can seem particularly devoid of physical pleasure when a person's diet is restricted, mobility is limited, smoking is prohibited, and sexual activity diminished or nonexistent. Breaking out against multiple constraints can serve as an act of vitality, flaunting the potential danger in exchange for a liberated feeling. The proclamation, "So what? I'm going to be dead soon, anyway," often accompanies defiant puffs on a cigarette and binges of favorite foods. Such people seem to seize upon a sense of entitlement to the last days of life, even if these actions serve to reduce the number of their remaining days.

Family members are often able to pose powerful challenges to such blatant disregard for health and death. A daughter can say "Mom, when you binge on those salty potato chips, I get scared you'll have a stroke and die. I want you to live for a long time." Family members can also plead with a loved one to give anti-depressant medication a chance, pointing out that the pills may help mobilize the very changes which would lead to real freedom: "Dad, these medicines might give you the energy to quit smoking. If you breathe better, you'll be able to go fishing again." Linking improved self-care with longevity and freedom may wake someone up to the importance of following medical advice.

Abusing Alcohol

Alcohol may be functioning as self-medication for depression. When approaching an older person's alcohol use, it is important to distinguish between lifelong abusers and those who began drinking in response to later life losses. Lifelong abusers are deeply accustomed to blocking out painful feelings. They may never have learned how to tolerate anxiety, boredom, hurt, or frustration. In addition, the extent of their physical addiction may make it dangerous for them to try to stop drinking without medical supervision. Hospital-based alcohol treatment, covered by Medicare, is often the best option in these instances.

In contrast, those who have not previously used alcohol as a means of survival tend to reach old age with a repertoire of coping skills. Having been able to endure life's normal hardships, they turn to alcohol only after health limitations interfere with their strengths, or when an event of sufficient magnitude overwhelms them. Studies have shown that caregiving, retirement, death of a spouse, and disfiguring surgeries are the most common causes of becoming dependent on alcohol for the first time in later life. Receiving help which specifically addresses these underlying problems may prevent the need for alcohol treatment and may set someone on a healthier course for bearing their difficulties. (See "When Self-Care Fails: Abuse and Neglect," pp. 36–41.)

Family members exasperated by their relative's self-destructive behavior may nevertheless have difficulty removing themselves from the rescuer role. For example, a man on a fixed income may spend so much on whiskey that he is left with insufficient money for food and utility bills. His adult children may react with rage each time they give him money for food or pay his electricity bill, yet they go on helping him: "We can't let him starve or freeze to death." One strategy is to offer to hold a portion of the person's income until the last week of the month. Another is to bring over food and to pay utility bills directly, rather than give cash which can be used for alcohol.

Requesting professional help with handling an older relative's abuse of alcohol is often a family's best recourse. A phone number for the state's adult protective services division should be listed in the community services section of the phone book. Caseworkers may be able to offer the older person referrals to alcohol treatment. If the person refuses treatment, they may be able to work with the family toward setting limits on their role as rescuers. Many people will not accept alcohol treatment until family members stop protecting them and they are forced to confront the consequences of their alcohol abuse.

Losing the Will to Live

Loss of the will to live is one of the most frequent underpinnings of self-neglect. Some people let their lives lapse during a bereavement or in the wake of too many losses, and then find themselves stuck in a state of lassitude long after their grief should have lessened. They become exhausted by a self-defeating cycle of feeling unable to go out and do things, facing a deadening sameness every day, and then losing still more of their drive to take care of themselves or reach out to others because nothing fresh is going on in their lives. Letting friendships and involvements recede then triggers a further loss of hope.

When asked "What would make life worth living for you?", some people respond with clear statements about wishing they could be useful or that they had a pet or a garden to look after. Their replies are full of clues as to the origin of their self-neglect and the prospects for reawakening their spirit for life. Others are unable to answer such questions, either because they are unaccustomed to thinking in these terms or because they have lost faith in themselves, in God, or in other people. It is often helpful to offer specific ideas to such people, even if they vehemently reject these options as unsuitable or unrealistic.

In their very vehemence, some people reveal themselves. Listening carefully during their flood of negativity may yield ideas. Residual shreds of motivation or desire may become evident as one option after another is rejected: "I don't want to sit all day with a bunch of old duds at day care, not doing anything, not learning anything, just existing." Doing and learning may be central to any intervention created for people who are appalled by the absence of activity and novelty in their lives.

No one can presume to know what would make life worth living for another person. Without such dialogue, able-bodied relatives and professionals can easily overlook a solution which would mean a great deal to someone living in reduced circumstances. Small changes can lead to large rewards in a life which has been devoid of provocation or stimulation. For instance, a woman who never leaves her apartment may find that having help getting down to the lobby once a week to see a bit of the world may give her something to look forward to and a reason to start taking her blood pressure medication more faithfully.

This process of challenging older people to describe what would help inspire their self-care is both respectful and potentially effective. Creativity may be the most important element in designing interventions which are truly responsive to the clues which have been provided in this fashion. People who neglect themselves already tend to fall outside the range of standard solutions or they would not be so difficult to assist.

Professionals may have to spend more time with such individuals, first locating the core motivation upon which to base their interventions and then trying out one idea after another. Family members may be helpful in this regard by providing information about what previously gave their relative something to live for. Generally, however, there is no substitute for spending time with the person and passing ideas back and forth until something sparks. The next section gives specific ideas which can get the process moving.

INTERVENTIONS TO RELIEVE DEPRESSION

Prior to carrying out interventions, it is important to consider anti-depressant medication. In many instances, medication gives older people the boost they need to be able to experiment with the ideas suggested by family members and professionals. Once they feel activated by the medication, many people will resume activities which previously gave them satisfaction or will try something new that may increase their interest in living. For some, knowing that the medication can be stopped once this revival is achieved may make anti-depressants tolerable to them. Others may need to learn how many millions of people use these medications at some point in their lives. Assuring them that they are not to blame for being unable to "snap out of it" may reduce their sense of shame.

Instituting a "Sabbath"

Having a psychological sabbath, one day a week different from the rest, can help restore a homebound person's zest for life. For this reason, family members who want to make the most of limited time will find that providing their relative an assured weekly outing is better than several spontaneous visits to the home. In looking forward to the outing, the older person gains a reason to keep track of the passage of time. Most importantly, anticipation of the coming eventful day helps enliven the intervening monotonous days. There are reasons to get out of bed on the other days, if only to maintain strength and mobility for the one day which will be unique.

A weekly change of scene can also improve a person's ability to look beyond herself. Fresh sights and sounds promote alertness, spark memories, and give someone new things to talk about. An outing requires more effort of family members than dropping over, but pays off when they discover that their relative's interest in their lives is reawakened along with her renewed engagement in life as a whole. The return of her vitality may in turn inspire family members to spend more time with her, less as an obligatory contact to be endured than as an relationship to be appreciated.

Instituting a regularly occurring pleasure at home also serves as a sabbath, a break from the routine of being ill or disabled. By encouraging their relative to recall activities enjoyed in the past, family members can begin to find ways to make these endeavors accessible in the present. For instance, being in contact with nature through a garden, sitting outside in the sun, or looking at the night sky may be experiences that someone confined to a wheelchair sorely misses. Having a ramp built over the front steps may be well worth the expense and the disfigurement of a yard, if the person's spirit for life resumes along with the capacity to go outside at will. Easily available pleasures lift a person's focus away from what has been lost, toward aspects of life still at hand.

Making the Most of Touch

Paying attention to the need to be touched may also help revive someone's spirit. Opportunities to touch their relative abound in caregiving situations. Placing a hand on their relative's arm during medical tests and examinations may be most welcome. More powerful than words of assurance, touch is one of the most calming responses that can be offered to fear. Giving someone who is in pain a footrub or a backrub may help the person release physical tension, thereby lessening the pain. Urging spouses to continue sleeping together, rather than establishing separate beds or bedrooms, may be a vital encouragement, if backed up by family members' willingness to allow the healthier spouse to take naps during the day while they tend to their ill relative.

Service providers who have physical contact with older people as part of their work should remember to make the most of opportunities to touch those who lack other means of receiving contact. For instance, home health aides have extensive opportunities to touch older people. Helping someone bathe provides virtually endless excuses for contact. To someone hungry for touch, having their hair washed, their back rubbed with soap, or their hair toweled dry may be more comforting than any amount of talking.

Physicians and other health-care providers can also help by prescribing touch as part of the care rendered by friends and relatives. For instance, the wife of a man paralyzed on one side by a stroke could be instructed to caress his paralyzed arm, both to stimulate a return of sensation and to help him accept this changed body part. His son could be encouraged to hold him up in a standing position for several minutes a day to relieve his wheelchair restlessness and to give him close physical contact.

Giving Back Control

Family members feeling resentful of their relative may be relieved to realize that rigidity is often an expression of a need for control, rather than a sheer urge to tyrannize. One strategy is to ask the older person to choose a few tasks over which he will maintain complete control in exchange for letting family members use their discretion in other areas: "Dad, I can't do everything the way you want me to, but I'd like to do at least a few things exactly how you tell me to do them." For instance, an older man may choose to have his son manage his bill paying precisely according to his instructions, while agreeing to back off from detailed requirements about how his socks are to be folded.

In returning power to an older person, the concept of symbolic control may be especially useful to family members. Carrying a wallet filled with money may symbolize manhood for a man who no longer leaves the house, just as having car keys in his pocket may reassure a man who never actually drives his car. Similarly, planning menus may give a woman who can no longer cook a sense of being back in charge of her kitchen. As with all symbolic activity, a single action takes the place of the many facets associated with it. The wallet, the car keys, and the menu planning each stand for abilities that may be slipping away but which can be retained in a small way.

Encouraging Contributions

Standards for meaningful activity shift as the person's number of choices declines. Family members need to be careful not to overlook forms of participation in the household or community that they perceive as trivial, but which would satisfy someone who fears having nothing left to give or produce. A woman with severe arthritic deformities in her hands may derive a sense of satisfaction from answering the phone and taking messages for family members. The fact that her handwriting is occasionally difficult to read may be less significant than the confirmation provided by this task that she continues to be a functional adult. In the same way, a man disabled by a stroke may find that using his "one good hand" to stuff envelopes for a charity affirms his capacity to be useful and allows him to maintain a link with the wider community.

Finding something useful for an ill or disabled person to do may require creative thinking, experimentation, and patience. The idea is to take advantage of any remaining capacities, while avoiding activities which would emphasize what has been lost. A man whose vocal cords were removed as part of cancer surgery may find that he enjoys volunteering as a crosswalk guard, using hand signals and whistle blasts to get the job done. Allowing a bedbound person to fold laundry or a wheelchair-bound person to cut up vegetables may be more satisfying to that person than family members realize and therefore well worth the time added to accomplishing these tasks.

Making Progress Visible

Achieving small successes also helps relieve depression, yet slow or quiet increments of victory are easily overlooked. For instance, a man recovering from a stroke may do his rehabilitation exercises halfheartedly, and then cite his minimal progress as evidence of the futility of continuing. A progress chart (see p. 200) can be used to shift a person's focus to measurable results. Through comments such as, "I see that on Monday you were able to do only three sit-ups and now you can do six," family members can reinforce both the continued effort and the perception of making headway. As time goes by, they can take out charts from past weeks to remind the person how far he has come in his efforts. The family's interest in these small triumphs can make them more rewarding to someone who would otherwise focus only on the tedium and pain necessary for improvement. By making a practice of looking at the chart at each visit or asking about it during each long-distance phone call, family members underscore the scale within which such achievements become visible.

By putting on music and exercising along with their relative, family members may discover the benefits of mutual encouragement. Someone recovering from a stroke may get great satisfaction from cheering his caregivers on and helping them reach their physical goals. Caregivers can mark their progress on similar exercise charts. The whole enterprise of recovery is aided by tactics which enhance the pleasurable aspects while deflecting attention from the discomfort.

Even without a specific rehabilitation program, exercises can be designed as a context for achieving small successes. For example, a route within the person's home can be designated as a lap, and a progress chart can be used to monitor the number of laps walked each day. As an initial activity for a person who has become immobile, houselaps have the advantages of not requiring changes of clothing, the negotiation of physical barriers such as steps, nor coping with extremes of weather. A helper's presence is usually not necessary to ensure safety, since handholds and resting places tend to be readily available within a home. The first week can be set up to be an easy success, such as the goal of two laps before each meal. Motivated by family members' interest and appreciative commentary, the person may spontaneously increase his number of daily laps. The combination of visible progress with caring witnesses almost always gives someone a boost out of weariness.

There are times when people sustain so many losses that they can barely revive themselves from one before another comes. Those who have lost a lifelong partner or friend, who have had to part with a home of many years, or who have had to give up beloved activities due to physical problems are especially vulnerable to depression if additional losses occur before their grief has subsided. Helping someone renew their motivation for life in the face of accumulated losses is a slow and sensitive enterprise not limited to the province of professionals. The ideas presented in this chapter may stimulate family members' empathy and creativity as they strive to help their relative regain a spirit for life.

WAYS TO MAINTAIN MOTIVATION

Institute a weekly outing for mental stimulation, a sense of anticipation, and mood elevation inherent in a change of scene. A ride in the car may be enough to break up the monotony of remaining in a known environment.

Restore areas of control. Since many illnesses result in a loss of the the ability to direct areas of life previously managed independently, an effective countering strategy is to find specific ways for an older person to exert control over as many choices as possible.

Focus on small successes as a way of helping the person change self-defeating beliefs. As small, readily observable successes build on each other, feelings of powerlessness tend to recede.

Devise contributions to the household, the family, or the community that satisfy the need for purposeful activity. The older person's past sources of meaning can provide clues.

Establish regularly occurring pleasures. No matter how narrow in scope, reliable pleasures give the person something to look forward to.

From Wendy Lustbader and Nancy R. Hooyman, *Taking Care of Aging Family Members* (New York: The Free Press, 1994). Copyright © 1994 by Wendy Lustbader and Nancy Hooyman; copyright © 1986 by The Free Press.

SUGGESTED RESOURCES

Articles

Frierson, Robert. "Suicide Attempts by the Old and the Very Old," *Archives of Internal Medicine*, 151 (1991), 141–144.

> Based on a survey, the author identifies risk factors of the elderly who have attempted suicide. These include being male, suffering from major depression, a high degree of premeditation, and solitary living arrangements. Strategies for reducing some of these factors are suggested.

Lamy, Peter. "Actions of Alcohol and Drugs in Older People," *Generations*, 12 (1988), 9–13.

> Readable overview of age-related physiological changes that affect the body's ability to absorb and dispose of drugs and alcohol.

Books

Billig, Nathan. *To Be Old and Sad: Understanding Depression in the Elderly* (New York: Lexington Books), 1987.

> The author emphasizes that depression is not inevitable and is treatable. Reviews the signs of depression, effective treatments, and frequent causes of misdiagnosis.

Frank, Arthur. *At the Will of the Body: Reflections on Illness* (Boston: Houghton Mifflin Company), 1991.

> The author explores his own experience of illness with great insight and honesty. The book challenges, inspires, and suggests ideas that may help an ill person out of depression.

Knight, Bob. *Psychotherapy with the Older Adult* (Newbury Park, CA: Sage), 1986.

> The author stresses the need for special knowledge in the areas of chronic illness, disability, death and dying, and the role of ethnic identity in later life. The themes of empowerment and life review are emphasized throughout.

Genevay, Bonnie, and Renee Katz, *Countertransference and Older Clients* (Newbury Park, CA: Sage), 1990.

> The authors address how practitioners' attitudes and feelings toward their older clients can affect their helpfulness to older people. Through a series of case examples, they illustrate how reactions to disability, dementia, death, sexuality, and substance abuse can influence professional effectiveness.

Lustbader, Wendy. *Counting on Kindness: The Dilemmas of Dependency* (New York: The Free Press), 1991.

> Examines what it means to be dependent from the dual perspective of the dependent person and the caregiver. This context provides a framework for building on "what is" and reducing feelings of resentment, depression, and anger as both the caregiver and the dependent person seek to balance their needs.

Osgood, Nancy. *Suicide in Later Life: Recognizing the Warning Signs* (New York: Lexington Books), 1992.

Useful to both professionals and family members, this book reviews the warning signs of suicide and is oriented toward prevention of unnecessary loss of life.

Organizations

Alcoholics Anonymous (AA). P.O. Box 459, Grand Central Station, New York, NY 10163

AA is a voluntary fellowship of alcoholics whose purpose is to help themselves and each other get, and stay, sober. For information, write to the national office, or look in the phone book for a local chapter. The national office can also send you their free pamphlet, "Time to Start Living."

National Council on Alcoholism. 1424 16th Street, N.W., Suite 401, Washington, D.C. 20036. (202) 206–6770 or (800) 475–HOPE.

This organization provides support and information to people with alcohol problems in the family. Write to the national office, or look in the phone book for a local chapter. Many older people have found this group especially helpful.

National Depressive and Manic-Depressive Association. P.O. Box 1939, Chicago, IL 60690. (312) 642–0049.

This association has over 200 chapters across the United States and Canada which offer support to people with depressive illnesses and their families. It sponsors education and research programs and distributes numerous brochures, videotapes, and audio programs.

National Institute of Mental Health. 5600 Fishers Lane, Room 15C–05, Rockville, MD 20857. (301) 443–4513.

The "Depression Awareness, Recognition, and Treatment Program" offers several publications on depression, including one especially written for older people, *If You're Over 65 and Feeling Depressed . . . Treatment Brings New Hope.*

PROGRESS CHART			
	Morning	*Afternoon*	*Evening*
SUNDAY			
MONDAY			
TUESDAY			
WEDNESDAY			
THURSDAY			
FRIDAY			
SATURDAY			

10

Financial Strains in Caregiving

Most older people fear health care expenses more than other worries in their lives. Some omit prescribed medications, put off necessary medical procedures, and refuse to hire extra help in their homes due to the threat of rising costs and anxiety about not having enough money later to meet their basic needs. Others have no idea what their options are or they misunderstand the requirements for government programs that they hear about from friends and neighbors. This chapter first explains the programs which help older people pay for their medical expenses and those which provide supplementary income. Then, options for the management of finances are depicted. Finally, the costs of various long-term care alternatives are compared and the common reluctance to spend money on these options is discussed from the perspective of both older people and their heirs.

UNDERSTANDING MEDICARE

Confusion about Medicare produces considerable anxiety for older people and those who assist them with managing their finances. For instance, many people hold the mistaken belief that Medicare will cover all of their medical expenses, becoming distressed and outraged when they discover that their out-of-pocket expenses are quite extensive. Hospitals and other medical providers bombard older people with

201

DISTINGUISHING BETWEEN MEDICARE AND MEDICAID

	Medicare	Medicaid
Eligibility	Determined by reaching age 65 or remaining on Social Security Disability for two years	Determined by income and financial assets
Dispensing Agency	The Social Security Administration; monthly premiums are deducted from the Social Security check	The local welfare office of the state
Sources of the Funds	Federally funded and uniformly administered from state to state	Federal-state partnership, with eligibility requirements varying by state
Common Attitudes of Older People	Viewed as an insurance program	Viewed as welfare
Deductibles/ Co-payments	Annual outpatient deductible, hospital deductible, and small co-payment of outpatient bills	Varies from state to state; some permit an older person to qualify for assistance after "spending down" income on care
Coverage of the Cost of Medicines	Does not cover medicines	Pays for most prescriptions

From Wendy Lustbader and Nancy R. Hooyman, *Taking Care of Aging Family Members* (New York: The Free Press, 1994). Copyright © 1994 by Wendy Lustbader and Nancy Hooyman; copyright © 1986 by The Free Press.

computerized billing statements which are needlessly complex and which do not always clarify how much is likely to be covered by Medicare. It can be difficult to persuade someone receiving these computer-generated statements that the bulk of her mail does not equal the size of her debt. The list below and the section which follows explain what is covered by Medicare and may help reduce anxiety.

Major Differences in Benefits Between Medicare and Medicaid

Nursing home benefits:

Medicare pays for limited forms of care in nursing homes, only for brief periods of time.

Medicaid pays for nursing home care for the duration of the person's life, after eligibility requirements are met.

Home health care benefits:

Medicare covers the full range of professional services, but is limited to certain types of health conditions and specific time periods. Long-term assistance with bathing, dressing, and housekeeping is not covered.

Medicaid covers a smaller range of home health services, but is less limited in duration and in the types of conditions which qualify a person for service. In some instances, long-term assistance with basic activities of daily life is covered.

How Medicare Works

The gap between the actual amount a physician or other provider charges for medical services and what Medicare deems allowable is the key to understanding the limits of Medicare. The following example, depicted in the "Medicare Vocabulary" chart, makes these limits clear. An older person is charged $120 by Dr. Smith and receives a check from Medicare for $80, because the allowable charge set by Medicare was $100 for this visit. If Dr. Smith had accepted assignment on this bill, the doctor would have received the $80 payment directly from Medicare and would have been permitted to bill the older person only for the $20 remaining of the allowable charge, not the $40 left on the original bill.

Families should encourage their relatives with limited incomes to check with providers before any services are rendered to determine whether they will accept Medicare assignment. In some parts of the country, medical referral services will supply the names of doctors, labs, and clinics which accept assignment. A senior center, senior information and referral hotline, or the local medical association may have information about such referral services. Some doctors accept assignment for all of their Medicare patients, while others do so on a case-by-case basis. An older person who asks her doctor personally to accept assignment will tend to get a better response than someone who asks the doctor's billing clerk, who may have been instructed not to accept assignment as a general office policy.

Several months may elapse between the date a service was actually rendered and the date Medicare sends the "Explanation of Benefits" listing what was paid. The only way to match Medicare's statements with billing statements from providers is through the dates of service, rather than the dates of the billings. In order to ease the matching process, it helps to highlight the dates of service on both the Medicare statement and the bills received from doctors, hospitals, and labs. Discarding duplicate bills while saving the itemized bills is another important step, as this reduces the size of the pile considerably. Supplemental insurances often require a copy of the itemized bill and the Explanation of Benefits. Duplicate bills are useless, unless they show payments made while waiting for Medicare reimbursement.

Medicare Supplemental Insurance

Most supplemental policies would pay only twenty dollars on the above claim, the difference between what Medicare paid and the allowable charge, rather than the full amount owed after the Medicare payment. Not realizing the limits of such insurance, many older people respond to advertisements from insurance companies and end up paying monthly premiums on policies which do not translate into significant protection against high medical costs. Frequently, people take out several policies at once, hoping that more insurance equals more protection, but this is usually not the case.

The state insurance commission or local senior services may offer assistance with making sense of various policies and determining which is the best buy in particular circumstances. Since some supplemental policies are worthwhile, existing policies should be examined carefully before they are discontinued. For example, policies which

MEDICARE VOCABULARY

Provider	Date of Service	Original Charge	Allowable	Medicare
Dr.Smith	Feb. 5	$120	$100	$80

Provider	The doctor, hospital, lab, clinic, or medical equipment supplier.
Date of service	The date that services were actually provided, as opposed to the billing statement's date.
Original charge	The provider submits a charge to Medicare which is usually more than what Medicare will pay. In this example, $120 was billed to Medicare.
Allowable charge	This is the charge Medicare sets for a service or procedure. Medicare pays 80% of the allowable charge, not 80% of the original bill. In this example, the allowable was $100.
Medicare payment	Medicare paid $80 in this example, leaving $40 still owed to the doctor
Assignment	By accepting assignment, a provider agrees to accept the allowable charge as the full charge. In this example, only $20 would have been owed if the doctor had accepted assignment.
Itemized bill	The first bill received from the provider, detailing charges item-by-item. This bill should be saved for supplemental insurances.
Explanation of benefits	The statement sent by Medicare explaining each payment made to providers. These should be saved for supplemental insurances.

pay the full hospital deductible are often a wise purchase for people who tend to go into the hospital at least once a year.

Learning how to fill out the forms correctly and which documents must accompany the claim can speed reimbursement and ensure that the older person receives full value from the supplemental policy. It is important to avoid sending the original copy of an Explanation of Benefits or an itemized bill to an insurance company, as replacing these can be difficult and such items are often misplaced during processing. A doctor's billing clerk or a hospital's billing department may be willing to make copies of these documents and assist with filling out the forms correctly.

Keeping Track of Medicare

Medicare statements, itemized bills, duplicate bills, and statements from supplemental insurances often turn into a threatening pile of unopened envelopes. These items arrive in such quantity and in such a bewildering array of computerized drivel that many people allow them to accumulate in shoe boxes or shopping bags rather than attempt to decipher them. The following "Medical Bill Accounting System" form is a tool for transforming this heap into an orderly and intelligible collection of statements. The system can do more to relieve anxiety about medical expenses than any amount of verbal reassurance.

The hardest part of this system is getting started. Older people and their financial helpers should begin by collecting and matching all the Medicare statements and itemized bills from dates of service during the past year. Documents from previous years should be set aside and duplicate bills containing no new information should be discarded. This process of separating out a reduced pile of documents for consideration makes the initial task seem less daunting.

The next step is to list dates of service in chronological order on the accounting sheet, filling in names of providers and amounts of original bills. The blank form can be enlarged before copies are made to ease its use by people with low vision or hand tremors. The final step is to fill in the amounts Medicare paid for each date of service and to note personal checks already sent to providers. When completed, the accounting page can serve as a cover sheet, with relevant documents clipped in order behind it. As additional documents arrive, such as statements from supplemental insurance, missing amounts can be filled in the appropriate spaces.

MEDICAL BILL ACCOUNTING SYSTEM

Date	Provider	Original Charge	Allowable Charge	Medicare Payment	Supplemental Ins. Payment	Notes

From Wendy Lustbader and Nancy R. Hooyman, *Taking Care of Aging Family Members* (New York: The Free Press, 1994). Copyright © 1994 by Wendy Lustbader and Nancy Hooyman; copyright © 1986 by The Free Press.

Keeping track of medical bills in this orderly fashion builds a sense of clarity and control where before there was confusion. Expenses for medicines, equipment rental, and medical supplies can also be listed, making the system valuable for tax purposes or for documentation supporting a Medicaid application. Above all, it reduces worry by making Medicare less mysterious and the array of paperwork more accessible.

Medicare in the Hospital

Fear of large hospital bills causes many older people to refuse to go into the hospital for necessary surgery or diagnostic procedures. Some do not realize that Medicare usually covers the entire hospital bill, less the hospital deductible. Most supplemental policies will pay the deductible, leaving those who possess this coverage with no bill at all. For people without supplemental insurance, the hospital deductible itself often becomes the obstacle to their accepting vital treatment. They may be unaware that Medicaid will cover this payment, if they meet the qualifying conditions for state medical assistance. (See "Understanding Medicaid," pp. 210–214.)

Understanding how Medicare reimburses hospitals is another important piece of the health-care puzzle. Medicare pays for a hospital stay according to the diagnostic group to which a person is assigned, called a "Diagnostic Related Grouping" (DRG), rather than according to the number of days the person actually stays in the hospital. For instance, if a broken hip places someone in the category for which Medicare will pay the equivalent of two weeks of hospital care, it is in the hospital's best interest to get that person out of the hospital in less than two weeks. The hospital gets the same reimbursement whether a particular person with a broken hip remains in the hospital ten or twenty days.

The fact that a hospital makes money on a stay under the DRG limit and may lose money on a longer stay means that a family cannot be assured that their relative's best interests are always the hospital's first priority. For example, a daughter may hear on a Monday afternoon that her mother is being discharged "tomorrow," even though she cannot take time off from work on such short notice nor arrange for home care services with so little lead time. She may also observe that her mother's medical condition, despite some improvement, is still too unstable to be managed at home. Knowing what to do in such instances is vital for family members wanting to obtain the best possible care for their relative and to arrange a safe and comfortable situation at home.

Older people and their families have the right to request a written document, called a "notice of noncoverage," which states the hospital's opinion that the care can be safely rendered in another setting. Requesting this notice gains the family forty-eight more hours before the discharge takes place or before the older person may become financially liable for further hospital care. The family should then meet with their relative's doctor, voicing their disagreement with the hospital's opinion and describing their concerns about the care situation at home. With or without the doctor's support, the family can request an immediate review from the "Professional Review Organization" (PRO) authorized by Medicare to review inpatient hospital services in their relative's area. Their phone number should be included with the "notice of noncoverage" or can be requested from the hospital. This organization, not the hospital, decides whether further hospital care is medically necessary. If it is deemed necessary, the hospital cannot bill the older person for the further care which has been authorized.

Unfortunately, financial incentives or administrative pressures on doctors to get older people out of the hospital as quickly as possible may mean that families cannot count on doctors to be their advocates in every instance. Medicare's cost-cutting efforts through DRGs have thereby damaged an historic trust. Unaware of this shift, many family members may go against their own judgment and scramble to pull together some semblance of safety for their relative at home "because the doctor said so." Professionals should teach older people and their families that they have the right to say "no" to an impractical or risky discharge from the hospital, even if this means finding another doctor who is willing to put their needs above these pressures.

Medicare at Home: What Role Does Long-Term Care Insurance Play?

One of older people's needs is for assistance with basic care at home over the long run, but Medicare is geared toward short-term, skilled home health care. For instance, an older woman recovering from surgery may qualify for the services of a Medicare-funded nurse and home health aide for eight weeks following her hospital stay. When her acute needs resolve, she may still need help with bathing, meal preparation, and household chores, but Medicare will not continue to cover the services of a home health aide after the nurse's skilled care is no longer required. This means that the older woman or her family will have to pay the cost of an aide on their own, do without these services, or try to qualify for other government-funded services. (See "Medicare-Funded Home Health Services," pp. 232–234.)

Long-term care insurance has evolved in response to these needs and is constantly changing. It is one of the most complex of all insurances. There are policies which cover only nursing home stays, some which cover home care, and some which cover both. Such insurance is not for everyone, since it basically functions as asset protection for people whose financial resources are much greater than the cut-off for government-funded services. To avoid the possibility of having to spend down their assets before they qualify for Medicaid and other programs, people with significant assets count on long-term care insurance to cover their needs the way government-funded programs cover the needs of people without financial resources.

To choose a long-term care policy wisely, it is necessary to examine the policy's "gatekeeper" clauses, the sections detailing the conditions under which coverage is restricted or excluded. An insurance company can sell a policy which provides lump sum coverage, to be spent as the policyholder chooses, or coverage based upon reimbursement for certain types of services, with a limit as to the total benefits paid. The following chart provides basic questions for comparing long-term care insurance policies.

Long-term care insurance is not a substitute for a Medicare supplemental policy and it is not advantageous for everyone. If a person's assets are modest and the price of premiums is high, a long-term care policy may be more of a financial burden than a benefit in the long run. (See "Suggested Resources" at the end of this chapter for obtaining further information on these issues.)

UNDERSTANDING MEDICAID

Many Medicare recipients with low incomes have difficulty paying their monthly Medicare premium and the bills left over after Medicare makes its payments. They may be unable to afford supplemental insurance. They may also be burdened by the high costs of medicines and other necessities that Medicare does not cover. Medicaid, medical

BASIC QUESTIONS FOR COMPARING LONG-TERM CARE INSURANCE POLICIES

What kinds of home care services are covered? Skilled nursing care? Aide or homemaker assistance with bathing, meal preparation, or household chores? Physical therapy? Other rehabilitation services?

What kinds of care are covered outside the home? Adult day care? Adult foster home care? Residence in an assisted living facility? All levels of nursing home care?

When do covered services begin? Under what conditions? Must benefits be related to a specific illness or injury? Do covered services begin only after a certain number of days in a nursing home? Do benefits begin as soon as the person is unable to perform certain activities of daily living, regardless of whether an acute problem exists?

Who decides whether the person's condition qualifies for benefits? Do specially trained, independent case managers make these decisions? Do "gatekeepers" employed by the insurance company base their approval of coverage on clearly stated, specific guidelines?

What are the benefit ceilings? Is there a "lump sum" limit on the total costs of benefits, or a maximum benefit period, such as three years? Does the policy pay a set percentage of approved services, the actual cost up to a daily maximum, or set dollar amount per day, regardless of the actual cost of services?

Who is authorized to provide covered services? Must the care be supplied by certain physician groups, nursing homes, home health care agencies, or other health care providers?

Are inflation protection options available? Is there a cost of living option based on the Consumer Price Index, or a percentage that the daily benefit will increase each year on a compounded basis?

assistance administered by the state, serves in these instances as a supplement to Medicare, covering Medicare's monthly premium, copayments, and hospital deductible, as well as most medicines, eyeglasses, and some additional services. The catch is that the person's income must be less than a specified level and the total value of the person's bank accounts and other assets must fall below a certain limit to qualify for this assistance.

How To Obtain Medicaid Benefits

For those who are proud of having survived a lifetime without "handouts" from the government, applying for medical assistance from the state can seem humiliating. Others who have lived through economic hardship most of their lives may have considerable mistrust for a system which seems to grant and withdraw benefits arbitrarily. In many states, elders must apply for medical assistance at their local welfare office, standing in the same lines and confronting the same bureaucratic procedures that demean and alienate applicants of all ages.

Overworked clerks and caseworkers often cannot spend sufficient time with low-income older people to help them handle the complicated paperwork and to assemble the required documentation. Elders who have problems with vision, hearing, hand tremors, English language fluency, illiteracy, mobility, or memory may be unable to work their way through the maze. Not surprisingly, many older people give up on obtaining the Medicaid benefits they deserve. As a result, vital prescriptions may remain unfilled and necessary medical procedures delayed until life-threatening symptoms develop.

The following questions and answers serve as a basic introduction to Medicaid, but state-to-state variations in the rules require that advocates be found in the person's local area. Some legal assistance clinics and senior case management programs offer help with obtaining Medicaid benefits. Older people receiving home health care can request the services of a visiting social worker for assistance with handling a Medicaid application. Ironically, older people who find themselves hospitalized for a condition they neglected due to lack of Medicaid benefits tend to receive immediate help with the paperwork while in the hospital. It is in a hospital's best interest to ensure Medicaid reimbursement to cover the large hospital deductible remaining after the Medicare payment and to ease the transfer of an older person to a nursing home should Medicare benefits run out before the person can be returned home.

QUESTIONS AND ANSWERS ABOUT MEDICAID (STATE MEDICAL ASSISTANCE)

1. How is eligibility for Medicaid established?

Each state determines its own income and asset limits for eligibility. At this writing, several states use $2,000 for individuals and $3,000 for couples as the cut-off point for assets. This means that a couple with $4,000 in the bank would be ineligible for assistance, no matter how low their monthly income and how severe their medical expenses. It is often difficult to convince older people to spend down their savings accounts to get them to the eligibility level, despite the many benefits they would gain by doing so.

2. What is the Qualified Medicare Beneficiary (QMB) program? Why are some people eligible for this program but not for the Medicaid program in their state?

The Qualified Medicare Beneficiary program is a federal program, with the same eligibility rules in every state. Many people have income which exceeds their state's Medicaid limit but which is below the limit for the QMB program. The problem is they are unaware of the QMB program or they fear that the application process is too complicated. At this time, any Medicare beneficiary whose income is under $570 a month and whose resources are below $2,000 can qualify. The person meeting these requirements must contact the state's Medicaid office and request QMB status. Once granted QMB, the person's monthly Medicare premium will be automatically paid by the program, as well as most medications and the 20 percent copayment on outpatient care.

3. What are the legal ways to spend down a savings account to meet a state limit on assets for medical assistance?

It is not legal for an older person to give away money from a bank account to relatives in order to qualify for medical assistance. A legitimate basis for achieving eligibility is depleting assets through the payment of household and medical expenses. For instance, paying for the construction of a wheelchair ramp and other necessary home adaptations contributes to a person's health and safety. When the need for state-funded assistance is anticipated, older people should be encouraged to retain receipts for what they spend on medicines, medical supplies, and other items not covered by Medicare. Receipts can be saved in an envelope and kept with the medical bill accounting system described earlier.

4. What documents should be assembled in advance of a Medicaid application?

Generally, all sources of income and all assets must be verified with documents, such as copies of Social Security, veteran's, or private pension checks. The cash value of all liquefiable assets must be similarly certified with bank statements, letters from life insurance companies stating the cash value of policies, and brokerage statements regarding the value of stocks, bonds, and money market funds.

5. If someone already has Medicare coverage, what is the benefit of assistance from the state?

The state's assistance functions largely as a supplement to Medicare; it does not replace Medicare. In essence, the state pays what is left over after Medicare pays its portion of claims. The chief value of state assistance, or Medicaid, lies in its coverage of medicines and some other health care expenses not covered at all by Medicare.

6. Why do some medical providers refuse to accept patients with Medicaid coverage?

Providers must accept assignment on Medicare claims when a patient is also covered by state medical assistance. They are not reimbursed for the full amount of their fees, but rather up to the allowable charges set by Medicare. This often means a loss of income from patients with Medicaid coverage, compared to patients who can be billed for the full amounts owed.

UNDERSTANDING THE SOCIAL SECURITY SYSTEM

Older people and their families often feel stymied when facing the confusing array of programs run by the Social Security Administration: Social Security retirement benefits, Social Security Disability Insurance (SSDI), and Supplemental Security Income (SSI). The following section presents some of the most frequently asked questions about each of these programs. Since eligibility requirements are subject to change, older people and their families should verify specific information by phoning their local Social Security hotline listed in the phone book. When in doubt about eligibility for SSI or SSDI, an inquiry is generally worthwhile, if only for the peace of mind of having pursued all options.

QUESTIONS AND ANSWERS ABOUT SOCIAL SECURITY RETIREMENT BENEFITS

1. What benefits does a widow receive from Social Security?

Most of the women currently reaching retirement age collect benefits on the basis of their husband's earnings record rather than their own, due to their discontinuous work histories and lower salaries. A widow may start to collect surviving spouse's benefits when she reaches age sixty, but she then loses 28.5 percent of what she would receive if she waited until age sixty-five. If she elects to receive this lesser amount at age sixty, her benefits will not increase to the full amount when she turns sixty-five. For a surviving spouse to collect benefits, the marriage must have lasted at least nine months. Widows under age sixty who are not disabled and who do not have disabled or entitled children under age eighteen in their care cannot receive Social Security benefits.

2. Can a divorced woman collect under her exhusband's earnings record?

A woman who is divorced after at least ten years of marriage and who reaches age sixty-two may collect 37 percent of her exhusband's retirement benefit when he turns sixty-two, if she remains single. At age sixty-five, she may collect 50 percent. If she has paid into Social Security and her benefits at retirement would be greater based on her own earnings record, she will receive her own benefits instead. A widowed or divorced woman who remarries loses her former husband's benefits and cannot collect on her new spouse's benefits until married at least a year.

3. If a person collects Social Security benefits before the age of sixty-five, what are the consequences?

At age sixty-two, 20 percent is deducted from the monthly entitlement that would have been received at age sixty-five. When a person reaches age sixty-five, this level of payment is not increased to what it would have been. A prorated formula is applied to calculate this deduction for each month nearer to the age of sixty-five that the person retires.

4. What is the relation between Medicare benefits and Social Security? Can Medicare be obtained prior to age sixty-five?

Medicare is administered by the Social Security Administration and is made available at the time that someone turns sixty-five. Someone electing to receive Social Security retirement benefits prior to age sixty-five still must wait until age sixty-five to receive Medicare benefits. The only way to obtain Medicare prior to age sixty-five is by receiving Social Security Disability Income for two years (see below).

At age sixty-five, the person must choose either hospital benefits (Part A) or both hospital and outpatient benefits (Part B). It is advisable to accept Part B benefits from the beginning, as adding them on later can cost a great deal more. The cost of the monthly premium increases by a penalty of 10 percent for every year the person delays receiving Part B. The exception is someone who declines Part B while still covered by a group policy through employment or a spouse's employment. This person is permitted a special enrollment period for Part B when the group coverage is terminated, without penalty.

5. How does someone apply for Social Security Retirement benefits?

A few months prior to the time when benefits are desired, the person should phone the local Social Security office listed in the phone book. The person's Social Security number will be requested, as well as that of the spouse if benefits are to be based on a spouses's earnings record. Any necessary forms to be signed are then mailed to the applicant. A personal interview at the Social Security office is not necessary in most instances.

6. How much can someone earn without losing their Social Security retirement benefit?

For someone receiving Social Security under the age of sixty-five, $7,680 can be earned per year or $640 per month. Beyond these amounts, the Social Security benefit is reduced by one dollar for every two dollars earned. For someone age sixty-five, up to age seventy, $10,560 can be earned per year or $880 per month. Beyond these amounts, the benefit is reduced by one dollar for every three dollars earned. After age seventy, any amount can be earned without penalty.

Those earning more than the annual exempt amount must file an annual report with Social Security by April 15th of the following year. Failure to do so results in a penalty of one month's benefit. For the first year of retirement, the rules differ. For instance, if someone age sixty-five retires in June, having already earned $20,000 that year, earning even one dollar over the $880 exemption in a month would result in his losing the full amount of his Social Security check that month.

QUESTIONS AND ANSWERS ABOUT SUPPLEMENTAL SECURITY INCOME (SSI)

1. What is the difference between SSI and Social Security retirement benefits?

Social Security retirement benefits are based on a person's earnings record, while SSI eligibility is determined by meeting certain income and asset limits. Thus, SSI can be received as a supplement when Social Security retirement income is below the SSI standard, a set amount which varies depending on where someone lives. Funding for SSI comes from general U.S. Treasury funds, while Social Security retirement benefits are paid out of a fund from workers' and employers' contributions.

2. At what income level is it possible to receive SSI in addition to Social Security?

The SSI standard varies from state to state and is computed on the basis of local living costs. The standard is meant to reflect the minimum amount of money necessary for housing and food in a particular area. For instance, at this writing, the SSI standard in Washington state is $462. An older person with a Social Security income of $400 a month could receive $62 from SSI monthly.

3. How much can a person have in the bank or own and still be eligible for SSI?

At this writing, individuals can have assets up to $2,000 and couples $3,000. Stocks, bonds, checking and savings accounts, and other cashable assets are included in this limit, except for a home, the value of one car, and household goods with a total equity value of $2,000 or less. The cash surrender value of insurance policies and of any real estate beyond a primary residence also count.

4. What happens if an SSI recipient inadvertently allows a bank account to exceed the asset limit?

Should deposits bring a person's account balance over the asset limit, the SSI payment ceases entirely until the account is reduced below the limit. For instance, if the Social Security office discovers through routine bank verifications that someone's account had exceeded the limit for a ten-month period, that person's monthly check will cease for the ten months necessary to pay back SSI for the period when the person had been ineligible. At such junctures, it may be advisable to phone the local Social Security office to discuss a repayment schedule that does not leave someone entirely without income.

5. Can a person earn money and still be eligible for SSI?

The first $65 in earnings per month does not count against the SSI payment; half of the earnings beyond $65 are deducted from the monthly SSI payment. Any other income above $20 a month, such as gifts received from relatives, counts against the SSI payment.

6. How are Medicaid benefits obtained when someone receives SSI?

SSI recipients automatically receive Medicaid benefits. For this reason, it is worthwhile to apply for SSI when someone is eligible for a small payment, because the accompanying Medicaid benefits may be of substantial value and there is no arduous application process to obtain these further benefits.

7. Can someone choose to give up income in order to qualify for SSI and automatic Medicaid?

Many people receive a small pension check, such as veteran's benefits, in addition to Social Security, which brings their total monthly income over the SSI limit. They are not permitted to decline this additional income in order to become eligible for SSI, even if the extra payment brings them only slightly beyond the SSI standard. This becomes particularly frustrating to older people who lose their SSI when a small

Social Security cost-of-living increase puts them over the SSI limit by just a few dollars.

8. If a person goes to live in their son or daughter's house, will they lose their SSI?

Whenever an SSI recipient's living arrangements change, their SSI eligibility is reevaluated. This apples both to their moving in with relatives and to relatives' moving into their home. In reassessing eligibility, a number of factors in the living situation are considered, including the number of people in the household and household costs. If the SSI recipient is not paying their fair share of living costs, reduction of the SSI payment will be made according to a set amount for "in-kind support and maintenance," currently $144.66.

9. How does someone apply for SSI?

A phone call to the local Social Security office begins the application process. If the person is found to be eligible, payments begin from the date of the initial phone call. Proof of all sources of income and bank balances will be required, but these documents can be mailed in. A personal interview at the Social Security office is not necessary in most instances.

QUESTIONS AND ANSWERS ABOUT SOCIAL SECURITY DISABILITY INSURANCE (SSDI)

1. If someone is under age sixty-five and unable to work due to medical problems, what is the process of establishing eligibility for Social Security Disability?

Social Security rules state that payments for disability may be made if "an individual is unable to engage in substantial gainful activity, because of a physical or mental impairment which can be expected to result in death or which has lasted, or is expected to last, for twelve months or longer." The applicant phones in a disability claim to the local Social Security office, and forms are sent to the providers of medical care for substantiation of the claim. If benefits are approved, a back payment is included in the first check, starting from the date of the initial phone call rather than the date of final approval; therefore it is important for those who believe they may qualify to make that initial phone call as soon as possible.

2. How long does it take for a decision on a disability claim and what can be done in the meantime for financial assistance?

In all cases, applicants must wait at least five months from the date of onset of their disability in order to receive a payment. For medical conditions in which the extent of disability takes longer to determine, the waiting period can extend well beyond five months. For example, the degree of impairment from a stroke often cannot be assessed until after several months of rehabilitation. In the meantime, a person left without income should inquire with their state's health and human services division regarding financial support until the claim is decided. Payments received from the state during the waiting period are later deducted from the large back payment from Social Security, once the claim is approved. The Social Security program thereby reimburses the state for its coverage during the waiting period.

3. What can a person do if her claim is denied by Social Security and she believes she meets the criteria for eligibility?

A request for reconsideration must be filed with the Social Security office within sixty days of the official denial. It is advisable to file an appeal in most instances, since many denied claims are reversed through the appeal process. A common reason for denial is insufficient detail in the supporting documents, particularly regarding the specific impairments that interfere with employability. Appeals cases are heard by administrative law judges retained by Social Security for this purpose. Their judgments are independent of the original decisions and permit the inclusion of additional evidence to support the claim.

4. Should a person hire an attorney to assist with the appeal?

The burden of proof is on the claimant to show that the Social Security administration mistakenly denied the disability claim. The assistance of someone familiar with the appeal process can be crucial in some instances. Many communities have legal aid organizations or senior advocacy programs willing to assist with Social Security appeals at little or no charge. Private attorneys are often willing to take cases in exchange for a percentage of the cash award from Social Security, if the chance for a favorable appeal is good. Nonlawyer representation at Social Security hearings is also permitted.

5. Why can't the Social Security office give a person an estimate of their monthly payment before the claim is approved?

Disability benefits are determined according to the number of quarters that a person contributed earnings to Social Security, as well as the total contributions over a person's work life. Workers in local offices do not have this information available. A booklet entitled How to Calculate Your Benefits, with formulas for estimating disability benefits, can be requested.

6. What if it is too difficult for a person to get to the Social Security office to file a claim?

Field representatives can come to the home, if medical problems interfere with visiting the office. Although claims can also be filed by telephone, a face-to-face contact gives the Social Security worker a firsthand view of the person's functional problems, which may add credibility to the disability claim.

7. If a person is almost sixty-two and disabled, should he wait until age sixty-two to file for Social Security retirement benefits or file a claim for Social Security disability?

If someone has worked five out of the ten years prior to his disability, he should file for Social Security disability rather than Social Security retirement. A disabled person draws the same amount as he would at age sixty-five and qualifies for Medicare two years after receiving Social Security disability benefits. In contrast, if the person waited until age sixty-two to apply for regular Social Security, he would receive only 80 percent of full payment and would have to wait until age sixty-five for Medicare.

8. Can a disabled widow or widower qualify for disability benefits?

A disabled widow or widower, fifty years or older, may receive disability benefits even without sufficient work credits of their own, as long as their deceased spouse had enough work credits at the time of death. The survivor's disability must have occurred before their spouse's death or within seven years after the death. A divorced person can collect survivor's benefits only if the marriage had lasted at least ten years. For survivors, however, the term disability is defined more strictly than if their spouse had applied for benefits. To receive benefits, a disabled surviving spouse must be unable to perform any gainful activity, rather than no substantial gainful activity before benefits will be paid.

THE MANAGEMENT OF AN OLDER PERSON'S FINANCIAL AFFAIRS

Given the complexity of these programs, many older people need assistance with paying their medical bills and managing their financial affairs. This is particularly true for older people with memory problems, declining vision, limited English fluency or loss of dexterity in their hands. Most prefer assistance which allows them to retain as much control as possible over how their money is spent and who has access to private information. Often, older people view dependence on someone else to manage their money as an admission of weakness or vulnerability. Family members and professionals should be sensitive to such feelings when discussing options for money management. Helping someone manage their finances while preserving their control or privacy can be a delicate balancing act, as depicted in this section.

QUESTIONS AND ANSWERS ABOUT MONEY MANAGEMENT

1. What is the difference between putting someone's name on an account as an "additional authorized signature" and "joint ownership with a right of survivorship?"

Listing someone's name as an additional authorized signature enables that person to sign checks in the event that the owner of the account is unable to do so, or for the sake of convenience to help with bill paying. By retaining the checkbook, the older person still controls withdrawals from the account. Putting someone's name on the account as a joint owner with a right of survivorship means that this person will own the account upon the older person's death. Many people do not realize that this designation on an account supersedes what is written in a will.

2. What does it mean to grant someone Power of Attorney?

Power of Attorney can be limited to specific transactions and responsibilities, such as the payment of bills. It can also be general and far-reaching, such as empowering someone to enter into contracts on the grantor's behalf. In granting Power of Attorney, a person does not lose the right to manage his own affairs, but rather extends this right to someone in addition to himself. The person granting Power of Attorney must be mentally competent and must fully understand the written agreement.

3. Are a lawyer's services necessary for granting Power of Attorney?

Forms are available in banks and stationery stores that can be completed without a lawyer's assistance. The form must be signed in a notary's presence and filed at the County Auditor's office. When specific limitations must be written in, however, a lawyer should be consulted for the precise wording in order to ensure maximum protection.

4. What is a "durable" Power of Attorney?

The heading "durable" refers to a clause which specifies that the agreement continues should the grantor become mentally incompetent. A Power of Attorney can be written to go into effect upon its signing or only if the grantor becomes incompetent.

5. What can an older person do to make things easier for her family in the event that she suddenly becomes incapacitated?

Compiling a list of vital information, putting it in an envelope, and informing family members of its location is a useful strategy. The list should include: sources of income, insurance policies, bank accounts, location of titles pertaining to property, location of a will, rent or mortgage payment information, safety deposit boxes, Social Security number, and the names of accountants, brokers, and lawyers.

6. What does the term "representative payee" mean?

Social Security benefits can be paid to someone else on the older person's behalf. A representative payee application can be obtained by phoning the local Social Security office. A "physician's statement" form is mailed directly to the person's physician after the application is submitted. The physician must then assess the older person's capacity to manage their benefit payments in their own best interests.

7. What is guardianship and under what circumstances is it obtained?

Guardianship is usually sought when an older person is unaware of or unwilling to acknowledge their loss of competence, in contrast to a competent person voluntarily relinquishing financial control by granting a Power of Attorney. Limited guardianship removes only the rights and responsibilities specifically delegated to the guardian. Full guardianship removes all the person's legal rights as an adult, such as the right to vote, marry, enter into contracts, write checks, buy or sell property, provide consent for medical treatment, or operate a motor vehicle. In both forms of guardianship, an attorney prepares the papers and files for a hearing, and a physician submits a report to the court including a medical assessment and an opinion regarding the person's ability to manage his affairs. Legal expenses and the time involved in the process of going to court often make this option unattractive to family members.

8. What is a revocable living trust?

A living trust is operative during a person's lifetime, in contrast to a testamentary trust, or trust under will, which is not in effect until a person dies. A living trust can be changed or revoked during the person's lifetime, and can pass on to heirs without going through probate. Trust provisions supersede what is written in a will and are less vulnerable to legal contest than a will. Also, an "incapacity" clause can be included which allows the trust to continue if the older person becomes incapacitated. This clause eliminates the cost and stress of guardianship.

9. When does it make sense to set up a living trust?

Banks levy an annual charge of between one and one-and-a-half percent of the value of the assets to be managed. They also have minimum charges which generally make it feasible to open a trust account only if assets exceed $100,000. Older people cashing out the equity of a long-term home may suddenly find themselves with a large amount of money to manage, especially if this cash is added to sizable life savings. Those lacking experience with money management may gain more from their assets by establishing a living trust than they could by managing their new wealth on their own. The income they earn from professional financial management may more than cover the fees incurred for such services. A spouse who has successfully managed finances throughout a long-term marriage may nevertheless choose a living trust in order to spare his partner worry and confusion in the event of his becoming ill.

Other advantages of a living trust reside in family politics. Assigning financial management tasks to a neutral third party avoids accusations of favoritism that can arise when a particular family member is chosen for the role. Also, a third-party manager can help mediate competing requests from adult children for loans and gifts from the trust: "Talk to my trust officer. I'm not the one in charge."

10. What services do trustees generally offer in addition to overseeing investments?

A list of services included in the basic trustee fee should be obtained when the trust is established, as well as a list of charges for additional services. Fees vary widely, depending on the nature of the services and who manages the account. Services may include tax return preparation, bill payment, recordkeeping, assistance with hiring extra help in the home, and other more personalized services.

11. Is it less expensive to have a lawyer, friend, or financial planner be the trustee rather than a trust officer in a bank?

The fees charged by a lawyer may be less than a bank's. A friend or private financial consultant may charge still less for the same services. Increasingly, private financial planners are offering more extensive services at lower cost than banks are able to offer. The advantage of a bank's trust department is long-term institutional continuity. For some older people, this lends an additional sense of security to the prospect of third-party management of their finances.

Resistance to Spending Money on Necessary Services

People who have lived frugally and saved carefully over the years tend to be uncomfortable with spending large amounts of money on their care needs in later life. They are likely to want to try to "get by" or "make do" with the least expensive alternatives. This reluctance to spend money may be deeply ingrained and may lead to angry reactions when family members exert pressure by asking, "What are you saving it for?" When such a long-standing personal style is challenged, defensive responses are inevitable.

Most of the current generation of older people vividly remember the Depression, which fuels their fear of dipping too deeply into their savings and then facing either poverty or reliance on government support. Anxiety about money may also be increased by government cutbacks on services and threats to limit outlays of Social Security and Medicare. Newspaper stories or friends' accounts of older people left penniless by the expenses of long-term care may intensify this determination to avoid spending money, even when doing so adversely affects immediate health and safety.

Spouses usually have the most reason to worry about depleting their savings for long-term care. For example, a woman who has been a homemaker most of her life may have a small Social Security income from her limited employment history, while her husband may have both his Social Security income and a private pension. If her husband has not elected survivor's benefits under his private pension, her income upon his death will be equal to the amount of his Social Security check. If they were to spend a large portion of their savings on hiring help to care for him at home, she would be unable to maintain her accustomed standard of living after his death.

Some older people have intended their life savings for purposes other than paying for home helpers or costly medical treatments. They hope to leave an inheritance for grandchildren to be able to obtain a college education or a first house, or for something equally valued. The idea of depleting their savings on their own care appalls them, especially if they regard their present existence as useless or unsatisfying. For instance, when a person is being maintained at home through the costly services of a private-duty nurse, she may tell her relatives, "I wish I would die soon," thinking painfully of the discrepancy between the cost of her care and the value she now places on her life. Family members tend to reply to such feelings with statements such as, "Don't say things like that, Mom," while privately agreeing and consequently feeling guilty, especially after their relative dies.

Openly admitting the truth is a preferable approach for family members: "Sure, there's lots of things we could do with the money, but as long as you're alive, we want to make you as comfortable as possible." Some families find that being able to laugh at the absurdity of the exorbitant expenses can remove their guilt and allow them to speak freely. A remark such as, "Gee, at this rate, you could be staying at a top-class hotel in Bermuda" may relieve the older person through humor and honesty.

Watching their adult children disagree over how care expenses are to be handled may be another source of financial distress for the older person. The expense of nursing home care often creates intense conflicts. Some family members may prefer to use the less expensive home care options while others would rather "get it all settled at once" in a nursing home, despite the resulting depletion of their inheritance. During heated discussions of what is best for the older person, conflicts about the inheritance may remain unspoken and therefore unresolvable until they are verbalized. (See "Worrying about the Inheritance," p. 71.)

What a service is worth often depends on how intensely it is needed. Each family member participating in the care of an ill relative tends to have different needs and therefore individual opinions as to whether paid help should be sought. Fear also mixes in with decisions about money. The future is, by definition, uncertain. As a concrete, countable reality, money in the bank is appealing. A tired caregiver may tell herself, "I can make it one more day," putting off the moment when she has to dip into her life savings to pay for services or spend down meager resources in order to qualify for government programs. More than any other factor, money determines the number of care options available to older people and their families, and feelings about money determine how these alternatives are used or resisted.

SUGGESTED RESOURCES

Articles

"The Traps in Long Term Care Insurance: An Empty Promise to the Elderly?" *Consumer Reports* (June 1991), 425–442.

> This report rates ninety-four policies and explains what consumers need to know in order to compare policies. Reprints are available through: C. U. Reprints Department, 101 Truman Avenue, Yonkers, NY 10703.

Organizations

American Association for Retired Persons (AARP). 601 E. Street, N.W., Fulfillment Department, Washington, DC 20049. (202) 434–2277

> AARP has many useful publications. Call or write for a list of all their publications. The following are only a sample of those relevant to financial matters.
>
> "Before You Buy: A Guide to Long-Term Care Insurance," D12893.
>   Explains how to choose a policy
>
> "Knowing Your Rights." D12330.
>   Explains Medicare beneficiaries' rights about the length of hospital stays
>
> "Medicare: What it Covers, What It Doesn't," D13133.
>   A summary of Medicare benefits, including the appeals process
>
> "Medigap: Medicare Supplemental Insurance," D14042.
>   Provides guidance on policy comparison and a glossary of terms
>
> "The Social Security Book: What Every Woman Absolutely Needs to Know," D14117.
>   Gives the facts

Commission on Legal Problems of the Elderly. 1800 M Street, N.W., 2nd Floor, Washington, DC 20036. (202) 331–2297.

> The commission works to improve the quality and quantity of legal services for older citizens. It refers requests for services to appropriate agencies or groups.

National Association of Insurance Commissioners. 120 West 12th Street, Suite 1100, Kansas City, MO 64105. (816) 842–3600.

> The insurance commissioner's office in most states provides assistance with understanding Medicare supplemental policies and long-term care insurance. Check the phone book or contact the national office.

National Senior Citizens Law Center (NSCLC). 1815 H Street, N.W., Washington, DC 20006. (202) 887–5280.

> The center is a public interest law firm with attorneys who specialize in serving low income elderly individuals. Publishes a pamphlet, "Medicaid Division of Assets and Rules for Long-Term Care," which explains the rules for avoiding spousal impoverishment.

COMPARISON OF LONG-TERM CARE COSTS

Type of Care	Description	Daily Cost	Monthly Cost
In-home nurse's aide	$10–15/hour, minimum 4 hours for help with bathing, dressing, meals, and medicines	$40–60	$1,200–1,800
Overnight aide	Flat rate (aide can get some sleep) Hourly rate, minimum 8 hours (aide often awake)	$50–100 $100–140	$1,500–3,000 $3,000–4,200
Live-in helper	Hired and supervised by family members; two days off per week provided by the family Hired and supervised by an agency	$35–50 $100–140	$1,000–1,500 $3,000–4,200
Retirement home	Apartment, meals, linen, housekeeping, recreation; fee depends on size of apartment and whether additional services are needed	$40–60	$1,200–1,800
Assisted living	Apartment, meals, linen, housekeeping, recreation, and personal care service; fee increases according to services needed	$40–90	$1,000–2,800
Adult foster care	Care in state-licensed private homes; room, meals, housekeeping, and personal care; fee depends on care needs	$40–70	$1,200–2,100
Nursing home	Fee depends upon the level of care needed; this is determined by the facility	$90–160	$2,700–5,000

From Wendy Lustbader and Nancy R. Hooyman, *Taking Care of Aging Family Members* (New York: The Free Press, 1994). Copyright © 1994 by Wendy Lustbader and Nancy Hooyman; copyright © 1986 by The Free Press.

Social Security Administration. (800) 772–1213.

This national toll-free number enables callers to obtain answers to questions about Social Security and Medicare. A free publication, "Your Medicare Handbook," will also be sent upon request.

U.S. Internal Revenue Service. (800) 829–3676.

Call this national toll-free number to order a free pamphlet, "Tax Information for Older Americans," Publication #554.

11

Bringing Services into the Older Person's Home

Most families do not fully use the community services that could support them in their care tasks. They may be unaware of services, or not know how to maneuver within what appears to be a complex and rigid system. Both older people and their families may be confused by eligibility requirements and paperwork. In addition, many feel uncomfortable accepting government-funded services. Another important factor may be resistance by either the caregiver or the older person to a worker entering the home, an issue discussed in depth in the pages which follow. Worry about the expense of paying privately for services may be another barrier. This chapter presents specific community resources and techniques for using them to extend an older person's ability to remain in her own home.

LOCATING COMMUNITY RESOURCES

Finding the time to phone around to agencies when feeling pressured by caregiving can be difficult for families. A useful starting point is contacting the senior information and referral hotline in the older person's local community. If the number is not prominently displayed in the service directory at the front of the phone book, an operator can easily obtain it. The people who answer this hotline have access to extensive listings of services and can save family members considerable time.

231

Before phoning agencies directly, families may find it helpful to make several copies of the following "Community Resources Phone Search Guide." The guide prompts family members to ask all the necessary questions at once, rather than their having to call back later to fill in missing pieces. Also, keeping track of information and comparing various options is easier if the guide is completed after each call.

MEDICARE-FUNDED HOME HEALTH SERVICES

A common misperception is that Medicare-funded home health services will meet all of an older person's care needs. When confronted with the actual service limitations, people holding this expectation become disappointed and angry. For instance, Medicare does not cover a nurse's aide to stay with the older person all day while a family member goes to work. Aide services are usually two hours at a time, one or two days per week and for a limited time period. If further services are needed, the older person and her family must explore other community resources or purchase private-pay home care services.

Another frustration is that the circumstances which permit someone to qualify for Medicare's home health coverage are narrowly defined. Above all, the older person must be homebound, e.g., have a medical condition which makes it difficult for her to obtain services outside her home. Next, the older person must be in need of skilled nursing or rehabilitation services, rather than simply requiring personal care or assistance with a chronic, unchanging condition. Finally, a physician must approve each type of service received.

Home health agencies in an older person's community can be found easily in the phone book, but only some are specially certified to provide Medicare-covered services. When a family member phones an agency, the first question to ask is whether the agency is certified. If so, the intake person will ask certain screening questions to help determine whether the person meets Medicare's requirements. Family members should have handy a list of the older person's medications, her physician's name and phone number, and a summary of her current medical problems. The agency will then contact the physician for approval of services and send out a nurse to conduct an initial assessment. Family members can request that the nurse contact them after completing the assessment to inform them which services will be provided, how long they will last, and how frequently visits to the home will be made.

The Medicare-funded services which home health agencies can

COMMUNITY RESOURCES PHONE SEARCH GUIDE

Agency Name_____

Address _____

Phone _____

Date of call_____

Person spoken to _____

Services the agency can provide/cost of services:

_____

_____

_____

_____

_____

What are the eligibility requirements?

_____

_____

_____

What is the waiting period? How much lead time is needed?

_____

_____

Name/number of person to contact if services are desired:

_____

_____

General impressions/notes:

_____

_____

_____

_____

_____

_____

From Wendy Lustbader and Nancy R. Hooyman, Taking Care of Aging Family Members (New York: The Free Press, 1994). Copyright © 1994 by Wendy Lustbader and Nancy Hooyman; copyright © 1986 by The Free Press.

offer, once someone is found to be eligible, are listed below. The range of services offered in a particular instance depends upon the older person's medical condition and the physician's approval. Family members can request a specific service beyond those which are initially offered, but the agency and the physician must then determine whether the additional service is medically justified.

Family members wishing to meet personally with home care staff during visits to the home should contact staff a few days prior to the anticipated visit. Because of unavoidable scheduling problems in home care, exact visiting times are difficult to arrange. Family members do best to allow a morning or afternoon for awaiting the visit. For family members who are employed full time or live at a distance, phone conferences can be arranged if the professional is given enough notice to schedule the call.

HOUSEKEEPING AND PERSONAL CARE SERVICES

In many instances, older people need someone to help them for a few hours once or twice a week with housekeeping, grocery shopping, and other tasks. Some people need help more frequently because they are unable to bathe without assistance or cannot get dressed independently. As described earlier, if the person's condition does not require skilled care from a nurse or a physical therapist, Medicare's home health benefit cannot be used to meet these ongoing needs. Instead, programs sponsored by the older person's state, county, or city may be available, but these tend to be limited to older people with low incomes or those meeting other eligibility requirements. This section details government-funded programs and then explains how to use private-pay services when no public services are available.

Government-Funded Services

Housekeeping and personal care services subsidized by local governments are offered in many areas, but these programs differ widely in their application procedures, range of services offered, eligibility requirements, and even the terms they use to describe these services. Calling the local senior hotline may yield the names and phone numbers of the various programs, as well as a quick review of which services are subsidized and how someone qualifies for them.

Most programs require an initial screening over the phone. If the older person's monthly income or total assets exceed the program's

---

HOME HEALTH SERVICES COVERED BY
MEDICARE (under certain conditions,
for limited time periods)

Nurse: supervises the care provided by the home health aide; reviews the older person's use of medications; teaches caregivers to do dressing changes or other skilled tasks; maintains contact with the physician as the older person's condition changes

Home health aide: assists with bathing, personal care, housekeeping tasks, and meal preparation

Occupational therapist: evaluates the home and provides adaptive devices; teaches skills of daily living, such as getting dressed independently

Physical therapist: establishes a home exercise program to enhance mobility and independence; teaches caregivers transfer techniques and safe methods for assisting with exercises

Social worker: offers referrals to other community services; assists with financial stresses, disunity among caregivers, and obtaining rest for caregivers; helps the older person cope with illness

Speech therapist: facilitates recovery from problems with speaking and swallowing; teaches the use of adaptive devices and communication techniques

Nutritionist: reviews dietary habits and makes suggestions for improvements; offers information about special diets

---

From Wendy Lustbader and Nancy R. Hooyman, *Taking Care of Aging Family Members* (New York: The Free Press, 1994). Copyright © 1994 by Wendy Lustbader and Nancy Hooyman; copyright © 1986 by The Free Press.

limit, the person will be immediately disqualified. If the person qualifies, a worker will be sent to the home to do an assessment interview and to evaluate the need for services. Questions will be asked about how the older person currently accomplishes the activities of daily living, such as cooking, cleaning, laundry, grocery shopping, and personal care. Generally, some deficiency in one or several of these areas is necessary before government-funded services are approved. Proof of the older person's income and assets may also be required.

Once services are approved, an in-home worker will be assigned directly from the government agency or from an agency in the older person's community which subcontracts with the government. In either case, the older person does not have a choice among workers but rather must accept whoever is assigned. Should the worker fail to work the scheduled hours or to perform the required tasks, the older person can then contact the worker's supervisor and request another worker.

The number of approved service hours is determined according to the older person's functional abilities. Some older people are apportioned more hours than they know how to use effectively. They may have difficulty letting someone else do the tasks they have always done on their own, despite their need for assistance due to frailty or illness. They may mistrust having a stranger in their home and may not feel comfortable delegating tasks involving the handling of money, such as grocery shopping. Some simply do not know how to supervise an in-home worker. In these instances, family members may have to help the older person adjust to the situation. (See pp. 243–244.)

Private-Pay Services

Since publicly-funded services are limited, many people have to resort to expensive private-pay services or go without. The cost of home care services through private-pay agencies often comes as a shock to older people and their families. The hourly rates are high, and there are usually three- or four-hour minimums for services in the home. For example, an older woman needing help with bathing may find that the services of a home health aide cost $10 an hour and that the agency requires her to have the aide come out for at least four hours at a time. Her bath will cost her $40, unless she can make full use of other services the aide can provide during the remaining time.

In some communities, there are nonprofit agencies with lower hourly rates and fewer minimum hours for services in the home. It is often worthwhile to call around to the agencies listed in the phone book, asking about rates, hourly minimums, and any flat-fee options that may be available, such as a $20 fee for bath assistance rather than an hourly charge. Prices can vary widely, especially when overnight aide services are needed. Some agencies offer a flat fee, such as $80 for the night, while others charge by the hour and require an eight-hour minimum.

Another key factor in choosing private-pay services is how the gradations of services are determined. Companion services may be priced at $7 an hour, but if the worker has to help the older person to the bathroom occasionally, the agency may require a more expensive level of service, such as the aide rate at $10 an hour. The following chart depicts the typical structure of private-pay services, with the cost usually increasing by one or two dollars for each gradation from companion through nurse. Since agencies vary in how they structure their service levels, family members may need to take careful notes as they do price comparisons among agencies.

To save money, many families hire in-home help through newspaper ads, word-of-mouth referrals, employment listing services, or posting signs on bulletin boards. Conducting interviews and checking references are time-consuming, but the cost savings can be substantial. For instance, a worker hired this way may charge only $6 an hour for companion services and may not ask for a higher wage if she occasionally has to assist the older person in the bathroom. Free of the constraints imposed by agencies, the hired helper and the family can work

---

GRADATIONS OF SERVICES FROM PRIVATE-PAY AGENCIES

Companion: social contact, accompaniment on walks or errands (not including housekeeping, meal preparation, or personal care)

Chore: housekeeping tasks, grocery shopping, laundry (not including meal preparation or personal care)

Homemaker: all of the above chore services, with the addition of meal preparation (not including personal care services or help with medications)

Home health aide: all of the above chore and homemaker services, as well as help with personal care needs such as bathing, dressing, help with medications, and the management of incontinence (not including skilled services which a licensed nurse must perform)

Nurse: skilled services such as wound care, injections, and intravenous feeding.

From Wendy Lustbader and Nancy R. Hooyman, *Taking Care of Aging Family Members* (New York: The Free Press, 1994). Copyright © 1994 by Wendy Lustbader and Nancy Hooyman; copyright © 1986 by The Free Press.

out a mutually acceptable arrangement regarding minimum hours and the types of tasks performed. The chief disadvantage of not using an agency, in addition to the initial hiring effort, occurs when the worker cancels on short notice. Family members may have to scramble to arrange coverage, while an agency tends to have ready substitutes at hand.

CARE MANAGERS

Increasingly, many communities have private geriatric care managers who can spare families the time involved in searching for services on their own. These managers are listed in the Yellow Pages under "Senior" or "Elder." Some may charge a flat fee for going out to the home, assessing the older person's situation, and recommending appropriate services. Others may charge on an hourly basis, according to the actual time spent. Still others offer ongoing monitoring and support for a monthly fee, once the older person has had an initial assessment.

Checking the qualifications of these private managers is important. Family members should ask about the educational background of the person who will do the assessment, as well as the number of years the person has done this work and their familiarity with local services and public programs. Experienced professionals can accomplish much more in one visit than newcomers can in several. Since this information affects the ultimate cost and quality of the service, family members have a right to assess a professional's level of knowledge and experience. Verifying the care manager's reputation in the community can be accomplished by phoning references or contacting local social service organizations.

Care managers vary in the range of services they offer, as well as their pricing structure. For example, a manager may offer a service package for a single monthly fee, including daily check-up calls, one monthly visit, access to a twenty-four-hour emergency phone line, and service coordination with the older person's physician, nurse, and in-home workers. Other services may be available on an add-on basis, such as assistance with handling medical bills and insurance claims. Determining exactly what is included in the basic fee allows family members to choose judiciously among care managers.

Confidence in the care manager's judgment and a liking for the manager's personality are other selection factors, especially for family members who live at a distance from their relative. There may be instances later when decisions are looming and family members will have to rely on the care manager's description of the situation. A competent manager should be able to communicate clearly, using a minimum of professional jargon and displaying patience when answering questions. The older person should also feel comfortable talking to the care manager, since their contact will be frequent and may eventually serve as a lifeline.

HOME-DELIVERED MEALS

Difficulties with cooking, the loneliness of eating alone, or forgetfulness can cause older people to snack or skip meals rather than eat nutritiously. Meals on Wheels is one of the most frequently used community resources for homebound older people. Typically delivered weekly, these government-subsidized frozen meals are less expensive than frozen dinners of equivalent nutritional value in grocery stores. In addition, they are suitable for low salt diets. Some programs may also offer delivery of liquid dietary supplements by the case and selected grocery items along with the frozen meals.

An extra benefit of home-delivered meals is regular and predictable social contact. For a homebound individual, the knock at the door and the conversation during the delivery may come as a welcome relief from isolation. The delivery person cannot stay long, but can easily check on the older person's welfare while putting the meals in the freezer. For instance, if the previous week's meals have not been eaten, the delivery person may question the older person about her health status and insure that proper referrals are made.

Obstacles to the use of frozen meals include insufficient freezer space, freezers which are not cold enough, and inoperable or nonexistent ovens. In such instances, neighbors may be willing to store meals in their extra freezer space and then deliver individual meals daily. Countertop ovens can be purchased to heat the meals, offering the advantages of accessible heat controls for low-vision or wheelchair-bound people who cannot manage conventional ovens. Countertop ovens with loud buzzers which can alert the person to remove the cooked meal are especially useful.

Memory loss is a more complex obstacle to using Meals on Wheels. An older person may have trouble remembering to phone in her order every week or to set the timer on her oven. Unless reminded, she may forget to use the frozen meals altogether. In some home-delivery programs, the phone staff keep a list of those who need reminders to place orders or help choosing meals compatible with their special diets. The older person who burns food may need to have a family member or friend provide phone cues for putting food into the oven and taking it out on time.

Boredom or repugnance are common reactions to frozen meals. In such instances, people can be encouraged to use the frozen meals as a backup, storing them in their freezer in the event of emergencies or unexpected situations. Since the taste of cardboard in the food is often a legitimate complaint, people can be urged to replace the cardboard covers with foil when heating the meals. The addition of seasoning, such as mild herbs, sauces, or garnishes can also make the food more appetizing and varied without interfering with dietary restrictions. If, despite these modifications, the commercially produced meals still fail to stimulate an older person's appetite, neighbors or family members can freeze individual portions of their own meals and deliver these to the older person's freezer.

WHEN IN-HOME SERVICES BY HIRED WORKERS ARE RESISTED

One of the greatest obstacles to the use of in-home services is the older person's resistance. This may be expressed directly, with outright statements of refusal, or indirectly, such as when an older person sabotages arrangements made by family members. Family caregivers who need time off may react with anger, viewing their relative's resistance as a lack of consideration for the many pressures on them. Common sources of such resistance are explored in the discussion which follows.

Maintaining the Illusion of Independence

Older people often declare that they are managing on their own when family members are in fact providing numerous services. A daughter may drop over at lunchtime with several bags of groceries for her mother, which she puts away while catching her up on family news. She may throw in a load of wash before preparing lunch, knowing that the clothes will be ready for the dryer by the time she finishes washing the lunch dishes. As the drying cycle finishes, she may vacuum the living room and scrub the bathroom. Later, her mother may describe the visit to a friend with the remark, "My daughter came by and we had a nice lunch together," omitting any reference to the tasks her daughter performed for her. She may see her daughter as an extension of herself, speaking truthfully when she claims that she is "independent" and does not need in-home services.

Over time, people tend to accept more and more assistance from family members without noticing how dependent they are becoming. They may view the help from their family as occasional "favors" offered to make their lives easier. In contrast, services from a stranger make the fact of needing help too prominent to be denied. If the daughter in the above example insisted on hiring someone to do the chores, the hired worker would suddenly become an emblem of the incapacities of aging.

Acknowledging dependency is painful. In dealing with these feelings, it is important to give the older person as many choices as possible within the limits of practicality. If the family has funds to hire a private-pay worker, the person can be involved in writing the newspaper ad, interviewing applicants, and making the decision of whom to hire. Even when the older person is restricted to government-funded workers, she can maintain some control over the situation by implementing the supervisory techniques described later in this chapter.

Fearing Reduced Contact with Family Members

As in-home workers are hired to replace the help of tired family caregivers, some older people fear that they will see family members less often. Regular routines of contact with family may, in fact, become disrupted once hired workers take over these chores. Whether consciously or not, older people in this situation may seize upon excuses to prevent the feared loss: "A woman down the block got robbed by her worker. I just won't have a stranger in the house." These justifications may be spoken with such urgency that family members do not realize that reduced contact with them is dreaded more than the reasons stated.

In such situations, family members should listen carefully to the feelings behind their relative's protests, not just to the content. Offering frequent phone calls at prearranged times and setting dates for family outings may assure the older person that she will continue to see family members on a regular basis. Such assurances are most persuasive when family members put their need for rest in personal terms: "Mom, I'll be much better company when I don't have to wash your dishes and do your laundry while we visit." By stating directly that their intention in hiring help is to prolong their ability to give care, family members show the older person that their actions are the very opposite of abandonment.

Worrying about the Depletion of Savings

Paying for such services not only makes their necessity more prominent, but may also evoke worries about running out of money. The fact that the state will pay for in-home services when an older person's savings balance drops below a certain level usually does not comfort someone accustomed to financial self-reliance. Those who have accumulated substantial amounts of money "for a rainy day" may steadfastly refuse to pay for in-home services, to their family's frustration and bewilderment. Beginning to spend even a plentiful savings account can be experienced as financial vulnerability and an acknowledgment that the final stage of life has arrived. Family members may feel less angered by the older person's refusal to spend money on needed services if they recognize that the dread of poverty or fear of death may lie behind the refusal.

Whatever the basis of the fear, the need to hold onto money is an inclination which is not easily dislodged. Family members' teasing comments such as, "You can't take it with you," may only serve to increase the older person's stress without affecting his inflexibility. One possible strategy for dealing with financial fears is to multiply out the cost of services for a defined number of weekly hours over a year's time to demonstrate exactly how much of the person's savings would be spent. Comparing the size of this sum to the person's total assets helps promote the idea that ample funds will remain for "the future," despite this opening of the financial spigot.

An older person's wish to leave savings intact to ensure a sizeable inheritance for family members is often paramount. The person may insist, "I worked hard all my life and I want to know when I leave this world that my family is secure." In effect, some older people transfer their need for financial security to their family. Viewing the inheritance as a measure of their success as a parent, they would rather maintain a disheveled household or perform unsafe tasks than reduce their estate. Occasionally, family members can convince a relative with such concerns that this stockpile of cash should be used to give them peace of mind now rather than luxuries in the future. (See "Resistance to Spending Money on Necessary Services," pp. 225–227.)

Lacking Supervisory Skills

A common frustration to both older people and their families is hired workers' poor performance. Many people do not know how to give clear instructions to in-home workers. For example, an older woman may stand by silently while a hired worker vacuums the open spaces of her living room without moving the coffee table to clean underneath. The dust remaining under the table may infuriate her as much as her failure to speak up humiliates her. Those who have had little experience with other people working for them can find giving instructions awkward until they learn how to do it. Once they become confident about their ability to supervise, they tend to use these services more willingly.

Devising a written checklist to guide workers can have a substantial impact on the older person's faith in herself as a supervisor. Each item on the checklist should include specific steps detailing how each task should be completed. Relieved of the need to remember and describe each task, the older person then uses the list as a step-by-step supervisory tool. For example, after a worker has cleaned the kitchen, the older person can give compliments and suggestions while checking off tasks on the list: "You did a nice job on the counters, but it looks like you forgot to sweep under the table." Instead of feeling angry and powerless, the older person becomes effective at helping workers do a good job.

Some people may need specific examples of how to give praise without being patronizing and how to offer correction without being insulting. Feedback about a tone of voice which is demeaning to workers or a style of speaking which curdles workers' pride may be necessary. Some older people cause their own unhappiness with successive workers by their dictatorial, nagging, or otherwise offensive supervision. As with any human interaction, decency and respect in a supervisory relationship go two ways. If older people create a comfortable working environment, they are more likely to elicit good performance. As a teaching tool, the following list of supervisory techniques can be used with older people who need to improve their skills in this area. Family members can help in the meantime by personally acknowledging the efforts of diligent workers who are not yet receiving proper respect and consideration.

INSTRUCTIONS FOR SUPERVISING IN-HOME WORKERS

1. *Make a list of the steps for each task.* Include preferences for specific cleansers and implements to be used, the location of these items, and other helpful suggestions, such as "Please separate out the white wash" or "Please be sure to sweep under the table."
2. *Avoid following the worker around the home.* Instead, ask to be notified after each room is completed. Then, acknowledge the tasks which have been done correctly, checking them off on the list and thanking the worker. Offer reminders of any tasks which have been omitted.
3. *Be sure to praise extra effort or thoughtfulness.* Do this even if what has been done is not perfect. It is important to build good will rather than focus on insignificant errors.
4. *Correct major errors by giving information rather than criticism.* Unless an error occurs repeatedly, assume that the person has been lacking information about how something should be handled within the home.

From Wendy Lustbader and Nancy R. Hooyman, *Taking Care of Aging Family Members* (New York: The Free Press, 1994). Copyright © 1994 by Wendy Lustbader and Nancy Hooyman; copyright © 1986 by The Free Press.

Fearing Victimization

The fear of being victimized is another source of resistance to in-home services. Receiving services from a stranger while alone in the home can be frightening to older people who perceive that they could be hurt or exploited in some way. Not only are there no witnesses to what occurs between the worker and the older person, but the worker may also gain access to costly possessions and items of sentimental value. Older people with poor vision, hearing, or memory may feel particularly vulnerable to the extent that their supervisory abilities are impaired by these deficits. They may continue to feel imperiled, even after family members assure them that the worker's references have been checked or that the agency provides ongoing supervision and training to their staff.

To begin addressing these fears, family members can offer to be present during a worker's first few sessions in the older person's home. This gives the older person time to develop enough trust in the worker to accept the service unaccompanied. In addition, this tactic permits family members to form their own impressions of the worker's reliability and competence. Often the greatest benefit from the family's presence is conveying to the worker that they will monitor the quality of the services and be concerned about the older person's security and satisfaction. Later, family members should make unplanned appearances to reinforce their role as observers.

To widen their protective role, family members should become familiar with the ways in-home workers do abuse older people. Some misuse their time, a problem which often can be averted through the use of the supervisory methods described earlier. Some workers kill time on easy tasks in order to avoid getting to the more demanding tasks. By using a checklist, the older person can restructure the sequence to leave the easiest tasks for last. Other workers may try to waste time by taking frequent cigarette breaks, making personal phone calls, or attending more to the television screen than to their work. As a corrective to these delay strategies, the checklist can be emphasized as a written record of what is accomplished, subject to the scrutiny of the older person's family or the agency supervisor.

The type of abuse which is hardest for family members to monitor occurs when a worker wins, and then takes advantage of, an older person's sympathy. An older person may deprive herself of needed services by doing "favors" for her in-home worker, such as signing for hours that the worker never provided, or regularly letting the worker arrive late and leave early. Some workers play upon an older person's kindness, telling their financial and family problems in vivid detail. Seeing herself as a friend rather than a victim, an older person may feel she is helping a person in need rather than being exploited when she signs for hours not furnished. The worker may even solicit cash "loans" which the older person extends out of this same concern. (See "When Friendship Verges on Exploitation," pp. 133–136.)

Stress from the growing realization that she is being abused may eventually manifest itself through sleeplessness or loss of appetite. Yet an older person who is being exploited may choose not to disclose the situation to family members. Feeling protective, she may worry about the worker getting fired if family members complain to the agency responsible for her employment. She may also want to retain this opportunity to be useful to someone else. Ashamed of her previous gullibility, she may blame herself for having been "taken" and yet be unwilling to admit that her role in the worker's life is a sham.

Fear of reprisal if the abuse is reported can be one of the strongest reasons for silence, especially if the older person has felt intimidated by the worker's friends or relatives who may have also entered the home: "If she gets fired because I tell on her, they'll break into my house." Check-up visits by family members during assigned hours are the best way to guard against abuse, because workers tend to curtail such activities if there are too many witnesses at hand. Neighbors can be particularly helpful in their capacity to visit at odd times. A worker who is aware that a neighbor may drop in at any moment is less likely to arrive late, leave early, or omit tasks.

Harboring Racist Feelings Toward Particular Workers

Racist feelings may be a further barrier to the acceptance of in-home services. Some people express their racism overtly, feeling entitled to their beliefs, while others are too ashamed to admit that this is their real reason for declining services. There are also those who do not suspect that they harbor such feelings, until a life experience brings their racism into view. For instance, many are astonished at their reaction when someone from a different race assists them with bathing or dressing. Having this person clean their house may be acceptable, but being touched by this person may evoke uncomfortable responses. Those who had always prided themselves on their tolerance may be embarrassed by this discovery.

Family members and professionals are often perplexed as to how to reply when an older person asks that another worker be assigned. One view can be summarized as, "You can't change lifelong beliefs, so why upset an ill person who has little time left?" Another is, "By going along with a racist reaction, you affirm it." Some take a middle ground, believing that racist statements should be corrected verbally, but that forcing an unwilling person to adapt is not productive for either the worker or the older person.

When family members differ in their beliefs about how their relative's racism should be handled, conflict can erupt that worsens the stress of the situation. One family member may express sympathy with the older person's feelings, while another may insist that racist remarks cease and that these preferences not be heeded. Around these issues, emotions often run hot and can therefore lead to painful family disunity.

A particularly frustrating situation is when an older person repeatedly sabotages in-home workers due to her racist feelings, but does not express them directly. She may harp on trivial errors or criticize the worker's cooking, making personal remarks which are actually fueled by racism. When confronted, the older person may deny that anything but the worker's job performance is at issue. She may enact a self-ful-filling prophecy by oppressing the worker so relentlessly with conde-scending comments and hovering suspiciousness that the worker responds with poor service, then use the evidence of poor service to justify her demand for another worker.

The dialogue below illustrates a potentially effective response to racist remarks. Recognizing the futility of arguing against nonrational feelings, this approach focuses on bringing global statements back to the immediate situation. Talking about an individual's specific actions is more constructive than trying to dispute someone's beliefs about an entire race's behavior.

> OLDER PERSON: Did you see how the chore worker left grease on the dishes? Her kind doesn't know the meaning of cleanliness.
>
> FAMILY MEMBER: Lots of people leave grease on dishes. Next time she comes, let's tell her she needs to use hotter water and more suds.
>
> OLDER PERSON: But they never learn, so what's the use? And if they learn anything, they're too lazy to do it right anyway.
>
> FAMILY MEMBER: She seems willing to learn and to work hard if we give her a chance, so let's try.

Some older people manage to put aside racist feelings after having regular contact with a particular in-home worker. While still retaining generalized beliefs, they may rationalize that an individual person is a lucky exception to the rule. The older person resolves the dissonance between her racist beliefs and the reality of an appreciated worker by adding a subgrouping: those who belong to a certain racial group but who manage to avoid absorbing the group's negative characteristics. After an older person experiences a succession of workers from vari-ous groups, she may begin to perceive that positive human traits have no connection to race.

Overcoming someone's resistance to accepting in-home services is no small achievement. Positive reports from friends and neighbors about their experiences may help an older person become more receptive, but even a single story of someone being robbed by an in-home worker can negate such encouraging influences. In many instances, families and professionals may be unsure of the reasons for someone's resistance, finding it hard to understand the person's apparent obstinacy. Knowing how to broach possible underlying issues may help assure the older person's care, family members' relief, and decent treatment of hired workers. Over the long term, using in-home services tends to be the most effective way to support an older person's wish to remain in her own home.

SUGGESTED RESOURCES

Articles

Fogel, Barry. "Psychological Aspects of Staying at Home," *Generations*, 16 (1992), 15–19.

> Discusses the meaning of "home" and its implications for both design of housing and for planning clinical interventions.

Koff, Theodore. "Aging in Place: Rural Issues," *Generations*, 16 (1992), 53–55.

> Briefly reviews some of the policy and program barriers to providing adequate services for rural elderly.

Stoller, Eleanor, and Stephen Cutler. "Predictors of Use of Paid Help Among Older People Living in the Community," *The Gerontologist*, 33 (1993), 31–40.

> Paid help was found to be more prevalent among elderly people with adequate economic resources who did not have family members and friends available to assist them. Household income has the greatest impact when older people have discretion regarding sources of help.

Yeatts, Dale, Thomas Crow, and Edward Folts. "Service Use Among Low-Income Minority Elderly," *The Gerontologist*, 32 (1992), 24–32.

> Based upon models in Texas, this article presents a practice-oriented framework for service use and strategies for overcoming barriers faced by low-income minority elderly.

Books

Carlin, Vivian. *Can Mom Live Alone? Practical Advice on Helping Aging Parents Stay in their Own Home* (New York: Lexington Books), 1991.

By describing creative ways that older people have found to remain in their own homes, the author illustrates how to modify the home, access services, and manage the finances of living independently. Provides a solid basis for informed decisions about housing.

Kane, Rosalie, and Arthur Caplan. eds. *Ethical Conflicts in the Management of Home Care: The Case Manager's Dilemma* (New York: Springer), 1993.

Sheehan, Susan. *Kate Quinton's Days* (Boston: Houghton Mifflin Company), 1984.

The author vividly describes an elderly woman's effort to remain in her own home following discharge from a hospital, particularly her experiences receiving services from a home care program.

Organizations

Elder Care Locator. (800) 677–1116.

This national toll-free number is designed to help identify community resources for seniors anywhere in the United States. The name, address, and zip code of the person needing assistance allows the Elder Care Locator to identify the nearest information and assistance sources in that person's community. Call between 9:00 A.M. and 8:00 P.M. Eastern Time.

National Association for Home Care (NAHC). 519 C Street, N.E., Stanton Park, Washington, D.C. 20002. (202) 547–7424.

NAHC monitors federal and state activities affecting home care and focuses on issues relating to home health care. They publish *Caring Magazine* on a bimonthly basis.

Professional Geriatric Care Managers. 655 N. Alvernon Way, Suite 108, Tucson, AZ 85711. (602) 881–8008.

This is an association of private practitioners who provide referrals as well as services. Call to determine if there is a care manager in the older person's local area.

U.S. Internal Revenue Service. (800) 829–3676.

Call this national toll-free number to order a free pamphlet, "Household Employees/Social Security Withholding Requirements," Publication #926.

12

Using Services Outside the Home

Mobility is freedom, and loss of mobility can lead to a discouraging sense of confinement. Taking care of everyday needs on one's own indeed hinges on having some form of transportation, yet driving may become too dangerous and using the bus, if available, may be too demanding. Even when other transportation options are available, many people have nowhere to go or they are repelled by activities designed specifically for older people. This chapter focuses first on the issue of transportation, particularly the effects of giving up the car keys and attempting to use alternatives to private automobiles. Senior centers, adult day centers, and support groups are then surveyed as options which can help remedy isolation and boredom, once barriers to their use are overcome.

GIVING UP THE CAR KEYS

For many older people, the ability to drive permits an active, independent lifestyle. Driving is particularly important in rural areas, where distances between communities are greater and public transportation options are scarcer than in cities. Depending on family members for rides may not be practical, especially if they have only one car, are employed full time, or live at a distance. In addition, the perception that asking family members for rides intrudes on their busy lives may be accurate. Even if family members are available and willing to provide

251

PROBLEMS COMMONLY EXPERIENCED BY OLDER DRIVERS

Vision problems: loss of night vision, depth perception, peripheral vision, and the ability to read signs with small print or insufficient contrast

Short-term memory loss: forgetting destinations, directions, and where the car is parked

Slowed reaction time: caused by sensory deficits, slower reflexes, muscular weakness and stiffness, or tremors in hands or feet

Heart problems: physicians may advise against the stress of driving and the danger of having a heart attack while driving

Problems from strokes: visual field cut, in which a section of the visual field cannot be seen; one-sided weakness that interferes with handling the wheel and pedals; reading or communication problems

Episodes of dizziness, drowsiness, or fainting: caused by neurological, respiratory, inner ear, and heart conditions, as well as from medications and insomnia

High blood pressure: in some instances, physicians may advise against the stress of driving

Back problems: spinal fractures and disk deterioration can be aggravated by driving

Arthritic changes: problems with manual dexterity; shoulder pain worsened by driving; reduced range of motion in the arms and neck

Diabetic problems: loss of sensation in hands and feet; episodes of low blood sugar resulting in confusion

rides, the freedom to leave the home at will, without needing to ask or wait for anyone, is a privilege few people willingly relinquish.

Even when driving becomes dangerous due to physical changes or health problems, many older people continue to drive. They cling to their car and driver's license with a tenacity both perplexing and frustrating to family members. Attempts to persuade an older driver to give up the car keys should be preceded by a close look at the specific problems the person is having and the reasons for the person's unyielding stance. Solutions short of a complete loss of driving ability may become apparent during this process.

Identifying an Older Driver's Problems

Driving ability is particularly vulnerable to physiological changes that come with aging. Vision, hearing, reaction time, manual dexterity, and memory are components of driving skills which typically diminish as people grow older. Even among people with adequate daytime vision, night blindness is common. Physical conditions which can impede a driver's safety are depicted in the preceding chart, along with their implications on the road. This chart can be used to help an older driver begin to identify and acknowledge problem areas that interfere with driving.

Attempting to compensate for any one of these problems, older drivers may adopt a rigid driving posture. They may sit forward in the seat, grasp the wheel tightly, and keep their gaze focused directly ahead in a kind of exaggerated concentration. This posture often contributes to a reduced ability to attend to events on the periphery, such as a pedestrian starting to enter a crosswalk or a car approaching from behind during merging. A woman who tenses her neck to compensate for poor vision and hand tremors may be unable to glance back to check her blind spot. Unaware of the near-accidents she causes by merging without checking to her left, she may continue to drive for years, leaving a host of frightened drivers and pedestrians in her path.

Understanding a Driver's Denial of Difficulty

Drivers of all ages make excuses for driving errors. Those threatened by the physical changes of aging, however, are even more likely to blame close calls on other drivers, poor brakes, or road conditions. As indicated in the above example, people can be oblivious to deficits which have come on gradually and almost imperceptibly, especially decreases in vision, hearing, and muscle flexibility. Denial may continue, even when passengers or other bystanders confront the person about blatant driving errors right after they happen: "It wasn't my fault, so back off."

In a common scenario, a wife may repeatedly warn her husband about his near-misses, only to be told that she is too critical or a "backseat driver." Caught in a bind, she may be terrified by his driving but also fearful of his wrath if she were to enlist her daughter's support in getting him off the road. To avoid being in the car with him, she may feign illness, but then be left worrying that he will injure himself or others. When a spouse complains about a partner's driving problems, courageous family members should get in the car with the older driver to observe her predicament firsthand. After this experience, they may be more determined than ever to stop his driving, yet find that they are at a loss about how to do so. Telling the spouse that they understand what she is going through, however, may be a welcome relief: "At least now I know I'm not crazy. You saw him do those things, too."

Feelings about masculinity may be an important aspect of an older man's determination to keep on driving. For instance, many older men express a sense of personal power behind the wheel and feel demeaned and emasculated when asked to stop driving. Control over an inanimate moving object may have become vital in a life devoid of other kinds of control. Some male drivers release aggression on anonymous people in other cars, having no other legitimate outlet for such feelings. In a traditional marriage, the man may have consistently assumed the driver's role, never accepting passenger status with his wife as the driver. Although his wife may be a competent driver, this role differentiation may be so deeply incorporated into his self-image as a protective, directive male that he resists becoming a passenger long beyond the point deemed safe by his wife and family.

Resistance may stem from still other sources. Possessing an attractive car may be the person's one remaining focus of identity, time, and money, especially for those who have experienced numerous other losses. Older men often derive considerable satisfaction from polishing and tinkering with cars. Simply having the car visible in the driveway may be more important to an older man than actually driving it around town, but the family's worry about his getting into an accident may have obscured the true basis for his wanting to keep his car.

Responding Constructively to Impaired Drivers

Sensitivity to both the symbolic and practical significance of driving helps family members channel their worries about an impaired driver into constructive responses. Often, the problem can be narrowed to specific roads or turns, such as an inability to merge safely onto freeways or to maneuver in congested city streets where too much is going on at once. Instead of asking their relative to surrender the car keys entirely, families can sometimes negotiate an agreement that driving be restricted to situations of optimal safety.

Asking a relative not to drive at twilight, or to park the car and take a bus into crowded downtown areas may solve many worries. Families can also help their relative find the safest routes to specific destinations. A parallel service road alongside the freeway might triple travel time but eliminate the problems of merging and lane-changing on the freeway. Similarly, an older person could follow a series of side roads, rather than the busy main arterial, avoiding the need to make risky left turns through traffic. In areas with disabled parking spaces, obtaining a disabled parking sticker permits the older person to park in specially reserved spots near a store's entrance, thereby eliminating the distracting search for parking spaces, the long walk to the entrance, and the need to remember where the car was parked.

Another strategy to increase their relative's safety on the road is for families to pay for a series of driving lessons. To overcome resistance to this idea, families can present driver retraining in the positive light of learning to compensate for normal changes of aging, as well as to brush up on driving skills and recent rule changes. Facing driving problems under a trained, impartial observer can be easier than receiving similar information from close family members. Outside the power struggles of his family, the older person may be able to approach his difficulties less defensively and learn some skills that actually prolong his tenure as a driver. If the instructor determines that no amount of training can surmount the older person's problems on the road, facing this in impartial company may make it less humiliating. The person may then decide on his own to withdraw from driving, without further prodding.

Once defensiveness about deficits is overcome, adaptations to the older person's car may be a further option. Hand controls, special steering wheel grips, additional mirrors, glare-reducing glass, extra warning signals, and adapted brake and gas pedals are examples of such modifications. Many older people and their families are unaware of the availability of these devices, or associate them only with severely disabled people. Families can contact their state's motor vehicle department or the occupational therapy department at their local hospital for referrals to agencies or car shops which specialize in such adaptations. Although these modifications may not solve all the older person's driving problems, they may add a margin of safety which extends the person's driving ability for months or years. In addition, during the process of testing for devices and learning their use, an older person who has resisted recognizing the extent of his impairments may become more receptive to examining them.

Despite these efforts, family members may have to go on mediating between their worries about safety and their relative's willingness to take risks for the sake of freedom. Unfortunately, many older drivers wait until a minor collision or a traffic violation from running an unseen stop sign convinces them that it is time to find other transportation options. Others may reach this realization when a beloved old car finally malfunctions or they fail the vision test for license renewal. For many older drivers, a physician's pronouncement that it is time to stop driving does convince them that they have to stop. In some areas, anonymous reports about impaired drivers can be phoned in to the licensing bureau, resulting in a mandatory driving test upon license renewal.

When a complete loss of driving is imminent, family members and professionals can help by identifying in advance the aspects of the person's life which will be most affected by this change. In rural areas and suburbs where public transportation tends to be limited, it is especially crucial to plan for alternate ways to meet practical and social needs. The following questions may be useful for advance planning:

Assessing the Impact of the Loss of Driving

1. *What basic needs has the older person met by driving?* (going to the grocery store, pharmacy, bank, and the doctor)
2. *What out-of-home activities will probably be forfeited once the older person can no longer drive?* (going to church, attending meetings of service clubs, going to the senior center, visiting friends in the hospital)
3. *What psychological needs may be left unmet once the person can no longer drive?* (time alone or away from a partner, the ability to render assistance to others, the stimulation of a change of scene, the role of protector)

Despite a family's careful efforts, an older person may become angry and depressed in reaction to the losses just depicted. Frustrated ex-drivers often turn into dictatorial passengers when they first give up driving. They may browbeat friends, family, and neighbors who are trying to be supportive by offering rides. Reminders that it usually takes time for former drivers to find other ways to exert control may lessen the helpers' hurt feelings. Families can try to emphasize the benefits of the change, such as increased exercise through walking or time to socialize with others while sharing rides. Gradually, as personal habits disrupted by the change fade from prominence, and as new routines fall into place, the older person's mood is likely to improve.

Expanding their relative's use of transactions by mail and phone can also help return a sense of control and independence. Many older people are accustomed to handling their banking, bill payments, and purchases in person. Unaware of other options, they do not benefit from the increasing range of business or domestic activities that can be taken care of at home, such as ordering home-delivered groceries, shopping via catalogs, or banking by mail. Family members can help by showing their relative how to prepare before calling in a phone order or by assisting with the paperwork of mailed transactions. In the absence of driving, many people derive satisfaction from continuing to conduct their own affairs as much as possible.

TRANSPORTATION OPTIONS

At the same time that health problems threaten older people's ability to drive, transportation alternatives may be unavailable or too expensive. Driving also entails the expense of owning, insuring and maintaining a car, costs which can be burdensome for those on fixed incomes. After giving up driving, many people feel socially isolated and deprived of useful activity. The following section surveys transportation options, examining problems and solutions associated with each. Familiarity with detailed aspects of these alternatives helps family members work with their relative toward overcoming barriers to their use.

Buses

Lack of prior experience with bus routes and timetables often discourages older people from trying out buses. When family members accompany their relative on exploratory trips, they help transform buses from alien conveyances to familiar and welcome options. The older person can practice mounting the steep bus steps with a family member standing by. Becoming comfortable with asking younger people to give up seats on crowded buses is another important adjustment. Learning that drivers can be asked to announce particular stops may relieve someone with poor vision or memory. Most communities offer a reduced-fare bus pass that greatly reduces the cost of this option and enhances the person's freedom to roam.

Cabs

Some localities subsidize taxi fares for getting to medical appointments and other necessary outings, which makes this option affordable for low-income older people. Professionals and family members can contact the senior information and referral hot line to determine whether such programs exist in the older person's community. Some older people in apartment buildings plan ahead to share a cab when they want to go to shopping centers, making this more economical and socially enjoyable than traveling alone.

Volunteer Escort Programs

Some communities sponsor programs in which volunteer drivers bring older people to medical appointments and grocery shopping. Unfortunately, such programs are usually limited to vital needs, leaving older people without rides to religious services or recreational activities. Occasionally it is possible to identify other participants who are willing to offer rides, such as through a senior center or church newsletter.

Van Service

Low-cost vans in some areas take older people to destinations of their choice. These van services tend to have geographic boundaries or "catchment areas" beyond which they will not provide transportation. A day's notice may be required for a pick-up, and considerable waiting may be required on the return trip. Some people who need frequent restroom access find that vans picking up as many as a dozen other people on one route can leave them squirming too uncomfortably. Despite these disadvantages, van services are easier for older people who cannot get to bus stops or need door-to-door service due to a disability.

Car Pools

Older people with destinations in common do well to car pool. Someone who is still able to drive and maintain a car may appreciate additional passengers for going to religious services, the grocery store, or recreational places, as long as the passengers share equally the costs of gas, maintenance, and parking. Car pools succeed only on the basis of fairness to both drivers and passengers. Taking care to pay promptly and to avoid keeping everyone else waiting are necessary courtesies. Family members and professionals can help older people arrange carpools by scouting out potential drivers and additional passengers through signs posted at the desired destinations.

Exploring transportation options with older people who have given up driving is pivotal in preventing their becoming homebound and isolated. Older people tend to seek alternatives which do not require their calling upon family members, instead preferring continued privacy and a feeling of control over their comings and goings.

OPTIONS FOR REDUCING LONELINESS

Even when transportation is not a problem, older people who feel lonely or who are craving meaningful activities may still resist attending programs targeted for seniors. Some dislike contact with their age peers or feel they have not yet crossed the line to join the population known as "those old people." Many who value work more than leisure prefer to stay home to devote themselves to useful projects, finding they have little desire to spend time mixing with others through dances, trips, and dinners. For others, the loss of lifelong friends may have created a fundamental weariness toward the idea of making new friends, blocking their interest in social activity. This section examines such barriers and strategies for overcoming them.

Disliking "Old People"

Older people who dislike spending time with their age peers often make derogatory remarks, such as, "Old people talk about nothing but grandchildren, aches and pains, and the price of milk." They complain that these conversations leave them feeling bored and alienated. Some refuse to participate in any activity or program with "senior" in the title, refusing to be associated with this label even if it is attached to employment programs or meaningful volunteer involvements. For them, the idea of living in a subsidized senior apartment complex can seem an abomination, no matter how low the rent. Similarly, the prospect of accepting discounts and other age-related benefits may offend their need not to feel segregated by an arbitrary chronological status.

Such attitudes often frustrate family members who are worried about a relative's loneliness. The loss of lifelong friends to death, incapacity, or geographic relocation can leave older people profoundly isolated. Family members may parade social options before them which seem stimulating, but only evoke indifferent or negative responses. They may plead, "Don't you want to meet new people?", believing that filling the gaps left by these painful losses is essential. Their relative's refusal to participate in "senior" activities may eventually anger them: "You say you're lonely, but you won't do anything about it. There's nothing wrong with these programs."

Understanding the layers of complexity underlying such refusals helps family members respond more constructively. For example, some people have been repelled by small talk all of their lives. Reminding them that "old people" are simply people who have grown older, family members can point out that the full range of human possibility continues throughout the lifespan. In any group of "old people," there are likely to be some who never venture beyond chitchat and others who are eager to talk at a more substantive level. Trying out activities like book discussion clubs, continuing education classes, and Elderhostel programs may generate contacts with older people who are interested in talking about something other than body functions and family doings.

For others, revulsion toward old age may have been absorbed directly from the surrounding youth-oriented culture. The common idea that anything "old" or "senior" is something outmoded and uninteresting is difficult to oppose through individual vibrancy, no matter how "young-at-heart" someone feels. It may be easier to avoid "senior" programs than to risk one's self-esteem. Frustrated family members may feel less impatient when they realize that their relative is guarding against a societal wrong rather than simply being stubborn.

Family members may also find it helpful to examine whether they are inadvertently contributing to their relative's aversion toward old age. In subtle ways, families often promote traditionally "senior" pursuits and steer older relatives away from activities they perceive as youthful and therefore inappropriate. Some adult children feel resentful at a parent's refusal to "act his age," reacting to an inner need to maintain separate identities and to keep the parent a parent and not a peer. Others hold youthfulness as an advantage over the parent, having looked forward to a time of life when they would be stronger or freer than the parent. Still others may be unaware that their relative has interests beyond those normally assumed for older people. For example, a man in his seventies who would have enjoyed attending a conference on nuclear disarmament with his twenty-year-old grandson may decline the grandson's offer to drive him to a lecture on foot care at his local senior center. The grandson may erroneously conclude, "Grandpa doesn't want to do anything anymore," never thinking to invite his grandfather to the conference with him.

Some older people who do not identify with their age peers may nevertheless be willing to be of assistance to "them." The role of helper bestows just enough separation for acceptable participation in senior programs. Playing piano at the senior center for the "old people" may be tolerable in a way that simply having lunch there is not. The volunteer cook, receptionist, or piano player may enjoy staying on for lunch and even attending an afternoon program, but only after the day's work is done and it is understood that they are "staff" rather than participants.

Weariness toward the idea of becoming friends with people who may soon get sick and die may be the widest gulf of all. Paradoxically, older people who have lost lifelong friendships of great depth and devotion may feel the least motivated to make new friends, knowing as they do how many conversations and shared experiences are needed to build a friendship even approaching this magnitude. The time ahead may seem too short and the kinds of activities they can do together may seem too limited. For any older person, getting close to someone who is reaching the end of their likely lifespan may seem too threatening: "Why should I have to keep going to funerals?" For some, the very sight of older people who have had strokes or a deforming physical problems makes them want to flee, as these conditions remind them of their own vulnerability and evoke their fear of aging.

Senior Centers

Stereotypes of senior centers prevent many from attending: "I don't knit or play bingo, so why should I go?" Family members can sometimes induce their relative to take a second look at senior centers by obtaining a calendar of events from the center nearest the older person's home. Some centers provide exercise and relaxation classes, writing groups, lecture series, action-oriented issue groups, and other educational programs, a far cry from knitting and bingo. Others have active volunteer task forces in which members bring meals to the homebound, help others with transportation needs, make specialized items for disabled people, and assist with running the center.

The opportunity for inexpensive, nutritious meals with others and weekly blood pressure checks and foot care by community health nurses can be other motivators for attending. Family members can place their relative's name on the center's mailing list as a way of highlighting these options and perhaps kindling interest. Accompanying their relative on an initial visit to the center is another way to overcome resistance. In such instances, families may want to phone ahead to ensure that center staff or volunteers are there to greet them. Staff can also help identify a neighbor to invite the older person to senior center events.

Adult Day Centers

For many older people, the severity of their frailty makes attendance at senior centers too difficult. Some need help with basic tasks like getting to the bathroom or handling utensils at meals. For these people, adult day centers provide meaningful activities along with necessary assistance, a combination of services which most senior centers are unable to supply. Adult day centers are organized as a structured environment for social contact, mental stimulation, exercise, supervision with medications, and nutritious meals. Depending on budget and space constraints, other possible services include round-trip van transportation, physical and occupational therapy, and nursing services for blood pressure checks, foot care, and other health needs. Quiet areas with beds are sometimes available for participants who need frequent rest.

Fees for adult day centers depend on the range of services offered and the extent to which costs are subsidized by government funding. Some centers use a sliding fee scale, which can reduce fees to a nominal amount for low-income people. For family caregivers who are employed outside the home, the cost of the center may be well worth their relief from worry about their relative's welfare during their workday. The cost tends to be much less than comparable hours paid for in-home hired helpers and gives the older person the additional advantage of getting out of the house.

Not all older people are eager to spend time at adult day centers.

Those with "day care" in the title suggest an equivalence with services provided for children which alienates many when they first hear about it: "I don't need to be babysat." Those entitled "day health centers" may fare better in this regard, until the older person is taken on a tour of the premises and sees participants with advanced memory loss or severe disabilities: "I don't want to spend the day looking at a bunch of people who are worse off than me. It's just too depressing."

A helpful strategy is for family members to plan to accompany their relative to the center for the first several sessions. As the older person develops familiarity with the other participants, staff, and program routines, family accompaniment can gradually be tapered off. Instead of seeing the others in terms of their physical problems, "that man in the wheelchair" and "that lady with the paralyzed arm," the new participant eventually starts to see the people behind the disabilities. The person may discover a welcome sense of usefulness in being able to assist those who have trouble holding a fork or who cannot see well enough to read the daily newspaper. Often, partners who start out providing accompaniment stay on as volunteers, having seen the needs firsthand and found satisfaction in helping to meet those needs.

Lack of transportation is another frequent problem. The day center may not own a van, or the person may live outside the van's catchment area. At times, family members can carpool with others who are transporting their relatives to the center, or can organize a system of neighbors, friends, and other relatives to rotate the driving.

A more difficult obstacle is when an older person lives alone and is unable to get dressed or perform other personal care tasks independently. Van or car pool arrangements may be available, but they are not of much value if no one is able to help the person prepare to be picked up. Although van drivers will often assist center participants with the finishing touches, such as buttoning a coat and getting down steps, they cannot be expected to supervise more extensive care needs regularly. In such cases, neighbors may be willing to assist with the morning preparation, especially if the older person's attendance at day care relieves them of the need to provide other forms of assistance during the remainder of the day.

Support Groups for Older People

Many older people claim that they would "never" participate in group therapy or join a support group. The fear of being called upon to "say something" that would violate their privacy is one of the most common reasons for this reluctance. Members of the generations which reached adulthood prior to the therapeutic explosion of the 1960's generally prefer to take in information without revealing their personal concerns. Lectures allow such passive anonymity, while support groups carry an expectation that individuals will personally contribute.

As an alternative, local chapters of organizations such as the Lung Association, Cancer Society, and Arthritis Foundation sponsor monthly educational meetings in which speakers address topics of interest to people coping with particular illnesses. Mingling casually after these presentations, people develop bonds from their monthly contact and from the discussions stimulated by the lectures. When such programs are skillfully led, members of the audience volunteer anecdotes and opinions without being pressured to do so. Shy people control the timing of their responses, and private people choose the content of their contributions. The larger educational and social format makes acceptable the "therapy" implicit in interacting with others who are dealing with similar physical problems.

When small support groups branch off from such educational programs, facilitators are able to build on the participants' comfort and safety with each other, and on their familiarity with coming to that particular setting. Support group participants do not have to define themselves as needing help, but rather as exchanging information. For similar reasons, support groups sponsored through senior centers and adult day centers tend to be much more acceptable to older people than those attached to mental health centers. Support groups associated with the mental health stigma tend to evoke reactions like, "You have to be crazy to go to a place like that."

Unfortunately, those most likely to benefit from an educational meeting or a support group are often those least motivated to attend. People immobilized by an illness or a bereavement may claim, "It's no use. Nothing can help me now." A persuasive response is to remind the person that experience is the best teacher and that others who have gone through the same experience may have valuable wisdom and practical ideas to offer. Few can dispute this argument. Some support groups are willing to send one of their members for a home visit to reach out to someone who still refuses to give the group a try. This personal contact, along with an offer to accompany the person to the first meeting, often breaks down the last vestige of resistance.

Hearing impairments deter many older people from attending lectures and groups. They should be encouraged to arrive early at lectures to obtain front row seats, thereby allowing for both lip reading and maximum volume from the speaker's voice. Group leaders can encourage all members to clearly enunciate their words and to speak slowly. Arranging chairs in close proximity may also help, when this is possible. Someone can be seated beside the hearing-impaired person to summarize inaudible portions of the group discussion. Professionals in these situations should be careful to convey a welcoming and easy attitude toward adaptations for hearing-impaired people, rather than giving any indication that the adaptations are a special effort.

Driving a relative to and from group meetings can seem to be one more burdensome task to family members, who perceive it as less vital than tasks directly related to the older person's physical health. Professionals can help by pointing out the many benefits that may arise as a result of their investing the extra time. Their relative's motivation to participate in rehabilitation efforts may improve, and this may in turn lead to better self-care. In addition, as family members talk informally with each other before and after meetings, supportive relationships among them may evolve. Car pool arrangements may eventually develop, as well as exchanges of health care equipment and tips about specialized community services.

Embarrassment about physical changes resulting from illness often deters people from all out-of-home ventures. Someone recently confined to a wheelchair may feel keenly self-conscious, preferring to remain home rather than risk others' stares at his partially paralyzed body. Someone needing to carry a portable oxygen tank and wear tubing in her nose may dread the curious looks of others on the street or in stores. Group meetings of stroke and respiratory clubs are ideal settings for breaking through such reticence, since everyone in attendance has firsthand experience with the same problems. Others' accounts of how they moved past social embarrassment often free those still encumbered by such fears. Observing people who go about their lives despite wheelchairs or oxygen tanks can have an inspirational effect that far surpasses the verbal encouragement of family members and professionals.

As family members and professionals often discover, the availability of services and special programs outside the home does not guarantee their use by older people. Family members may be repeatedly frustrated by their older relative's unwillingness to try out these programs, especially when the person has been complaining of loneliness or having too much time on her hands. Door-to-door van services or reliable buses may be available once someone gives up the car keys, but the person may have a hard time adjusting to the loss of control involved in using these alternatives. Working to overcome barriers to out-of-home activities tends to be worth the effort in giving a bored and lonely older person new kinds of freedom.

SUGGESTED RESOURCES

Books

Estes, Carroll, and James Swan and Associates. *The Long Term Care Crisis: Elders Trapped in the No-Care Zone* (Newbury Park, CA: Sage), 1992.

> Through a study of seven providers in twelve communities, the authors show the negative effects of prospective payment systems (DRGs) on community care. The no-care zone represents the gap between the acute care services available and what the elderly need, particularly in terms of social services.

Organizations

American Association for Retired Persons (AARP). 601 E. Street, N.W., Fulfillment Department, Washington, DC 20049. (202) 434–2277.

> AARP has many useful publications. Call or write for a complete list of publications. The following is only a sample of those relevant to this chapter.
>
> "Getting Around: There are Times When We Should Not Be Driving," D13849.

American Automobile Association (AAA). Listed in phone book.

> The Mature Operator Program is offered by local AAA clubs. It is an eight-hour classroom refresher course for persons age fifty-five and over to enhance driving knowledge and safety, and to promote awareness of new techniques for overcoming deficits.

Elder Care Locator. (800) 677–1116.

> This national toll-free number is designed to help identify community resources for seniors anywhere in the United States. The name,

address, and zip code of the person needing assistance allows the Elder Care Locator to identify the nearest information and assistance sources in that person's community. Call between 9:00 A.M. and 8:00 P.M. Eastern Time.

Elderhostel. 80 Boylston Street, Suite 400, Boston, MA 02116. 617–426–8056.

Offers educational opportunities through colleges nationwide and abroad.

Foster Grandparent Program (FGP). Funded primarily through AC-TION, 1100 Vermont Avenue, N.W., 11th floor, Washington, DC 20525. (202) 634–9108.

Matches volunteers over age sixty with disabled or troubled children. Check local phone book.

National Institute on Adult Day Care. Sponsored by National Council on the Aging (NCOA), 600 Maryland Avenue, S.W., West Wing 100, Washington, D.C. 20024. (800) 424–9046.

Publishes a directory of adult day care in the United States. Ask for order #2022.

Retired Senior Volunteer Program (RSVP). Funded primarily by AC-TION, 1100 Vermont Avenue, N.W., 11th floor, Washington, DC 20525. (202) 634–9108.

Links people over age sixty to volunteer opportunities in hospitals, senior centers, nutrition programs, and educational programs. Available in all states. Check the local phone book.

13

Living Together in the Caregiver's Home

Many families invite older relatives into their homes out of a desire to make caregiving more convenient. Maintaining one home rather than two often seems appealing. In other instances, living together is the least expensive alternative, especially if keeping the older person in her own home requires hiring costly overnight help. Some families make this decision on short notice, responding to a relative's need for extra support after discharge from the hospital or following a bereavement. This chapter identifies the benefits and drawbacks of giving care in a family member's home, offering suggestions for solving the most common dilemmas arising in these arrangements. Shared households can be satisfying to family caregivers and their older relatives when needs for privacy, respite, and support are adequately met.

DECIDING TO LIVE TOGETHER

Advantages to shared households must be weighed along with the drawbacks. For older people and family members with time for advance planning, this section surveys the territory ahead and demarcates both positive and negative considerations. Ideally, families would discuss these factors prior to making the decision to live together, but often such deliberation is not possible.

FACTORS TO CONSIDER WHEN AN OLDER PERSON MOVES INTO A FAMILY CAREGIVER'S HOME

Expense: Does a family member have to give up employment or reduce working hours to provide care?

Accessibility: Does the family's home require modifications, such as a wheelchair ramp?

Space: Is an extra room available to ensure privacy? Is a bathroom located near the older person's room?

Intimacy pressures: Will too much contact strain relations between the older person and family members?

In-Law relationships: Does the son- or daughter-in-law get along with their in-law?

Grandchildren: Has a grandchild been forced to give up a private room? Will any other changes be imposed?

Lifestyle discord: Do aspects of one generation's lifestyle cause distress to the other?

Future plans: Will long-awaited travel plans have to be disrupted? Will career goals have to be postponed?

Confinement: Which out-of-home activities will caregivers have to forgo? Is respite help available?

Cultural and personal expectations: Does the older person or family view in-home caregiving as a duty?

From Wendy Lustbader and Nancy R. Hooyman, *Taking Care of Aging Family Members* (New York: The Free Press, 1994). Copyright © 1994 by Wendy Lustbader and Nancy Hooyman; copyright © 1986 by The Free Press.

Advantages of Shared Households

Saving money is a prime benefit of living together. After investigating the costs of hiring a live-in worker, paying hourly aides, or helping to pay for a retirement home equipped with the necessary services, families often determine that living together is considerably less expensive than the other options. Due to financial limitations, many families find that they have no choice. Once their relative's care needs become extensive, sharing a household may become the only viable alternative to nursing home placement.

If the family is experiencing financial troubles apart from care expenses, living together may be a way to gain financial relief. Merging the older person's income with the family's may be a welcome exchange for the assistance provided. Additionally, an older person who is able to cash-in the equity on a home owned for many years may be able to compensate family members for employment they have forfeited in order to provide care or to pay for substitute helpers while family members are at work.

For many families, taking an older relative into the family's home is regarded as fulfilling a basic responsibility rather than an extraordinary sacrifice. This expectation may have been shaped by childhood experiences of living with a grandparent. To the extent that this experience was positive, family members may want to give their children similar contact with an older person's guidance, nurturance, and storytelling. If their relative is particularly beloved due to the help and support she rendered earlier in life, or if the present relationship is one of great affection, her living with the family may also serve as an expression of gratitude and the pleasure of having her around on a daily basis.

With increasing numbers of women in the work force, another advantage of moving the older person into a daughter's or granddaughter's home may be the potential for child care. Especially for low-income or single parent families unable to afford day care, the ability to leave young children at home with the older person may be a key motivation for sharing a household. Even older relatives who cannot provide extensive help with housekeeping due to physical limitations can contribute their presence when children arrive home from school, an advantage that working parents and their children may highly value. A frail older person who cannot handle major child care duties may still be able to play a game or read to a child, thereby relieving the parents so that they can prepare meals or run errands.

An immediate gain for the older person in making such a move is increased contact with family members and their social networks. The daily commotion from these contacts gives a previously isolated person more to talk about and more reason to be alert and animated. The phone rings more often and people come through the home more frequently. These everyday experiences, such as watching children with their friends, are more stimulating than sitting alone watching television. Family members' friends and neighbors may develop their own bonds with the older person and be willing to spend time in the home, freeing the family for some out-of-home involvements.

The opportunity to contribute to the family's well-being may be another attraction for the older person. In addition to assisting with child care and chores, the older person may be able to answer the phone and take messages, do mending, or work on time-consuming projects such as furniture refinishing. In some instances, a satisfying emotional role in the family's life may evolve, allowing the relative to feel a greater sense of purpose and value. Some grandparents are able to serve as buffers between parents and teenagers, giving the advantage of their more detached perspective to both parties during times of conflict.

In contrast to her life alone, the older person living with family may acquire a more comfortable lifestyle. Her family's home may have features which she enjoys, such as a yard or garden, closer access to bus routes and safe places to walk, or more labor-saving appliances than her home. Sharing expenses may free a portion of her income. If she is able to get out, she may thereby be able to afford more recreational activities, such as shows or concerts. The ability to afford such "extras" may raise her spirits and lead to the formation of new friendships. For an older person subsisting on a minimal Social Security check, sharing a home with relatives may provide her with such basics as nutritious food and a well-heated home.

For some older people, the safety accorded by others' presence in the home, especially at night, may be the chief attraction of sharing a household. Those who have had frightening experiences with being unable to get up off the floor after a fall may regard others' presence in the home as a primary asset. For those who have a particular dread of dying alone, shared living arrangements may seem especially appealing. For example, someone on oxygen for advanced respiratory disease may view having others nearby as an advantage in the event of a respiratory emergency, which more than compensates for the loss of privacy and autonomy in a shared household.

Disadvantages of Shared Households

In deciding whether to offer their home to an older relative, family members often fear their own confinement above all other consequences. This fear may be justified when the older person's care requires someone's continuous presence in the home. Those in the midst of active careers may worry about burning themselves out by coming home every evening and weekend to caregiving demands. Middle-aged women eager to pursue their own interests after years of child-rearing may especially resent the disruption of their plans. Newly retired people may be frustrated by having to postpone long-awaited travel plans.

In many families, the emotional balance achieved at a distance is likely to be disrupted by close proximity. Lifestyle differences in child-rearing practices, choice of friends, and even food preferences can become areas of contention when living space is shared. Seemingly insignificant details of daily life, such as omitting prayer before meals or hurriedly setting the dinner table, can become sparks of conflict that would not have occurred with separate residences.

Another common dread is that the older person will meddle in matters that family members prefer to handle without interference. Family members may be reluctant to establish a situation in which their relative has unlimited access to information about their personal affairs. Parent-child control issues long ago laid to rest may be revived. Despite the span of years, for instance, a forty-year-old woman may find herself acting like a rebellious twelve-year-old around her mother. After extended time in the same house, she may discover that her boundaries as an autonomous adult have become shaken due to her mother's new access to details of her personal life. A natural reaction is to use verbal sparring to defend against a parent's attempts to give advice or make judgments. Unless such reactions are channeled into more productive responses, relationships between a parent and adult children can be injured when they share a household.

In making the decision to invite the older person into the household, the adult child and her spouse may differ regarding the necessity or desirability of doing so. The spouse who already resents time spent on caring for an in-law may view a shared household as a further violation of both time and privacy. In addition, the spouse may be concerned that his own parents may feel slighted by "the other side" moving in, or he may fear that his parents might need care while his energies are diverted for his in-laws. Whatever the disagreement's source, marital conflict over this decision can be a major obstacle to its success.

Grandchildren may also have doubts about their grandparents moving into their home. If they are forced to give up their own room to make space for the grandparent, as is often the case, the feeling of being intruded upon may outweigh their affection for the grandparent. The prospect of sharing a room with a younger sibling or using a pull-out bed in a den without a door to close is reprehensible to most teenagers. Their private spheres may also be invaded in other ways.

They may resent their grandparent's expressed displeasure at their music, hair style, or clothes—generational differences to which their parents may have adapted. Some may remain outwardly silent about their resentments while simmering internally, unless their parents include them in the decision-making process and make it acceptable for them to express their negative feelings prior to the move.

A common fear, difficult for family members to face, is that they will change their minds about living together once the unforeseen realities of the situation become evident or the care becomes more taxing. It can seem that the decision cannot be altered once their relative moves in with them. From the start, it is helpful to include the older person in discussions where family members honestly assess their own capabilities and openly share their concerns about future problems: "Mom, I'll do my best, but I'm worried about my bad back and how long I'll be able to help you." Such honesty may arouse the older person's anxiety, but may also motivate her to participate in physical therapy and other activities which promote self-care.

Older people also perceive numerous drawbacks to shared households. In exchange for anticipated benefits, they first must contend with leaving their own homes. A deep attachment to the dwelling itself may be compounded by fondness for belongings which cannot be moved to a family member's residence. Familiar walks and views, a beloved garden, or neighbors of many years' duration are among the losses experienced during such a move. Sorting through and packing possessions and distributing items among family members can be heart-wrenching. (See Chapter 14.)

Loss of personal space can also be a difficult adjustment. After years in her own house or apartment, an older person can feel claustrophobic in a single room. Common areas of the family household may be more cluttered than she would like, or used for entertaining guests whom she would rather avoid. Some family members may indicate, either directly or through embarrassed glances, their preference that the older person stay in another area of the home while certain guests are present. As a result, the older person may spend most of her time in her room, the one household area over which she can exert control. These reclusive tendencies may frustrate those family members who do attempt to make their relative feel welcome in the rest of the home.

An older person's seclusion in such situations may be partially due to disruptions of her daily routines. Accustomed to eating and sleeping at certain times or watching particular television programs, she may be forced by majority rule to concede to the family's patterns of eating, sleeping, and watching television. Noise during evening hours may be especially disruptive to her need for quiet at that time. The sense of abandoning her previous daily habits for the family's preferences can make an older person's desire for the private domain of her room more intense. It may also account for unexplained or atypical grumpiness.

The older person's new proximity to family conflicts may be another unfortunate consequence of a shared household. Marital stresses, discipline problems with teenagers, and other strains become unavoidably visible. Adult children who are preoccupied with their parent's care needs may not be aware of the extent to which their own problems become a burden to the parent. The older person may dislike being drawn into family disagreements, compared to her former safety as a distant observer. The temptation to give advice or take a stand may be too powerful to restrain, despite an older person's wish to remain separate from the upheaval: "I'm just too old for this kind of thing." Avoiding such frays is yet another reason older people living with family may choose to confine themselves to their rooms.

Occasionally, the family's expectations of their relative's contribution to the household clash with the older person's preferences and physical abilities. A daughter may count on saving day care costs for her children once her mother moves in, without realizing that her mother is apprehensive and unenthusiastic about coping with two active children. Despite her wish to be of use to her family, her mother may feel she lacks the physical stamina required by young children. Alternatively, the older person's desire to help may exceed her cognitive abilities. A grandmother in the early stages of Alzheimer's disease may insist that she can baby-sit. Her daughter is then placed in the bind of not wanting to hurt her mother's pride while worrying about her children's safety. The daughter may have to enlist a friend or neighbor to check on the well-being of both her mother and children.

No matter how much families try to make their relative feel welcome, many older people find that their son or daughter's house never feels like "home." Instead, feelings of uselessness and being in the family's way may arise. If family members rearrange their schedules to ensure that someone is home all the time, the older person may feel guilty about being an imposition. If a grandson graciously gives up his room for her, she may remain continually aware of his displacement. Money spent to adapt the home, such as for an additional bathroom or a wheelchair ramp, may weigh on the older person if she is unable to contribute financially. Despite her family's repeated assurances that they are pleased to have her there, she may attribute any missed out-of-home activities as evidence of her being a burden on the family.

PROBLEM-SOLVING STRATEGIES FOR SHARED HOUSEHOLDS

In intergenerational households, a major problem is maintaining each member's separateness. Patterns of daily life are initially unclear, with both younger and older generations uncertain if they are intruding on the other's privacy. An older woman in a basement apartment may wonder how often to accept her daughter's invitations to come upstairs to join family dinners. She may be unable to tell whether she is invited out of guilt or a real desire for her presence at the dinner table. When she declines an invitation in order to give the family privacy, she may worry that her daughter's family misinterprets this as disinterest or rejection. With such uncertainty, families and their older relatives often compensate by spending more time together than either finds comfortable or desirable. Both sides may be unable to think of a way to broach the topic without hurting the other's feelings.

Maintaining Private Time

One way to resolve such awkwardness is to create a structure in which periods of private time occur automatically. Instead of uneasy guesswork, the older person and family can establish scheduled routines of contact and separateness. For instance, a parent in a downstairs apartment can plan to join the family for dinner every Tuesday and Thursday evening on an ongoing basis. Similarly, a parent living within the main part of the home can agree to spend the first hour after dinner with the family and the rest of the evening "on his own." With routine arrangements, the family can stop feeling guilty about taking their private time, and the older person need not worry about intruding.

Setting up such expectations as soon as the older person moves in is usually easiest. The mutual benefits of separateness, however, can be negotiated at any point in shared living situations. A daughter can say, "Mom, I've been thinking that we'll all be better off if we make a schedule of who's doing what and when. Then you'll know what to expect, and no one has to worry about hurting anyone's feelings." Several different ways of dividing evenings and weekends can then be discussed, with all household members included in choosing the most convenient plan. A grandson may insist, "I need to have quiet to do my homework after dinner," with the result that a 9 p.m. snack time is selected for after-dinner contact. Even if arrangements have to be readjusted frequently, at least the right to private, autonomous time for each household member becomes established.

The need for privacy has more significance than the organization of time. Family members may want to have phone conversations out of the older person's earshot, but feel awkward in moving to a more private area of the home to talk. Instead, they hold stilted conversations with veiled meanings while their relative tries to appear not to be listening. It is better to establish the practice that all family members will seek privacy while on the phone, no matter who is nearby. The same expectation can hold when visitors come to the home, with family members allowing each other the private use of common areas when needed.

Interfering or Contributing?

Keeping silent while a bystander to family conflicts is often a challenge to older people. For example, an older woman may fall into a mediator role between her son and his teenage children, yet she may have limited tolerance for their displays of hurt and anger. In addition, she may have her own ideas about how a parent should handle adolescent defiance. Her son may feel his role usurped when she injects her opinion into the fray, leaving him in the bind of feeling angry yet not wanting to upset her.

Third parties "butting in" to arguments generally serve as a lightning rod, draining off the anger onto themselves. A strategy to protect the older person from such stress and to reduce the adult child's sense of interference is to ask the older person to reserve her input until after the immediate conflict is over. Removing herself from the area when a conflict erupts, she can then become a silent observer for a later time when she will contribute her observations. Going to the physical periphery, such as moving into the living room when the argument is in the kitchen, can enable an older person to remain on the emotional periphery. When spouses fight, it is especially critical for the older person to avoid taking sides or taking on the mediator role. In a family with daily eruptions, for instance, a son may agree to set aside one evening per week to solicit his mother's views, in exchange for her keeping silent the rest of the time.

Giving the Older Person a Role in the Family

The recognition of an older relative as a legitimate part of the family system is inherent in these approaches. Segregating an older person's input differs from degrading it as "meddling." Intergenerational households often have difficulty accepting the ways an older relative's presence alters the balance of relationships, especially without traditional matriarch or patriarch roles. In the absence of models for how members of extended families should live together, the role of silent observer is a workable compromise. Such agreements respect the nuclear family's autonomy, without stripping the older person of the dignity inherent in an active role in the family.

The older person's place in the family can also be affirmed through her inclusion in the formative stages of household decision-making. Without giving up final control, for instance, a son could review with his mother the pros and cons of having the house painted vs. doing the work himself. He can invite her opinion without promising to follow it. The less trivial the decision, the greater the importance of including the older person as a contributing adult. Whether to accept a job in another part of the country or to send a child to a private vs. a state college are examples of decisions with geographic and financial implications which could seem demeaning if announced after the fact to the older person. Family members may need to remind each other periodically to consult their older relative on family matters. As indicated in Chapter Nine, allowing an older person to contribute to the household can be a powerful antidote to depression, even when these contributions are largely symbolic.

Devising concrete contributions to the household can be more difficult for families than permitting their relative a verbal role in household affairs. Traditional older women may have a particular need for doing household tasks as a way to affirm their identities as homemakers. In some instances, adult children may feel uncomfortable at the sight of a frail parent vacuuming the living room or scrubbing the bathtub. Afraid that she may harm herself by working beyond her capacities, they may plead with her to rest. Her housekeeping preferences may seem absurdly detailed to her children, who are more concerned with her health than the gleam on porcelain fixtures. Another problem arises when family members are pressed for time and become impatient with an older relative's slow and meticulous cleaning methods. As with other areas of tension, the best strategy is to settle these differences before they develop into larger conflicts.

Housekeeping plans promoting peaceful cohabitation could begin with the premise that household members each have control over their private rooms. For an older person newly confined to a small room, having control over that personal space is especially crucial. Even a daughter's well-intentioned "straightening up" in her mother's room can be felt as a violation, leaving her mother with only her own body to manage. When the older person is also disabled and cannot manage her body independently, her ability to direct details within her room becomes still more vital. In exchange for the older person's autonomy in this sphere, families can request noninterference in their control over other household areas. Designating specific tasks for the older person to participate in, such as folding laundry or mending, can often satisfy an older person enough to prevent her from trying to help in areas family members prefer that she avoid.

Money can underlie or add intensity to many of the problems described above. An older person may be unable to rid herself of the feeling of being a burden unless she pays room and board to the household. Some older people will restrict what they eat, unless family members allow them to contribute to the weekly grocery bill. To continue to feel they belong to the realm of adulthood, many older people need to retain an economic function: "I'll pay the heating bill, since I like the house very warm during the winter." Those too disabled to help with concrete tasks may especially appreciate being allowed to chip in some cash to the household. Rather than avoid discussing money, family members should explore their own and the older person's attitudes.

ARCHITECTURAL OPTIONS

Many families find that structural changes in their home ease some of the difficulties inherent in shared households. Architectural choices include basement apartments, "mother-in-law" apartments, mobile homes, duplexes, and additions to existing structures. Families often obtain the funds for these adaptations through the sale of an older family home, turning the equity into living options for the older person. Occasionally, siblings resent their potential inheritance going into home improvements for one member of the family, until they calculate the comparative cost of nursing home care over several years' time.

Basement Apartments

Turning a basement area into a fully equipped apartment is often the least expensive way to create more living space in an existing home. One problem is that such arrangements can be confining to an older person who has trouble managing steps. Also, noise from active household areas above the basement may interfere with an older person's desire to go to bed earlier than anyone else in the family. A further difficulty is the fact that basement windows tend to be smaller and higher than those on upper levels. The inability to look out at street activity, limited daylight, and often inevitable dampness can make a basement apartment a depressing place to live, despite lovely furnishings or modern fixtures. In homes where the basement steps, noise, and lack of windows do not present problems, the installation of bathroom and kitchen facilities and a comfortable heat source are generally worth the investment.

Mother-in-Law Apartments

A more expensive option which solves the obstacles of steps, noise, and windows is to build an addition onto the home. Limited yard space, zoning restrictions, and insufficient funds may preclude this alternative. Building a vertical addition may be possible, but this may not eliminate the problem of steps. Instead, a small prefabricated home in the backyard known as a "granny flat" may meet space and financial constraints. Since such structures can be disassembled when no longer needed, an exception to zoning restrictions may be granted. Problems can arise from neighbors complaining that such structures are "too tacky for the neighborhood," or from modular pieces being too large to fit through the narrow pathways to the backyard.

Mobile Homes

House trailers and small mobile homes can be a practical and economical option for housing an older person near the family, but may also invoke neighbors' displeasure. A common scenario is for an older relative to park a mobile home on the side of the driveway for an extended visit. Eventually, the visit becomes a permanent arrangement as the older person discovers that proximity to family compensates for the confined living space. Such situations are most common in rural areas with spacious yards and distant neighbors. Another way to use this option is for an older person to offer his home to his adult children or grandchildren and then move into a backyard trailer, gaining family support in exchange for unneeded living space.

Duplex Apartments

An increasingly popular option is for newly retired adult children to move from a large family home to a duplex, thereby gaining the ability to rent the other half until one of their older relatives requires care. They may also anticipate their own later years when one of their children may move into the other half to care for them. In addition, duplex apartments provide the possibility of renting to nonfamily members at reduced rates in exchange for assistance with housekeeping, yard work, and other needs. In this light, a duplex can be an investment in the potential both to give and receive care.

Other Adaptations

Architectural options of a lesser scale include adding a bathroom, soundproofing a bedroom, and dividing den space to make another bedroom. Adding a wall and a door to a den can sometimes make it habitable for a teenager, who would then be willing to give up his private bedroom for a grandparent's use. Building a separate entrance into a street level room or installing a refrigerator and sink in a laundry area to create a kitchenette are examples of adaptations that may be relatively inexpensive. Professionals can assist families and older people with generating creative ideas for home adaptations to solve problems of privacy and noise, thereby minimizing the stresses of increased proximity. (See also "Modifying the Home," pp. 171–176.)

THE NEED FOR TIME AWAY

Even with such changes, family members generally find that their relative's constant presence in their home heightens their need for periodic relief, or respite. Opportunities to run errands, to go out to dinner, or just to have time alone become especially precious in their scarcity. Although families differ in the amount and frequency of their need for time away, respite is critical for sustaining care over the long run.

What Other Family Members Can Do

Family members outside the immediate care situation can aid primary caregivers in a number of vital ways. One contribution is to perform tasks that relieve some of the caregivers' pressures. For example, picking up medications at the pharmacy or providing transportation for the caregivers' children are forms of concrete help not directly related to the older person's care but which can significantly reduce the caregivers' stress. Directly asking the caregivers what would be helpful to them is the best approach.

Another aid to primary caregivers is for family members to accompany their relative to medical, dental, and other out-of-home appointments. A dual function is served by removing a major task from the caregivers' list of duties and providing them with private time while the relative is out of the home. Since such appointments are usually scheduled in advance, the caregivers can plan ahead to make optimal use of the time off.

Providing large blocks of respite time on a regular basis is perhaps the most useful way for other family members to assist primary caregivers. A sibling who works full-time could relieve his sister and her husband one evening per week by taking his mother out to a leisurely dinner. Another option is for the older person to stay at another family member's home one or two weekends a month, thereby allowing primary caregivers to take a weekend trip or use the time for their personal needs. If the older person cannot easily be moved from one home to another, family members could trade homes for the weekend. Out-of-town family members could come to spend a week in the primary caregivers' home, allowing them to appreciate the care tasks firsthand while caregivers take a much-needed vacation.

Unfortunately, family members may not be willing or able to provide such crucial support to primary caregivers. Outright refusals or passive avoidance of chances to be helpful may be accompanied by the defensive assertion that nursing home placement is the better solution: "If you're going to keep her in your house instead of putting her in a home where she belongs, that's your business." Other family members may resist contributing funds to help pay for substitute help, claiming that respite care is an expensive luxury. Those who have never been caregivers themselves may have no idea of the strains involved and may not realize how vital it is for caregivers to rest. They can sometimes be persuaded to contribute, with the argument that home care by family members achieves significant savings over the nursing home expenses that would otherwise drain the inheritance.

Other Respite Options

Neighbors can be a valuable resource for quick bursts of relief. Living nearby allows them to help caregivers on short notice, when unexpected needs arise. Although assistance from other family members and hired helpers usually has to be scheduled in advance, neighbors may be willing to step in for an hour or so on a spontaneous basis. In this way, neighbors can help reduce the caregivers' overall level of stress. Professionals can assist family caregivers with identifying neighbors likely to help and with overcoming the family's reluctance to ask for such help. When deciding which family members should take the older person into their home, the presence of supportive neighbors should be a key factor in the choice. (See "Neighbors, Friends, and Other Helpers," pp. 125–138.)

If space is available in the home, a further respite alternative is to find someone willing to spend time with the older person in exchange for free or low-cost room and board. Having to cope with yet another person in the household often discourages such arrangements, although the loss of privacy is often worth the freedom gained. With such arrangements, the specific time expectations of the live-in should be negotiated in advance. (See pp. 287–290.)

Formal respite services include in-home companions, nurse's aides, and homemakers who can be hired through agencies or obtained through special state-funded programs if the older person qualifies. In some communities, religious and service organizations coordinate volunteers to provide respite free of charge, although recruiting and maintaining volunteer respite workers is difficult. Respite services in the home have the advantages of keeping the older person in familiar surroundings and avoiding transportation problems. Since public funding for in-home workers is limited, cost is often the major obstacle for families.

Out-of-home respite care includes adult day centers and nursing homes with beds designated for short stays. "Respite care beds," if available, can be reserved in advance, thus enabling the family to plan a true vacation. Nursing homes without an established respite bed system may still be willing to negotiate a short placement, if the cost of the full private-pay rate can be met through a cash advance. Respite in a nursing home has the advantage of providing trained staff twenty-four hours a day, thereby assuring a high level of care and emergency medical backup. As a result, caregivers may feel more at ease about going away on a vacation than they would leaving their relative at home with hourly workers coming in for part of each day.

The major obstacles to the use of respite beds in nursing homes are the excessive cost and the scarcity of respite beds. Families often face long waiting lists for beds which are not covered by Medicare or private insurance. In addition, the older person, especially if cognitively impaired, may be disoriented by the temporary move to a nursing home. Others may resist going because they do not believe that the family actually intends to bring them back home after a month or two. The use of this option can be eased by including the older person in the decision as much as feasible, describing the facility in detail, and emphasizing a predetermined date for returning home.

Living together in the caregiver's home is the situation in which caregivers are most prone to exhaustion. Professionals should emphasize that if family members fail to take care of themselves, they will eventually erode their ability to give care. The weekly cost of hiring paid substitutes, if funds are available, is only a fraction of the nursing home charges which would result if they deplete themselves. If funds are not available, professionals should assist the family in exploring ways that community programs, neighbors, and other family members can relieve the primary caregivers. When caregivers get sufficient rest and privacy, caring for a relative in the family's home can be one of the best arrangements for all concerned.

SUGGESTED RESOURCES

Articles

Lang, Abigail M., and Elaine M. Brody. "Characteristics of Middle-Aged Daughters and Help to their Elderly Mothers," *Journal of Marriage and the Family*, 45 (1983), 193–202.

> Daughters who are older and share households feel intense caregiving responsibility. Being married and being employed compete with demands of parent care. The article emphasizes the need for a family-focused social policy.

Soldo, Beth J., and Joana Myllyluoma. "Caregivers Who Live with Dependent Elderly," *The Gerontologist*, 23 (1983), 605–611.

Situations where care is provided to a dependent, unmarried relative appear to be the most vulnerable to dissolution because one in four of these households is headed by a woman for whom employment is an economic necessity. Home care benefits need to be targeted to such households.

Books

Carlin, Vivian, and Vivian Greenberg. *Should Mom Live With Us? And is Happiness Possible If She Does?* (New York: Lexington Books), 1992.

This book is intended to help middle-aged children and their aging parents who are thinking about living together. Addresses issues such as privacy, communication, social obligations, and safety.

Organizations

Family Service America, Inc. 11700 West Lake Park Drive, Milwaukee, WI 53224. (414) 359–1040.

FSA is a network of nonprofit counseling agencies serving families throughout the United States and Canada. Their member agencies provide individual and family counseling for caregivers, as well as other services. Contact the national office for local referrals.

National Home Caring Council (NHCC). 519 C Street, N.E., Washington, DC 20002. 202–547–6586.

Write for the free pamphlet, "All About Home Care: A Consumer's Guide."

U.S. Consumer Product Safety Commission. Publication Request, Washington, DC 20207. (800) 638–2772

Write for a free copy of "Safety for Older Consumers: Home Safety Checklist."

14

Alternative Living Situations

Many options exist between living alone in a private residence and going to a nursing home. Yet older people and their families often dread a nursing home as a last resort without learning about the choices in between. The first part of this chapter discusses how to hire live-in helpers. Home-sharing arrangements are then depicted, followed by a section which explains the other care alternatives: retirement homes, assisted living residences, subsidized apartments, and adult foster homes. The profound resistance felt by older people as they face leaving a home of many years is explored. The chapter concludes with ways to help with the wrenching task of packing up a lifetime's accumulation of possessions and with adjusting to a new residence.

HIRING A LIVE-IN

Prior to seeking a live-in helper, it is important for families to appraise their relative's needs and to decide between finding a person to share the home and hiring a salaried live-in. Home-sharers expect to reduce their personal expenses by living with an older person, usually planning to attend school or work at the same time. The other type of applicant views caregiving as their employment, expecting a salary in addition to room and board. Although the distinction can become blurred in practice, starting out with this framework helps families weigh their relative's needs and finances against the realities of the applicant pool.

Deciding the Terms of Employment

As this distinction implies, home-sharing applicants seek a living situation different from that of salaried helpers. For example, an older woman needing only companionship at dinner and someone's presence in the house at night might be able to rent a room to a student at a discounted rate. If she later wanted the student to take over her household chores, she might offer free rent and a small cash payment. In contrast, a woman needing someone to prepare her three meals a day, along with helping her to the bathroom at unpredictable times, would not be able to attract someone with school or job commitments. She needs to seek a person who regards caregiving as their job, and offer a salary reflective of both the tasks required and the short supply of such helpers.

The degree of restriction on their personal freedom tends to be the deciding factor for home-sharing applicants as they choose a living situation. If an older person's personal care needs can be managed during the early morning and late evening, for example, these duties would not interfere with out-of-home daytime commitments. Similarly, if chores and errands can be performed on an impromptu basis, in and around other involvements, free rent may be an acceptable compensation. But if the care tasks require intermittent daytime availability, such as administering medications and cleaning up after incontinence episodes, most applicants will not accept the arrangement without a salary.

When family members realize that paying a salary is unavoidable, they next face the reality that financial compensation is only one of the factors considered by applicants choosing a live-in situation. Since the demand for live-in helpers tends to far exceed the supply, families usually need to work to make their relative's situation as attractive as possible. The following chart can help family members identify the advantages and disadvantages of the situation they are offering.

Of these factors, family members and friends' support is often most important to live-in applicants. They want to be able to rely on substitute help coming promptly on their days off, as well as someone to relieve them when they have a personal emergency. Experienced live-ins prefer situations in which families espouse a spirit of partnership in the care, rather than an attitude of dumping all responsibilities on the

---

FACTORS THAT PROSPECTIVE LIVE-INS CONSIDER IN CHOOSING EMPLOYMENT

Privacy of the living accommodations: Is a private room available? How separate is it from the older person's living area? Is there a private bathroom? Use of kitchen facilities? Space for having own guests?

Nature of the care needs: Does the older person need assistance or wander during the night? Is incontinence a frequent problem? How much lifting is required?

Household cleanliness and order: Is the home pleasant to spend time in? Are there odors or areas of clutter?

The older person's personality: Is the person demanding or manipulative? Is the person respectful and pleasant toward others?

Availability of transportation: Are family members able to drive the helper to and from the home? Is public transportation nearby? Will the helper be expected to provide transportation for the older person?

Degree of support from family members and friends: Will the helper be left in a lurch if the care suddenly becomes more difficult? Are people available to be called upon in emergencies? Will there be regularly scheduled days off?

From Wendy Lustbader and Nancy R. Hooyman, *Taking Care of Aging Family Members* (New York: The Free Press, 1994). Copyright © 1994 by Wendy Lustbader and Nancy Hooyman; copyright © 1986 by The Free Press.

helper. Live-ins find that the availability of next-door neighbors who will step in for an hour or two while they run errands, exercise, or tend to incidental needs is especially appealing. Family members can demonstrate their supportiveness in this regard by providing a list of nearby friends and relatives willing to assist the live-in helper.

Days off are a key issue for prospective live-ins. Most insist on two twenty-four-hour periods per week when they can leave the residence and be released from all responsibility for the older person's needs. Some will request weekends off, while others will ask only for two consecutive days. Families who show applicants an organized plan for substitute help will tend to have more hiring success than those unprepared to deal with this problem. Experienced candidates may have been previously burned by families who did not plan for substitutes and then forced them to give up their days off.

An unspoken concern many applicants have is whether the older person is likely to die soon after they move in. They may ask family members detailed questions about the older person's health status, without divulging this concern as the motive behind their questions. It is helpful for family members to be prepared to address this issue, perhaps by asking applicants to state their ideal length of employment. While some prefer short-term commitments, others desire a situation in which they can settle in for a long stay. Family members may also want to offer final candidates for the live-in position a chance to discuss these concerns with a health care professional who is involved in the care situation, such as a visiting nurse.

Prior to placing ads and setting up interviews, a final step is to determine whether the older person has strong racist feelings that will complicate the hiring process. Some older people are explicit with family members about their racist attitudes, while others express their feelings covertly by sabotaging the hiring of certain individuals. In some localities, for example, a large proportion of the applicants for such positions will be newly arrived immigrants with minimal English-speaking ability. However uncomfortable the issue may be for family members, advance awareness of the older person's attitudes can prevent awkward or hurtful moments for the applicants. A professional's skills can also be enlisted here to help the older person become more realistic about making adaptations. (See "Harboring Racist Feelings Toward Particular Workers," pp. 246–247.)

The Mechanics of the Hiring Process

Senior information and assistance hotlines, senior centers, or home health agencies often maintain lists of people seeking salaried live-in positions. Occasionally, job programs at community colleges or state unemployment offices will accept such listings. Posting notices in neighborhood laundromats and supermarkets may reach applicants interested in living in particular neighborhoods. Another effective means is placing ads in community newspapers, church or synagogue bulletins, and advertising supplements with local neighborhood distribution.

SAMPLE AD

Older woman recovering from a stroke needs a LIVE-IN helper. Salary plus room and board. Private room. Family nearby. Two days off per week. Personal care, meal prep, chores. No lifting. Call 683–9162, 7–9 pm, Mon.–Thurs.

Becoming adept at screening applicants over the phone and eliminating inappropriate callers is a time-saving skill. The following questions can help families identify which people they want to interview.

Questions for Screening Live-In Applicants Over the Phone

1. What are your reasons for wanting to live with an older person? Have you done this before?
2. What employer and landlord references do you have in the local area? Can you give me their phone numbers?
3. Do you drive? Do you own a car? Do you need access to a bus route?
4. What are your usual bedtime and waking hours?
5. Are you a smoker? Do you use alcohol?
6. Do you expect to have friends visit you in the home?
7. (Read off a specific list of tasks and expectations.) How do these sound to you?

The sample ad shown above may be useful to family members as a basis for devising their own. Generally, ads for salaried live-ins should stress the family's support, days off, and the nature of the care tasks. Other phrases to help applicants screen themselves may include "non-smokers only," "experience necessary," and "must have local references." Since waiting at home for calls can be a nuisance, the ad should designate a narrow time period: "Call between 7:00 and 9:00 P.M. weekdays." Telephone answering machines ease the intrusiveness of this process, but discourage applicants who are uncomfortable with leaving messages. Those who are currently in live-in positions, for instance, usually do not have a private phone number to which a call can be returned.

Some older people fear that prospective live-ins who tour their homes are "casing" the house for a break-in. In these instances, setting up initial interviews at other locations is advisable, such as meeting family members for coffee at a restaurant. Conducting initial interviews in this way also allows applicants to ask questions they would have withheld in the older person's presence, thereby giving family members a glimpse of their attitudes towards older people. Once applicants are narrowed down to a few finalists, second interviews can be held at the home to include both a detailed tour and a chance for the older person to interview the applicant.

It is helpful for family members to have a list of questions for the interviews. Possible topics include the applicant's family background, past job experiences, places lived and traveled, food and music preferences, favorite television programs, uses of leisure time, and other nonintrusive yet personal areas of discussion. Having the older person ask these questions establishes an immediate involvement in the hiring process and conveys to the applicant that the family respects their relative's judgment and supervisory role.

Watching how applicants respond to the older person often reveals more about them than the content of their answers. For example, those who persist in directing their responses to family members, as if the older person was incompetent or insignificant, show inherent disrespect for older people. Likewise, candidates who fail to ask the older person questions about her life history or personal preferences demonstrate their lack of interest. Those who speak directly to the older person and ask her respectful questions are likely to be the better caregivers.

A serious red flag is an applicant who supplies names of references who cannot be reached by phone, or references whose prior relationship with the applicant are only vaguely linked to employment. People who have legitimate references tend to supply accurate phone numbers and useful suggestions as to how these individuals can best be contacted. Even in circumstances with no other available applicants, it is preferable for family members to extend their search efforts rather than risk hiring a skilled con artist. To hire someone without checking references, no matter how engaging and trustworthy this person appears, is to put a vulnerable older person at risk.

Another issue which may arise during the hiring process is whether Social Security contributions are to be deducted from salary payments. Some salaried live-ins prefer that payments not be filed with the government, while others insist upon proper deductions and reporting. These stipulations may conflict with family members' preferences, such as those who want to maintain careful legal records for tax purposes or those who view the paperwork needed for legal filing as a nuisance. To determine legal requirements, families can phone the local Social Security office listed in the phone book and inquire about the salary level at which payments to household employees must be declared. The form for obtaining an employer's identification number can be obtained by calling the Internal Revenue Service. After the first filing, forms are mailed in quarterly to the IRS and are relatively easy to complete.

The following form shows a sample agreement in which the terms of employment can be specified. Although many families are inclined to believe the relationship will work on good faith, putting expectations in writing avoids misunderstanding, prevents future problems, and lends an organized formality to the hiring process.

When the Older Person Resists Live-In Help

Some older people express indignation when they learn that a live-in helper is to be paid a salary as well as room and board. Those who do not perceive the full extent of their care needs or cannot see the disadvantages of their living situation from a live-in's perspective may believe that family members are foolishly throwing away money by offering a salary: "That's crazy to have to pay her to live in a nice home like this." If the salary is to be paid from the older person's funds, these perceptions can become a major obstacle during the hiring process. In some instances, a professional's experience in this area may convince an older person that the salary level is indeed realistic and that the outlay is well worth the services to be rendered.

An older person who has never lived with anyone but a partner, parents, or siblings may also feel frightened by the idea of living with a stranger. Worries about what this unknown person may do may escalate to the point where the older person tries to disrupt the hiring process, pleading with family members to drop the whole idea: "If I promise not to call you so often, can we do without this?" Family members can use the following list to enumerate the advantages that will accrue if the arrangement is successful, while pointing out that this person will be a "stranger" only a short while. Emphasizing that references will be carefully checked and that family members will come over frequently in the beginning may further ease the older person's anxiety.

SALARIED LIVE-IN HELPER AGREEMENT

1. *Room and Board*:
   Employer will provide three meals a day and a private room.
2. *Salary*:
   Employer will pay $_____ gross monthly. $_____ will be deducted for Social Security, leaving a net pay of $_____ per month.
3. *Time Off*:
   Employer will provide two twenty-four hour periods off per week, on _____ and _____. Live-in will give at least one week's notice if these days need to be changed.
4. *Extra Work Days*:
   If substitutes fail to arrive on live-in's days off, employer will pay live-in $_____ per day.
5. *Duties of Live-In Helper*:

   _____

   _____

   _____

   _____

6. *Termination of the Agreement*:
   Either party can terminate this agreement with two weeks notice. If a hospitalization occurs, normal pay will continue for _____ days. Thereafter, if live-in does not seek other employment, $_____ will accrue each day, payable in a lump sum once the hospitalization ends.

Employer_____   _____
                    (Signature)   (Date)

Live-in_____   _____
                    (Signature)   (Date)

Advantages of Successful Live-In Arrangements

- *Sense of security at night:* Having someone in the home during the night is comforting.
- *Improved nutrition:* Having company at meals increases both appetite and motivation to prepare interesting meals.
- *Increased visitors to the home:* The live-in helper's friends may make the home more lively and stimulating.
- *Financially practical:* The cost of hiring a similar amount of help on a per-day basis is much more expensive.
- *Prolonging the family's ability to help:* Having someone in the home spares family members from driving back and forth for incidental needs and reduces their overall stress.

Some older people interpret the family's desire to hire a live-in as a consequence of their excessive requests for help, while others regard it as an indication that family members are tired of them and want to have less contact. In these instances, the potential for hurt and misunderstanding is extensive. Family members can prevent strain by honestly explaining the advantages of a live-in from their perspective: "We wouldn't feel so worried about your loneliness if you had someone here with you," or "This way, we'll be able to actually visit with you instead being so tired from taking care of everything." When family members admit their own exhaustion as the true motive for hiring a live-in, the rest of their assurances then become more believable.

An older person's fear of abandonment by family if a live-in takes over care duties should also be discussed directly: "It's not that we'll stop visiting and calling you, but that we'll be less pressured when we do come over." Some of this fear can be reduced by pledging an evening each week for a family visit or outing. Another option is for family members to arrange to serve as substitutes on the live-in's days off, thereby assuring their relative of regular contact. When practical, such commitments convey the sense that the live-in will supplement the family's help rather than replace it.

The following vignette conveys a host of other worries that may account for an older person's resistance to live-in help:

Will I ever get to have solitude? What if she hovers around me all the time? I might not like her cooking. What if she eats me out of house and home? She might want to have a man stay overnight in her room. What if she brings over people I don't want to have in my house? What if she blasts her stereo when I'm trying to get some sleep? She might watch TV programs I don't like. What if she hogs the phone or runs up long-distance bills? What if she isn't tidy?

When people share a residence, friction is inevitable. One strategy is to ask specific questions during the interview process, allowing applicants to respond directly to predictable concerns: "How would you handle the need for privacy and solitude? Do you expect to have overnight guests?" Another way to relieve anxiety about potential conflicts is to enact a two-week trial period to go into effect as soon as the helper moves in. A trial period gives both people a chance to assess the situation and to attempt to resolve disagreements on their own. At the end of two weeks, family members or a professional can conduct a mediation session to ensure that grievances are being aired rather than held in as resentments. Negotiation techniques described in the section on family meetings may prove helpful in this regard. (See pp. 73–79.)

HOME-SHARING ARRANGEMENTS

As depicted earlier, the attitudes and expectations of people interested in sharing a home with an older person differ widely from those applying for employment as live-in helpers. In home-sharing, the older person is viewed as a housemate rather than an employer. Arrangements must be based upon a fair exchange of benefits rather than the imposition of preferences and requirements. The challenge is to determine in advance which benefits to offer and how much to expect in return. For instance, the older person might regard companionship as a benefit gained by both parties in living together, but the younger housemate might have competing social interests that make this expectation a burden rather than an advantage.

An important first step in finding a home-sharer is to assess the benefits that can be offered against the pool of available applicants in a particular community. For example, college towns usually have an abundance of students seeking inexpensive housing, which increases the likelihood that older people in these areas will have a choice of housemates while offering little beyond low rent. In other areas, the housing market may be such that older people must offer free rent and other benefits in order to attract any applicants at all. Starting out with a realistic assessment of the housing market saves time and ensures that the older person offers a reasonable arrangement.

In many communities, there are agencies that match homeseekers with those hoping to share their homes. A way to identify the location of such agencies and information about the services they provide is through the local senior hot line. Some agencies not only match older people with potential home-sharers but also assist with smoothing out disagreements during the initial adjustment period. If such agencies do not exist in the older person's area, hot-line staffers may nevertheless be able to refer family members to local professionals able to assist with the process of finding a home-sharer.

The following is a sample ad that can be adapted to individual circumstances. Home-sharing ads should emphasize the freedom to pursue outside commitments as well as any features of the residence that enhance personal privacy.

SAMPLE HOME-SHARING AD

SHARE A HOME with an older man. Free rent in exchange for household chores and evening companionship. Private living area with separate entrance. Call 426–8973, 6–8 pm daily.

The following list portrays the most common reasons that older people give for wanting to share their homes and ways to translate these into concrete expectations:

Expectations in Home-Sharing Situations

"Someone in the house with me at night"	Every night? Could the housemate go away on weekends? What time would you want the person home in the evenings?
"Someone to eat meals with me"	Which meals? How often? Who prepares the meals, and who cleans up afterwards?
"Someone to help with the chores"	Which chores? How often? Laundry? Food shopping? Who scrubs the bathroom?

Expectations in Home-Sharing Situations (cont.)

"Companionship; someone to talk to"	Do you expect the person to spend time with you every evening? Saturday and Sunday? Is companionship at the evening meal enough?
"Shared expenses"	Are utilities to be divided? How is the food budget to be determined? Which household items are split equally? Which are personal expenses?
"Someone to run errands and give me rides when I need them"	How available does the person have to be? Will you provide a car?

Homeseekers also need to be prodded during the interview process to spell out exactly what they hope to gain from the living situation. For instance, a woman with young children may identify "help with child care" as one of her goals in seeking a shared home. Does this mean that she expects the older person to be home when the child returns from school each day? How many evenings per week does she hope to leave the child in the older person's care? When both parties clarify their expectations, future conflicts can be prevented.

Some older people refuse to consider housemates considerably younger than themselves. Citing life-style differences, they claim that the gulf between the generations is too great. It can be helpful to ask the older person to identify the generational differences which seem most divisive and then to venture solutions to these hypothetical conflicts. For instance, the fear that "music will be blasting at all hours" can be countered with the suggestion of establishing quiet hours when both parties agree to minimize music and other sounds.

Conflict around issues of sexual activity may be a key problem dreaded by older people: "I couldn't stand it if my housemate had a man stay overnight in her room." For some, worry about overnight guests centers more on issues of privacy rather than sexuality: "I just don't want to step out of the shower and find a strange man in the hallway." These are the very issues which should be aired during the interview process. One way is for the older person to state her preferences clearly, allowing applicants with contrary intentions to rule themselves out. Another solution is for the housemate to stay overnight on weekends at her friend's house rather than violate the older person's sense of propriety or privacy.

When finalizing arrangements, expectations should be put in writing specifying the amount of rent to be paid, terms for a damage deposit, amount of notice to be given upon termination, and other pertinent issues. When services are to be rendered in exchange for free rent, these should also be itemized on the agreement. Prior to signing, older people should verify all information given by homesharing applicants. Checking applicants' prior landlord references and credit history adds to the security of these arrangements.

Older people who insist on finding someone their own age as a housemate generally face a limited pool of applicants. Since most older people prefer to remain in their own homes, a greater number of older people are seeking housemates than want to move to someone else's home. An older person with organizational skills and sufficient motivation could try to assemble a group housing situation. Offering reduced expenses, shared household tasks, and ongoing companionship, the older person could advertise for age peers interested in these advantages. Shared households may contain the additional benefit of potential caregiving should someone in the home become ill, as long as the housemates remain healthy enough to sustain each other.

Although home-sharing options are increasing in number and popularity, professionals and families need to be sensitive to the fact that some older people remain uncomfortable with the idea of shared living arrangements. Those accustomed to years of solitude may prefer to endure the costs of hourly help and the risks of living alone rather than accept intrusions on their personal habits.

RETIREMENT HOMES, ASSISTED LIVING, AND OTHER OPTIONS

Many older people and their families are confused by the many housing alternatives that have become available in recent years. They may assume that retirement homes are the same as nursing homes, or wonder how facilities advertising "assisted living" differ from ordinary retirement homes. Distinguishing among the options requires a clear understanding of the levels of service offered at each type of residence. This section explains the various types of housing and how to choose among them. A checklist is offered which can help families compare different options and ask the right questions while taking tours of facilities.

Subsidized Senior Apartments

In many areas, apartment complexes subsidized by federal and state funds have been built for older people. Most of these buildings were designed to be accessible for the disabled and are often located near shopping and other services. The rent is adjusted to a percentage of the older person's income, usually one-third. As asset restrictions vary, qualifying information must be obtained from the city or county housing authority in the older person's community. For example, having more than $20,000 in the bank disqualifies applicants from subsidized housing in certain regions.

These buildings tend to have emergency call buttons in the apartments, with a manager on duty twenty-four hours a day. Some buildings have a weekly van to nearby shopping areas. If needed, housecleaning services or assistance with cooking, dressing, and grooming must be obtained separately through public or private agencies. Generally, residents must be able to manage their daily lives with minimal assistance.

Retirement Homes

A great variety of housing options are grouped under the heading "retirement homes." Most facilities using this term offer meals in a central dining room, recreational activities, and weekly housekeeping. Assistance with medications and personal care is usually available at extra cost, but residents are expected to be able to transport themselves to and from the dining room independently. Facilities differ in the extent to which frailty or disability is tolerated. Since the costs, services, and the style of retirement homes vary so widely, a questions-and-answer section follows.

Assisted Living

Residences using the term "assisted living" tend to offer all the services of retirement homes, plus help with dressing and grooming built into the monthly rent. Availability of a nurse on the premises is usually greater than in retirement homes, and more severe levels of incapacity are tolerated. Some facilities offer services close to the level offered by nursing homes, while still maintaining people in their own private apartments. The purpose of assisted living is to offer supportive services without diminishing residents' privacy, dignity, and autonomy.

Adult Foster Homes

Often termed "residential care homes," these are private, state-licensed homes where older people receive care. Residents pay privately or, if they are on a low income, obtain state funding. Generally, these homes take care of two to four residents at a time, but some homes are licensed for more than four. The quality of care tends to vary from home to home, depending on the skill level and dedication of the caregivers. Families can obtain a list of licensed residences from the state's health and human services division responsible for long-term care.

Older people who meet the state's requirements for Medicaid nursing home funding usually qualify for state payments to adult foster homes. As with nursing homes, the monthly fee paid by states to these homes tends to be much less than private-pay rates. As a result, the better homes tend to avoid accepting state-funded residents. On the average, private charges range from $800 to $1,600 per month, depending on the geographical area and the level of care required. Adult foster homes can thus be significantly less expensive than private rates in nursing homes.

Before selecting one of these homes, family members should carefully interview the people who will provide the hands-on care. Later, they should follow up with frequent visits to ensure the quality of services. At their best, care in these homes is more personalized and homelike than in nursing homes. At their worst, older residents are vulnerable to abuse and neglect due to infrequent inspections and minimal licensing requirements.

QUESTIONS AND ANSWERS ABOUT RETIREMENT HOMES

1. What is a simple way to distinguish between a retirement home and a nursing home?

A definition which removes confusion is: "A retirement home is an apartment complex with extra services included in the rent." Some people hear the word "home" and picture a place where ill people lie in bed and receive nursing care. Emphasizing the fact that each resident in a retirement home maintains a private apartment helps dispel confusion, as does mentioning that nursing care is available only on a part-time basis in these facilities.

2. What are the "founder's fees" and "buy-in plans" offered by some retirement homes?

Some facilities require a large down payment, called a founder's fee or buy-in plan, which guarantees residents access to a nursing home or other services within the retirement complex. This is appealing for those who want to feel that all their needs are covered for the rest of their lives. Although the guarantee may seem attractive, such large initial fees are a gamble that later care needs will justify the investment. If the person dies without ever needing such care, the facility pockets the nonrefundable fee. In some cases, these fees do not cover the full cost of care, or the contract contains a clause permitting transfer to an outside nursing home if the facility's beds are full. In all cases, the older person and family members should read the contract carefully and ask questions about parts of the contract they do not understand.

3. What level of independence is required for admission to most retirement homes, and what happens if the older person's health condition deteriorates while she resides there?

As part of choosing a retirement home, family members should inquire as to the circumstances under which residents are requested to leave the facility or are not permitted to return after a hospital stay. Although most retirement homes are explicit about admission requirements, some are vague about their termination policies. An admission criterion for almost every retirement home is that residents be able to transport themselves to and from the dining room on their own. Residents who become frail may be permitted to use wheelchairs for long distances, but some homes do not allow wheelchairs under any circumstances. Another common admission criterion is the ability to dress and bathe independently. If severe health problems occur, some homes allow residents to hire personal care aides, whereas others insist that a resident needing such help be moved elsewhere.

4. What are the chief benefits of moving to a retirement home?

Having neighbors in close proximity and activities available on the premises can dramatically reduce loneliness and boredom. When meals are served in a common dining room, cooking tasks are elimi-

QUESTIONS FOR COMPARING HOUSING OPTIONS:

Senior Subsidized Apartments, Retirement Homes, and Assisted Living Residences

Location
- Close to family and friends?
- Access to public transportation?
- Safe places to walk nearby?
- Bank, pharmacy, grocery store nearby?
- Vans available for appointments? Shopping?

Meals
- Served on the premises?
- Cafeteria style or table service?
- Number of meals negotiable?
- Guests allowed on a per-meal basis?
- Fully equipped kitchen in each unit?
- Special diets accommodated?

Staffing
- On-site manager 24 hours a day?
- Nurse on duty? How often?
- Help with medications? At what cost?
- Infirmary on the premises?
- Someone to organize activities?
- Housekeeping services? How often?
- Physical therapy available?

Layout
- Laundry rooms conveniently located?
- Storage areas available?
- Activity room? Lounge area?
- Individual heat controls in each unit?
- Safety rails in the bathrooms? Hallways?
- Call buttons in each unit? Where?
- Soundproofing between units?
- Private phone service in each unit?

Costs
- Founder's fee? Initial down payment?
- Fee to remain on the waiting list?
- Extra fees for personal care services?
- Conditions for terminating the contract?

From Wendy Lustbader and Nancy R. Hooyman, Taking Care of Aging Family Members (New York: The Free Press, 1994). Copyright © 1994 by Wendy Lustbader and Nancy Hooyman; copyright © 1986 by The Free Press.

nated and the benefits of eating with others are gained. For a couple, a retirement home ensures that when one spouse dies, the surviving spouse can rely on established social networks during the bereavement and adjustment process.

6. Why do monthly rates of retirement homes and assisted living residences vary so widely?

Facilities owned by nonprofit organizations are generally less expensive than for-profit facilities. Rental rates are also affected by a facility's age, location, and the range of services included in the monthly fee. Rates sometimes vary widely within a single facility due to differences in apartment size and in the meal and care plans selected. When older people and their families decide in advance what they most want from a retirement home, they can more easily compare costs and services as they visit various facilities. For some, choosing the retirement home closest to a family member's residence is paramount, while for others cost is the deciding factor. The preceding table of questions helps older people and their families compare options.

RESISTANCE TO ALTERNATIVES

While searching for suitable alternatives to home care, family members often find that they are more enthusiastic and motivated than their relative. The older person may agree that she needs more help, a safer place to live, or the stimulation of being around other people, but she may claim that services, safety, and social contacts are just not worth the price of giving up her home. Inertia against a change of this magnitude may be intensified by devotion to a pet who cannot be brought along, attachment to a beloved garden, dislike of high-rise apartment buildings, and worry about living among a "bunch of old people."

In both emotional and practical payoffs, family members almost always stand to gain more initially than does their relative. For example, they may be eager to be released from the responsibility of maintaining their relative's house and yard. Acknowledging this up front, rather than pretending that the proposed move is entirely for the older person's benefit, often helps propel acceptance: "Mom, now we're taking care of your house and ours. It would be so much easier for us if you moved to a retirement home, because then we could take care of just one house and use the leftover time to spend more enjoyable time with you." The move then becomes something that the older person is giving to her family: "I'll move so that you won't have to do all that extra work."

No matter how they present the reasons for a move, family members may have to wait for a precipitating event that overcomes their relative's resistance. They may feel less frustrated if they anticipate the human tendency to make changes in response to distressing experiences rather than promises of future benefits. An older person who struggles daily with steep steps is not likely to find this sufficient reason to leave a lifelong home until she has a frightening stumble. Although family members may dread her breaking her hip in a fall, a close call may be necessary before her fear becomes strong enough to make a move more appealing. Occasionally, a less dangerous event such as the breakdown of a water heater or major repairs to a roof may serve as the "last straw," causing an older person to conclude that remaining in her house has become too difficult.

In addition to emotional inertia as a source of resistance, home ownership may be integral to a person's identity. A house and yard often function as an extension of the self. Those who have tended gardens for years may continue to derive considerable satisfaction from this form of self-expression. For others, the house itself may be something to show for years of hard work and mortgage payments. Frequently, a house provides older people with their only remaining ways of spending time meaningfully: "If I move to an apartment, I'll have nothing to work on." When a garden or a workshop is unavailable in the proposed residence, an older person's fear of idleness may outweigh the advantages of moving.

One of the most common reasons for reluctance arises from relationships with pets. Although many people maintain deep attachments to pets throughout life, pets can assume the heightened importance of sole companions for isolated older people. Ever available, affectionate, and noncritical, pets afford older people who live alone the opportunities to talk out loud and express emotion. Some actively chitchat with their pets and satisfy their need to nurture by spoiling their pets. For such older people, parting with a pet in order to move into a retirement home may constitute an insurmountable obstacle. A few facilities do permit pets, but they may be more expensive than the older person can afford or not located in the person's community. An occasionally successful strategy is for family members to find someone to care for the pet and to allow periodic contact so that the separation is not total. Unfortunately, some older people will not agree to move until a beloved pet dies, which then serves as a powerful precipitant of action.

As another reason for putting off a move, some older people refuse to accept an apartment more than a few floors above ground level. Although seemingly a stubborn pretext, people who have always lived in a house commonly react with discomfort to the idea of living "up high" away from green grass or shrubs. Those who have trouble with steps may dread depending on an elevator in the event of a fire or an elevator malfunction. Discussing this special need with the manager of a prospective facility is usually better than trying to argue away such feelings. The waiting period for a ground floor apartment may be longer than for other apartments, but a strong psychological obstacle to the move may be eliminated.

During first visits to retirement homes, the older person may dislike a certain facility because she sees someone using a cane or a group of people who appear to be "old." While the older individual herself may be in her eighties, she may be opposed to any identification with disability or aging. If a facility which has been rejected on this basis seems otherwise well suited to the older person's needs, family members can ask the management for the name of a particularly active resident who would give a personalized tour. Meeting someone who has maintained a lively spirit within the facility can often relieve these concerns about proximity to inactive people.

DISPOSING OF POSSESSIONS

The thought of sorting through years of accumulated possessions can be a major obstacle to an older person's moving. For some, packing up and giving away household items is symbolic of dying. The disposal process feels synonymous with throwing away the future as well as the past, as if the disappearance of the accumulation is equivalent to the person's disappearance. Parting from possessions that have been tied through memories to previous roles, such as wife and mother, is especially painful. By disposing of the tangible signs of such roles, the older person may react as if she is losing confirmation of her sense of worth.

In many instances, an older person who asks a family member to "help" with the sorting needs a listener more than an assistant. The older person may be unable to allow items to vanish into a box before explaining how they were acquired, their purposes over the years, or the memories attached to them. Such stories serve to make sense of life, permitting an older person to complete experiences through the telling of them. Transmitting these memories to family members is a means of passing on the past instead of seeming to lose it. By viewing the sorting process in this light, family members can transform what is otherwise a chore into a meaningful life event.

Because storytelling is central to the sorting process, however, it can slow progress to a pace that exasperates those who are giving assistance. No matter how much interest and respect a family member may feel for the process, time constraints are a reality which can produce legitimate impatience. A family member who flies out to use a two-week vacation to help a parent with the disposal of possessions may need to hurry the stories in order to make the most of limited time. To be both practical and respectful, family members can ask the older person to anticipate the importance of the longer stories and to make tapes prior to the actual packing time. A friend or neighbor can listen as the older person records the stories in advance of the family's assistance. Such recordings have the additional value of preserving stories for family members who are unable to help sort the household.

Further problems can arise when the older person agrees to a garage sale, but insists on prices that are too high. Aware of the items' original value, the older person may feel infuriated by the idea of selling them for a fraction of the cost. To deal with this, families sometimes accept the items as gifts, while privately planning to dispose of them. Instead of resorting to deception, family members can avoid future hurt by storing some items until after the older person is settled in her new residence. Once the emotions of moving have subsided and an acceptable future is assured in the new setting, the stored possessions may seem less important and the older person may be less upset by disposing of them at a low cost.

Still more complex dilemmas are generated when an older person attempts to make gifts of personally significant items. How such gifts are handled by family members may indicate to the older person how they will later treat their memory of her. A woman who gives a cherished heirloom to her son and then discovers it under a crate in his basement may feel that by dishonoring her memento, her son dishonored her. It may be helpful for family members to realize the loaded nature of such gifts and to ask the older person to explain their significance prior to accepting them. Citing limited space and a desire to give her mementos a place of honor, family members can then ask the older person to choose only the most precious items for this purpose. Another option is to rotate the display of certain items.

Overwhelmed by a mountain of small decisions, some older people are unable to find a beginning point in sorting through their possessions. The following decision-making categories can help set the process in motion:

Categories for Sorting

1. If I had just one box to fill, what would I take with me?
2. If I had room for ten boxes, what would I enjoy having with me in my new home?
3. What things do I want to keep, but I don't mind storing?
4. What am I ready to part with, but would prefer to keep in the family, if possible?
5. What am I prepared to give away, sell, or throw out?

The older person should be encouraged to make such categorized lists in advance of the need to start packing. Imagining the items to go in the first box can be a particularly helpful technique in freeing the person for the rest of the decisions. Having named the "necessary" items, the person may feel the confidence that, "If I had to, I could live without everything else."

Widowed people needing to break up a household previously shared with a spouse may experience a profound inertia when faced with the task. Items as mundane as a magazine rack may hold significance for the couple's past life together. Disposal of such items may seem disrespectful to the deceased person. Sorting through the spouse's clothing and personal papers can evoke unfinished grief, particularly if such items have not been touched since the death. Many bereaved older people leave the spouse's clothing hanging in the closet indefinitely and dread being pressured to part with it during the moving process. Family members can suggest that certain items of clothing be set aside for inclusion during the move, as this may relieve considerable anxiety.

For family members, the most difficult situations are when the older person refuses to participate in the choice process. Unable to feel enthusiasm for the new life ahead, some older people express feelings of despair through statements such as, "Do what you want with my things. It doesn't matter, anyway." Older people entering a structured living situation directly from a hospital may insist that they are glad to be spared the necessity of sorting through and grieving their life's accumulations. Family members should view this attitude as transitional, expecting it to change as the older person develops friendships and interests in the new setting. By renting a storage area for six months, family members spare themselves the responsibility for making these choices, and allow the older person to make decisions about personal belongings when his or her spirit for life resumes.

ADJUSTING TO NEW SETTINGS

During times of upheaval in life, an individual's particular style of dealing with change tends to come to the fore. Some people have dire reactions, magnifying their distress and seeing what lies ahead in all-or-nothing terms: "Moving to a retirement home is like dying. My life as I've known it is over." Others constrict into rigidity, becoming focused on the small details of life over which they still have control. The most fortunate are those who have always taken life as a series of transitions and have enough inner flexibility to ready themselves for the next challenges. In helping someone adjust to a new setting, it helps to keep in mind how the person has previously coped with change and to recognize personal styles of grieving. This section explores common reactions to moves of this nature.

Grief for What Has Been Lost

People who leave a lifelong home for senior apartments or retirement homes tend to adjust more slowly than those parting with a more recently acquired home. Arriving in the new setting, they may feel as if their connection to the past has been severed. The possessions which they took with them may provide little solace. As with any major loss, separation from a home of many years often requires a mourning period before the person becomes open to developing new attachments.

For those who have simultaneously left a known geographic area, the adjustment can be complicated by their missing friends and neighbors who are now out of reach. Visits from family members take on a heightened importance in the absence of these networks. The older person may have expected more time with her family: "I did this to be near my daughter and her family, but I only see them once a week." Yet expressing this disappointment may seem unreasonable in view of their relatives' busy lives.

Hoping for a smooth adjustment, family members are often puzzled when a relative holds back from making friends in the new environment. Resistance toward becoming part of the community can last for several months, depending on how intensely the person refuses to identify with "all those old people." The person may maintain a separation by rejecting neighbors' friendly overtures or by watching for experiences that confirm her derogatory perceptions of fellow residents. (See "Disliking Old People," pp. 259–261.)

Couples are especially prone to remaining aloof, since they constitute their own social sphere and may feel little impetus to reach beyond this comfortable domain. In many respects, they bring their previous world along with them to the new setting in the person of their partner. For some couples, tensions arise when one partner feels eager to reach out to strangers and the other prefers to huddle in the safety of the known.

A willingness to establish roots in the new environment usually evolves with time. Once they have accepted the change, people often become receptive to making new friendships. Some find that the sheer repetition of daily contact with tablemates in the dining room and neighbors in their hallway breaks through their resistance. Faces become familiar, and random chatter in the elevators and in front of the mailboxes gradually leads to more personal conversations.

Compared to home ownership, residence in a managed community requires considerable passivity. Waiting for a custodian to handle maintenance problems is as much a loss of control as it is a relief from responsibility. To someone accustomed to modifying his living space at will, a large psychological shift is required in receiving services from others. In a similar way, new residents usually miss their former control over when they had their meals and what they ate, even though the burden of meal preparation may have been a reason for the move. Being served in a central dining room entails such passivity that some older people insist upon occasionally preparing their own meals, if their apartment is adequately equipped. As with all the other changes, most people find that they grow accustomed to the loss of control over time, focusing avidly on the forms of control which remain.

Coping with the Loss of Privacy and the Rise of Gossip

Another major shift in these settings is the degree of access people have to each other's daily lives. Unaccustomed to strangers scrutinizing their affairs, those who previously lived in private homes are often unnerved by people in the lobby observing them as they come and go. Being cornered in the elevator by a nonstop talker or a particularly intrusive neighbor may rattle them more than those who have experienced apartment life previously. For some, needing to be aware of the volume of music and voices, as well as being subjected to the sound levels of adjacent apartments, are new irritations. In settings where meals are served in a central dining room, facing the same people three times a day can seem a drastic loss of privacy compared to former patterns of occasional meals with friends.

Within all communities, gossip flourishes when people have little else to occupy their attention. Who was seen leaving a neighbor's apartment at midnight and who leaves a urine odor behind after she occupies a couch are topics which can seem engrossing in the absence of larger concerns. Unless people stay involved in outside interests, petty aspects of their environment assume an unwarranted prominence. Friends within such a community can try pledging to one another not to indulge in these "easy" topics, but rather to push themselves to talk about political events or anecdotes from their experiences in the outside world, past or present. Acknowledging the effort involved in reaching for topics beyond their immediate circumstances, such friends can prod each other when they slip from broader conversations into gossiping.

To assert an adventurous spirit despite such scrutiny requires a secure sense of individuality and personal confidence. Without this, many residents of retirement homes and senior apartments have a difficult time achieving indifference to what others may say about them. Some residents may so intensely dread walking past observers in the lobby that they leave early in the morning for outings or omit them entirely. If the building has a back door, they will sacrifice convenience to avoid intrusive queries such as, "Where are you headed at this hour?" or "Gee, you're all dressed up." Since saying or doing things out of the ordinary attracts attention, many find safety in adopting bland conformity as their response to others' over-concern with their affairs.

The power of gossip to disrupt residents' sense of personal freedom in these settings needs wider professional recognition and intervention. When the majority of residents are homebound, insularity should be countered with planned infusions of information and experience from the outside world. Guest speakers, slide shows, and other regularly occurring programs can serve to relieve internal pressures by providing an external focus. Shared cabs and car pools for residents to go out to concerts and films can compensate for insufficient recreational staff or for lack of van services in certain settings.

When older people are grouped together, death looms as a presence more than in communities with a mix of younger and older people. Frequently, ambulances remind residents of their fragility and confront them with death and illness. These reminders can contribute to residents' feelings of captivity, as when a woman forgoes her weekly walk to the grocery store in reaction to a neighbor's breaking her hip while on a similar outing. In this regard, the constant talk about other people's ailments can be seen as a form of personal vigilance rather than idle curiosity.

On the other hand, many people who move into assisted living facilities and retirement homes begin enjoying them immediately. The services relieve them from worrying about the practical details of daily life. They welcome the social contacts and feel protected by others' scrutiny, knowing that neighbors will check on them if they fail to come to the dining room or the mailboxes. The ability to watch out for and help others provides a pleasing sense of community. Eating in the company of others increases their enthusiasm for meals and thus improves their general nutrition. Family members enjoy a similar freedom from worry, usually finding that the quality of their time with their relative improves in proportion to the extent to which they are themselves freed from responsibility. Family members can focus on the kinds of conversations and activities previously deferred when they were trying to maintain their relative in a private home.

Leaving a home of many years is a difficult decision under any circumstances, but it is especially taxing in later life when so many other sorrows may be accruing. Often, the risks involved in staying put seem worthwhile to the older person, even when family members continually assail the person with their worries. The chief benefits of alternative living situations are greater safety and less loneliness, benefits which family members may find themselves trying to "sell" to their relative in vain. By understanding what the options are and learning how each is viewed by older people, family members and professionals become more adept at responding to this resistance and instigating a genuine discussion of alternatives.

SUGGESTED RESOURCES

Books

Carlin, Vivian, and Ruth Mansberg. *Where Can Mom Live? A Family Guide to Living Arrangements* (New York: Lexington Books), 1987.

Reviews a wide array of housing options, including shared homes, accessory apartments, life-care communities, elder cottages, and home equity conversion. Presents guidelines to assist the elderly with making decisions.

Carlin, Vivian, and Ruth Mansberg. *If I Live to Be 100: A Creative Housing Solution for Older People* (Princeton, NJ: Princeton Book Publishers), 1989.

Provides an in-depth picture of a middle-income congregate residence that contains many advantages for the elderly. Includes information about other communal living options, suggestions for choosing congregate care, and a list of such facilities across the country.

McCamant, Kathryn, and Charles Durrett. *Cohousing: A Contemporary Approach to Housing Ourselves* (Berkeley, CA: Habitat Press), 1988.

Cohousing is intended to combine the autonomy of private dwellings with the advantages of intergenerational community living. This book vividly illustrates the cohousing concept through case examples, primarily from Denmark. It discusses obstacles to implementing the concept in the United States.

Porcino, Jane. *Living Longer, Living Better: Adventures in Community Housing for Those in the Second Half of Life* (New York: Continuum), 1991.

Oriented toward planning for housing options by the middle-aged and young old. Nontraditional communal living arrangements are reviewed, including specific case examples from around the country.

Raimy, Eric. *Shared Houses, Shared Lives: The New Extended Families and How They Work* (Los Angeles: J. P. Tarcher), 1979.

Streib, Gordon, Edward Folts, and Mary Anne Hilker. *Old Homes— New Families: Shared Living for the Elderly* (New York: Columbia University Press), 1984.

A comprehensive review of shared housing for the elderly, using case studies from different communities in the United States and Canada. Chapters on home-sharing, foster family care, and granny flats are especially relevant. Identifies policy implications for the future.

Organizations

American Association for Retired Persons (AARP). 601 E. Street, N.W., Fulfillment Department, Washington, DC 20049. (202) 434–2277

> AARP has many useful publications. Call or write for a complete list of publications. These are only a sample of those relevant to housing matters.
>
> "Consumer's Guide to Accessory Apartments," D12775.
>
> "Consumer's Guide to Home Sharing," D127774.
>
> "Continuing Care Retirement Communities," D12181.
>
> "Housing Options for Older Americans," D12063.
>
> "Resource Guide for Rental Housing," D12773.

American Association of Homes for the Aging (AAHA). 901 E Street, N.W., Suite 500, Washington, DC 20004. 202–783–2243.

> AAHA represents nonprofit organizations dedicated to providing health care, housing, and services to elderly people. Write or call for their pamphlet, "The Continuing Care Retirement Community: A Guidebook for Consumers."

The CoHousing Company. 48 Shattuck Square, Suite 15, Berkeley, CA 94704. (415–549–9980)

> This architectural and consulting firm maintains a national referral network for people interested in cohousing throughout the United States. They also provide financial consultation and assist with design of projects.

Gray Panthers National Task Force on Housing. 1424 16th Street, N.W., Washington, DC 20036. (202) 387–3111.

> The task force publishes a quarterly magazine, "Call for Decent Housing."

National Shared Housing Resource Center. 431 Pine Street, Burlington, VT 05401. (802) 862–2727.

> The center publishes a pamphlet, "Is Homesharing for You? A Self-Help Guide for Homeowners and Renters." They also serve as a resource center and offer technical assistance for 350 shared housing projects nationally.

15

Extending Family Caregiving into the Nursing Home

Few older people willingly choose to live in a nursing home, and most families arrive at this decision only after exhausting their home care resources. Placing a relative in a nursing home is one of the most painful decisions of people's lives. The pain stems partially from the catastrophic images harbored by older people and their families about nursing homes: "Going to a nursing home would be the end of me," or "Any family who puts their relative in a nursing home just wants to get rid of the person." These images do not have to become realities. In this chapter, an approach to nursing home placement is demonstrated that establishes a partnership between the older person and the family, beginning with the decision to seek placement and continuing through the adjustment period and ongoing life in the nursing home.

WHEN NURSING HOME PLACEMENT BECOMES NECESSARY

The nursing home decision is often made in reaction to a crisis, such as the older person's imminent discharge from the hospital. In other instances, the primary caregiver becomes ill and no one else is able to take on the care at home. Some families think about nursing home placement for months or years, waiting for an emergency to give them the momentum to enact these plans. Often, family caregivers keep

315

going until they are at the end of their rope, both physically and emotionally.

Setting Up a Trial Period at Home

Hospitalization is a common catalyst for nursing home placement. Increasingly, hospitals are discharging to home care or nursing homes people who in the past would have been kept in the hospital until they were medically more stable. Governmental incentives for shorter hospital stays have resulted in an increase in short-term nursing home stays for people recuperating from surgery or curable illnesses. Discharge planners often push family members to make their decision after physicians and other hospital staff pressure them to "get those beds open."

Family members who have long been contemplating nursing home placement may reason that their relative's home routines have already been disrupted and that going to a nursing home directly from the hospital is likely to be the easiest transition. Having access to a discharge planner who is familiar with local nursing homes may seem a welcome advantage in the timing of this decision. Problems arise when the older person does not agree.

When older people vehemently resist going to a nursing home from the hospital, a trial period back home may be the best strategy in the long run. Such periods allow people to test their capacity to live independently, especially in instances when their functioning has declined significantly during their hospital stay. Unless permitted this trial, some older people retain unrealistic beliefs about their capabilities and blame family members for prematurely relegating them to nursing home status: "You just don't want to help me anymore."

After returning home, people in dire need of nursing home placement are often able to see how much care they actually require. Those living alone may endure long nights without anyone to help them get to and from the bathroom or to administer medications. Those living with family members may observe how difficult it is for others to get them in and out of bed and how much more comfortable they were when trained aides assisted them with these transfers. When feelings of insecurity and physical discomfort mount during the trial period, those in need of twenty-four-hour care tend to become more amenable to the idea of moving to a facility where such care is available.

For families, however, these trial periods are often nerve-wracking. Their frail relatives are, in essence, choosing to take risks to find out if they can still make it at home. Families struggle over how much extra help they should offer while knowing that it may be better to hold back and allow the reality of the situation to sink in. Requesting a referral to a home health agency can be valuable during this time, since a visiting nurse or physical therapist can offer a realistic appraisal of the home care situation. Hearing the pronouncement from a professional, "This is too much to handle at home," often helps both older people and their families accept the need for a nursing home.

Recognizing the Red Flags for Nursing Home Placement

At times, the decision to pursue nursing home placement results from family problems that are not related to the older person's condition. In other instances, the care gradually becomes more difficult, until caregivers are drained or they begin to experience physical problems of their own. The following list depicts common indicators that nursing home placement may soon become necessary. Professionals should be alert to these circumstances, as families often try to cope with them long beyond the point when it is healthy to do so. Seeing their situation depicted on this list may help some families recognize that their ability to provide good care at home is nearing an end, and that the time is coming when they have to find ways to express their devotion in another setting.

Incontinence is a relentless source of weariness. Partners in long-standing relationships are most likely to sustain this burdensome level of care over extended time periods. Their physical exhaustion increases month by month from lifting and turning their partner to prevent bed sores and carrying endless loads of laundry. Hiring home health aides at high hourly wages, even on an occasional basis, is not affordable for most families. Live-ins employed for this purpose tend to resign, unless provided with ample family support and a competitive salary to keep them from securing an easier position elsewhere.

When the older person is too heavy for lifting, caregivers quickly wear themselves out. For example, strokes often result in the person's inability to assist with being lifted, making their body heavier with what is known as "dead weight." Transfer techniques and assistive devices can help, but often the caregiver's strength, size, and body weight are simply insufficient for the kind of lifting required. Older women are especially vulnerable to injuring themselves under these circumstances when they have not been trained in transfer techniques and are unable to admit that the lifting is too much for them.

RED FLAGS FOR NURSING HOME PLACEMENT

Burdensome incontinence: Strenuous effort is required to prevent skin breakdown.

Too much heavy lifting: The caregiver is unable to lift and transfer the person safely, despite having received training in special techniques and the use of assistive devices.

Caregiver is sleep-deprived: The caregiver's sleep is disturbed on a nightly basis and relief help is not available frequently enough or at all.

Caregiver becomes ill or injured: The caregiver tries to go on providing care while neglecting an illness or injury that requires medical attention or extended rest from caregiving.

Other stresses impinging on the care: The caregiver is going through a divorce, coping with another illness or a death in the family, or facing problems with finances, employment, or dependent children.

From Wendy Lustbader and Nancy R. Hooyman, *Taking Care of Aging Family Members* (New York: The Free Press, 1994). Copyright © 1994 by Wendy Lustbader and Nancy Hooyman; copyright © 1986 by The Free Press.

Situations in which the caregiver's sleep is disturbed every night also produce progressive exhaustion. Ill people who need to be assisted to the commode during the night or who call out at all hours for pain medication quickly sap their caregivers' strength. Those who reverse day and night sleep patterns may wake up family members by turning on the lights or by pacing noisily around the house. Sleep medications can occasionally resolve these problems, but frequently cause undesirable side effects such as daytime grogginess or the risk of falls. In addition, such medications do not solve the problem of the caregiver who loses sleep from having to get up to provide assistance, such as turning his bedbound relative. Paying an aide to stay overnight regularly can equal or surpass the cost of twenty-four hour care in a nursing home. Sleep deprivation often results in the caregiver becoming short-tempered, forgetful, and depressed.

Burdensome care itself can lead to the primary caregiver becoming ill or injured. Caregivers often fail to go to the doctor when they first experience symptoms. While they tell themselves that they are too busy to get help, their medical problems often worsen. Many conceal their symptoms from family members, afraid that they might be forced to go into the hospital if their illness or injury were discovered. The idea that their relative could enter a nursing home temporarily while they recuperate may never have occurred to them.

Outside stresses of major proportions are legitimate reasons for putting a relative in a nursing home, but many caregivers try to endure beyond their capacity. For example, trying to take care of her mother while ending a thirty-year marriage may tear an older woman apart emotionally. The conflict between her need to reassemble her own life and her need to give her mother good care may be devastating. Asking her mother to tolerate living in a nursing home for six months might give her time to compose herself and catch her breath, and her mother may be able to accept the move as a way to support her daughter during this difficult time.

Health care providers should watch for signs of family members' fatigue, stress, and depression. Speaking with them privately for a few minutes each time they accompany their relative to medical appointments is a good practice. When the care has become overly exhausting or stressful, professionals play a key role in helping family caregivers recognize when to let go.

HOW TO BRING UP THE TOPIC

As the decision to pursue nursing home placement evolves in their minds, family members frequently try to shield their relative from this impending possibility, reasoning, "It would only make her worry." While attempting to locate affordable help in the home, they may assure their relative that "everything's going to be okay." In the meantime, they may be secretly taking tours of nursing homes and putting their relative on waiting lists. The strain of this double life often becomes agonizing. Family members may sustain themselves with the hope that something will happen to spare them the terrible moment of telling their relative, "We've got a bed for you next week in a nursing home."

Mentioning the Unmentionable

The hope that they will not have to resort to a nursing home is only part of what prevents families from being open about their worries.

The deeper source is the guilt of admitting that they are unwilling or unable to restructure their lives sufficiently to keep their relative at home. A daughter may feel intense remorse as she imagines saying to her mother, "Mom, I just can't give up my job right now. I love you, and I hate the thought of your being in a nursing home, but I've worked so hard to get where I am." The need to retain a job rather than care for a parent can seem shameful to someone who values others' needs over personal ambition. Resolving such a dilemma may be the most profound struggle of someone's life.

Professionals can be instrumental in helping family members see that including their relative in this struggle is far better for both than being secretive. For instance, a visiting nurse or case manager can meet with an older woman and her daughter to educate them about home care options in their community. During the discussion, the professional can mention the unmentionable: "Sometimes families try out all these options and work as hard as they can to keep a parent at home, but nursing home care turns out to be the only solution." Once the term "nursing home" is out on the table, the older person and her family can begin to work together to try to avoid nursing home placement, while jointly recognizing its possibility.

Speaking the words "nursing home" may not immediately instill a spirit of partnership. The older person may instead try to exact bargains and promises: "I'll stop being so stubborn about getting a home health aide if you'll promise me you'll never put me in a nursing home." Rather than making a groundless promise, family members faced with such pleading should point to the practical realities: "Mom, we're going to do all we can to keep you at home. I promise you we won't leave a single stone unturned, but there could come a time when the resources are just too limited for your condition." The older person can then target her anger at the inadequacy and cost of home-based services, rather than feeling that family members are her adversaries. This is the beginning of a partnership.

An often unspoken backdrop to a family's exploration of community resources is the question of the older person's move into a family member's home. The older person may wonder whether she will be invited, while the family wrestles privately with their conflicting loyalties to their relative and their other personal commitments. As with all the other home-based options, family members should try to talk openly about the advantages and the drawbacks: "Asking Billy to give up his own room right now might not be the best idea for a sixteen-year-old obsessed with his privacy." The list of factors to consider before an older person moves into a family caregiver's home (p. 270) may facilitate frank discussion of why this is not a realistic option for the family.

An older person who is included all along in family members' attempts to surmount problems on her behalf is less likely later to feel she has been "dumped" into a nursing home. A father who joins his daughter in interviewing live-in applicants may realize how difficult it is to find reliable helpers, especially at the salary he is able to offer. A daughter who talks with her mother about the ways job pressures conflict with her desire to provide care will make her mother feel loved, even if she eventually chooses to continue her employment rather than assume full-time caregiving. Similarly, a son who admits that he is afraid that having his mother live with him would injure their relationship frees her to vent related concerns from her standpoint.

Differing Opinions

Despite family members' efforts, this spirit of partnership often becomes vulnerable to differences about what constitutes a "safe" or acceptable living situation. For instance, a person who falls frequently may insist, "Look, if I'm willing to lie on the floor until my neighbor gets home to help me up, that's my business." His son may respond, "Dad, I hate the thought of you lying on the floor like that. What if you were injured? In a nursing home, there'd always be someone around to help you." The degree of danger deemed acceptable depends on the motivation for tolerating it. In many instances, older people are willing to withstand threats to their safety because of their intense desire to stay home. Motivated by a different desire, that of peace of mind, their families may regard the same dangers as intolerable.

Unless conflicting views are openly acknowledged, the older person may begin to hide problems from family members. In the above example, the older person may ask the neighbor who assists him not to tell his son how often he needs help getting up off the floor: "They think it's too dangerous for me to keep living here alone, so you'd better not tell them I fell five times last week." Family members concerned about safety become a "they" with opposing goals. To avoid this tendency, families should admit when nursing home placement is largely for their benefit: "Yes, we're the ones who would be relieved, and you'd be giving up a lot for our sakes." The older person has less reason to conceal risks if his preferences are acknowledged and understood to be valid.

When professionals encounter adversarial positions in families over this issue, they can easily be drawn into choosing sides. The more productive approach is to mention that such conflicts are common and stem from opposite priorities between older people and their families. The following dialogue represents a distillation of these differences. Reading the dialogue aloud may bring relief to a divided family by illuminating the universal aspects of these issues.

FAMILY MEMBER: We love you and want you to be safe.

OLDER PERSON: Safe for what? I don't care how long I live; I just want to stay home.

FAMILY MEMBER: But we worry about you all the time. We'd never forgive ourselves if you got hurt here.

OLDER PERSON: So, I'm supposed to give up my home and go into a nursing home to make you feel better?

FAMILY MEMBER: Yes, if there were people with you at all hours of the day, we would feel better. That's all there is to it.

OLDER PERSON: I hate the thought of people with me all hours of the day.

The primary dread that older people have about nursing homes is that family members will abandon them. A son who says "Dad, it's going to be a hard adjustment, but we'll stick with you all the way" is more believable than one who says, "Dad, you'll see. It's not such a bad deal." Fake reassurances only make people feel more frightened. It is better to acknowledge that living in a nursing home does entail fundamental change in the boundaries of personal privacy and control over basic aspects of life in exchange for certain advantages.

Grasping the Advantages

In order to address anxieties about nursing homes, it is helpful to explore the images that someone holds from past experiences. The reality that some older people thrive in nursing homes may be entirely foreign to those unfamiliar with decent nursing homes. The idea that "not all nursing homes are alike" is difficult to convey if someone has had firsthand experience with a deplorable, understaffed nursing home. The following list, depicting positive aspects of life in decent nursing homes, can be reviewed by family members together with their relative.

POTENTIAL BENEFITS OF NURSING HOME LIFE

Better Family Relationships: Without the strain of physical care, families are released to enjoy their relative's company again. Relationships may improve.

Increased Social Contact: Roommate relationships are sometimes close and supportive. Sitting with the same people at meals can produce a small community. Nurse's aides often become close to those for whom they provide personal care.

Accessible Activities and Services: Musical programs, craft activities, discussion groups, and outings in the home's van may be regularly offered. Religious services and clergy may be available on the premises. Barber and beautician services may be offered on site.

Rehabilitation Services: Daily physical therapy, with access to special equipment, may be available. Specially trained aides may teach personal care skills, assist with daily exercises, and encourage the person's progress.

Improved Health, Security, and Comfort: Better management of nutrition, skin care, and medications may result in a better quality of life. The person's memory and alertness, as well as overall comfort, may improve. Having people around to talk to, and rely on, even in the middle of the night may be a great security.

From Wendy Lustbader and Nancy R. Hooyman, *Taking Care of Aging Family Members* (New York: The Free Press, 1994). Copyright © 1994 by Wendy Lustbader and Nancy Hooyman; copyright © 1986 by The Free Press.

A key benefit for the older person may be better relationships with family members. Removing the stress and tedium of physical care tasks, a nursing home opens up the possibility for family members and the older person to enjoy spending time together again. A daughter previously preoccupied by her mother's complex care may be able to enjoy her mother's memories and seek out her advice about family matters. The focused attention that was not possible under all the pressure at home may become the most valuable asset of their time together in the nursing home. Rather than being oriented to getting things done, visits in this context convey the feeling, "I come because I like being with you."

Having many people around in close proximity is not rewarding to everyone, but some find that their social life revives when they move into a nursing home. Sitting with the same people every day at meals, they develop enjoyable camaraderie. The most fortunate find a kindred spirit in their roommate and evolve a close friendship. If there is little staff turnover at their facility, some become close to the aides who take care of them. Many people find that they are much less lonely than they were at home where mobility problems limited their access to others.

The activities and services available on the premises of a nursing home may reawaken a person's interest in life. Someone who lost the will to work on knitting projects at home may find fresh motivation while showing others how to do particular patterns in the nursing home's craft room. Attending religious services as often as desired may be deeply comforting, and not having to ask for a ride to do so may be a great relief. Access to rehabilitation equipment on the premises, in conjunction with a physical therapist, may speed someone's recovery. Going on outings in the facility's wheelchair-accessible van may expand a disabled person's activities in the outside world, actually giving them more freedom than they had at home.

HOW TO CHOOSE A NURSING HOME

If nursing home placement occurs directly from a hospital, the older person and the family may have little control over the choice of a facility. The hospital bed may be needed for someone with more acute medical needs, or their relative may be exceeding the limits of insurance coverage. The discharge planner may insist that the first available nursing home bed be taken, whether or not the opening occurs in a place convenient to a family member's home or where an older person's friend already resides. Taking the person home to wait for a bed in the most desirable facility may not be possible, due to the severity of the person's care needs or the length of the probable waiting period. Moving the older person later to a preferred nursing home may be a possibility in some cases.

Funding is one of the central factors affecting choice of a facility. Older people and their families often first encounter the limitations of

Medicaid, the major source of public funding for nursing home care, when choosing a facility. Some homes are not certified for Medicaid-funded residents, but accept private-pay residents and then transfer them to Medicaid facilities when their funds are exhausted. This can mean that someone becomes accustomed to living in a nursing home and then is faced with a wrenching move to a new place. Understanding Medicaid funding is necessary before other factors can be considered in choosing a nursing home.

QUESTIONS AND ANSWERS ABOUT MEDICAID FUNDING FOR NURSING HOMES

1. Why is it often easier to obtain a nursing home bed for someone with private funds than for someone with Medicaid?

Each state determines the rate paid by Medicaid to its nursing homes. In most states, this amount is substantially less than the charges for private-pay residents. Because of this gap between what Medicaid pays and private rates for care, nursing homes try to maintain a balance of private and public-pay residents. Giving preference to private-pay applicants on their waiting list is a common practice in nursing homes, even in states where this practice has been prohibited by law.

2. What should we do if we have only enough to pay private rates for a limited time?

Selecting a nursing home that participates in the Medicaid program is important if the older person is likely to require Medicaid assistance in the future. Otherwise, when funds run out, transfer to another facility can be traumatic. Once admitted as a private-pay resident to a Medicaid-licensed facility, the older person cannot be legally transferred to another facility when private funds are depleted.

3. Does a Medicaid beneficiary have to contribute to the cost of care?

The Medicaid beneficiary must pay any income received to the nursing home. The home gives the resident a personal allowance from this amount, with the balance going toward the payment of nursing home costs. Medicaid pays the difference between that amount and the rate set by the state for that person's level of care.

4. Does the older person's home have to be sold as soon as she becomes a nursing home resident? Can an apartment be maintained using part of the person's income under Medicaid guidelines?

In some states, the Medicaid program permits a grace period during which a portion of the person's monthly income may be used to maintain a previous dwelling. The grace period's intent is to allow for the possibility of a resident's reentry into the community, if her physical condition improves or the placement is unsatisfactory. The state financial worker handling the application for Medicaid assistance should be consulted.

5. How can financial hardship be prevented for the spouse remaining at home?

A couple can sometimes split their assets in order for a nursing home resident to become eligible for Medicaid assistance without impoverishing the spouse. Since the rules vary from state to state, the couple should consult a lawyer or the local legal services office.

6. Are all of the resident's nursing home expenses covered in the Medicaid payment? What is normally included in a home's daily rate and what types of charges are extra?

The Medicaid payment schedule allows for a daily rate, which generally includes room and board, custodial care, skilled care such as medical consultation and nursing services, and most rehabilitation therapies offered by the nursing home. Dental services, some medications, beautician and barber services, and incidentals, such as facial tissues and hand cream, are not typically covered in the daily rate. Families of both Medicaid and private-pay residents should request a list of items included in the daily rate from the particular nursing home. The contract should also specify conditions for notification of rate changes, refunds, and holding a bed in the event of hospitalization.

7. How is an older person's level of care determined, and how does this affect the fees charged?

Medical staff determine the level of care on the basis of the older person's physical and mental status. For example, if two people are needed to transfer someone from bed to wheelchair, this person would be regarded as heavy care. Each state has its own gradations when Medicaid is the funding source. Family members handling private funds should ask homes to explain how they set fees for private-pay residents, as these tend to differ from one facility to another.

8. Can a nursing home refuse to admit anyone?

Some homes deny admission to certain types of patients because of staffing or facility limitations. Medical or behavioral problems, such as serious drug or alcohol abuse, and wandering or belligerence, can prevent admission.

9. What is the difference between nonprofit and proprietary homes? Is the quality of care the same?

Nonprofit homes, often sponsored by religious organizations, channel excess earnings back into the home to improve services to residents or for maintenance of the facility. In contrast, proprietary homes pay out excess earnings as profits to the owners, or to stockholders if the home is part of a corporation. With few exceptions, the differences between nonprofit and proprietary homes can be seen in the ratio of staff to residents, with nonprofit homes having more aides available to provide hands-on care. Nonprofit homes also tend to employ professionals beyond the minimum Medicaid requirements, such as a full-time social worker or physical therapist. Claims by proprietary homes that they provide comparable quality of care should be examined carefully, especially when a home is part of a chain of nursing homes owned by a corporation repeatedly cited for deficiencies. Asking a nursing home admissions person, "Who owns this home?" is the most direct way to determine whether a facility is nonprofit or proprietary.

10. What is the best way to compare nursing homes in a particular community?

Discharge planners in hospitals, social workers in home care agencies, and medical personnel in clinics that serve older people tend to have firsthand knowledge that can save families time. The county's Area Agency on Aging, senior information and referral hot line, and local Medicaid office can be contacted for lists of area nursing homes. The state's nursing home ombudsman program, an office which handles complaints about nursing homes, can indicate whether a particular home has been often cited for deficiencies. Other methods for comparing nursing homes are presented in the next section.

Comparing Nursing Homes

Residents in nursing homes who are visited regularly get the best care. This fact of nursing home life makes location the prime factor in the selection, after financial considerations. For instance, a nursing home located between a daughter's home and her place of employment should be chosen over a less conveniently-located home, even if the other facility has more attractive furniture and bigger rooms. Similarly, whether or not a nursing home is near a bus stop is a key consideration for someone whose spouse no longer drives or whose friends depend on bus transportation. Over time, visitors become the focus of nursing home residents' lives, with the more superficial considerations fading from prominence.

When more than one nursing home is convenient to family members' homes, the next most important selection factor is the people in the home who deliver hands-on care. Nurse's aides spend more time with residents than do other staff, helping with bathing, dressing, grooming, and using the toilet. The personal nature of their contact can produce intimate bonds or humiliation, depending upon how they perform these care tasks. Some of the nursing homes that appear on the surface to be the best channel their funds into expensive mortgages rather than into maintaining a favorable ratio of aides to residents. Overworked aides with too many people to serve cannot take the time to be nurturing or considerate, while aides with reasonable workloads tend to do the little "extras" for people in their care. For these reasons, a run-down home with outmoded furnishings can sometimes be superior to newer and fancier facilities, if the home's management has set a priority on good working conditions for staff.

Visiting a nursing home during the evening or on weekends often provides more information about staffing levels than observing the home during official weekday tours. Nursing homes can all seem the same from 7:00 A.M. to 3:30 P.M., Monday through Friday. Fewer staff are on duty on evenings and weekends, making these revealing times to observe staff attitudes and skills. Watching the way aides serve food to residents who cannot handle utensils and how they talk to residents as they escort them back to their rooms can help families distinguish one facility from another. Overworked and burned-out staff tend to talk to each other rather than to the residents they are serving, ignoring residents' needs for human contact. In contrast, staff graced with decent working conditions tend to joke with the residents, touch them, and keep a balance between their socializing with each other and paying attention to the people who need their responsiveness.

For people requiring rehabilitation services, the availability of registered physical and occupational therapists and appropriate equipment can be as crucial as general staffing levels. Some homes have extensive physical therapy equipment and can offer state-of-the-art therapy for recovery from strokes, instruction in the use of prosthetic devices, and other services deemed vital by the older person and his family. Asking admissions personnel how often a registered physical therapist serves the facility may be helpful, because many nursing homes use trained therapists as occasional consultants and have aides perform the bulk of hands-on physical therapy. This strategy saves money for nursing homes, but detracts from the quality of the rehabilitation program.

The home's attitude toward food can also be an indicator of how residents are treated. Families may want to inquire about menu variations, residents' access to snacks, coffee, and tea for themselves and their guests, and whether guests are welcome in the dining room. Some homes have refrigerators and storage bins for storing special treats brought in by family members, allowing residents to request their treats whenever they want to enjoy them. Some homes have small dining rooms on every floor, while others have large, centralized dining rooms.

Many other factors affect residents' quality of life in nursing homes. For an older person with strong religious or cultural ties, a nursing home with staff and residents from the same denomination or ethnic group can make a significant difference in the older person's level of comfort within the facility. For someone with an intense need for privacy, some homes have single rooms available on a waiting list basis for private-pay residents, while others have only two- and three-person rooms. Whether the outside environment has places to walk and sit, how well-equipped the activity rooms seem to be, and whether the home has a social worker to serve as an advocate for residents are factors important to some.

Finding a nursing home convenient for their relative's personal physician is a choice factor rated highly by some families. Most doctors have certain homes in which they follow patients after placement, because they prefer to visit several patients at a time to make these visits cost-effective. In such instances, family members may have to choose between their own convenience and the physician's preference. A doctor's long-standing knowledge of the older person's medical problems and personality style is especially useful during the adjustment period, when so much else is unfamiliar. Trust in their own doctor's concern and competence can be a great comfort to older people with complex medical problems. Since some homes require or strongly encourage the use of their in-house physician and some require outside doctors, family members should ask about the home's policy during the selection process.

THE ADJUSTMENT PERIOD

The first several weeks—sometimes months—of residence in a nursing home are the most difficult. Loss of control over personal hygiene, privacy, possessions, and medications are only a few of the changes to which residents must adapt. Eating mass-produced foods at set times, having a loudspeaker intrude on naps and conversations, and accepting help from people of different racial or ethnic groups may also challenge someone's capacity to accept the new environment. Grief for the home lost and personal routines vanished may be profound. Bearing their relative's sorrow and waiting for it to subside can sap the spirit of even the most resolute family members, unless they know what to expect and how to respond.

Handling Pleas to Go Home

During their first few days in a nursing home, older people often engage in desperate bargaining with their families: "If you take me out of here, I promise I won't call you so often." Even those who have entered the home fully agreeing that this is the most practical option may collapse into irrational pleading when faced with the reality of their choice. To be begged for release in this way is extremely painful for families. Guilt from the sacrifices they have chosen not to make may hurt so intensely that they are tempted to reverse their decision. They may find themselves making promises they cannot fulfill: "Mom, I'll take you home in a few months, when the doctor says it's OK."

By making groundless promises in response to pleading, family members put themselves in a deceptive role that can be more painful than gradually working through the truth of the situation. A better approach is to support the person's hope that her physical condition will improve and to focus her attention on her rehabilitation efforts: "When you're able to transfer in and out of your wheelchair independently, we'll talk about getting you back home." Even if attainment of a specific rehabilitative goal is improbable, maintaining this kind of hope is a way to ease the adjustment process. Most importantly, it places the person's focus on striving toward physical improvements rather than on trying to influence the family's supposed control over the situation.

Some people are greatly helped if family members agree to delay the sale of their home or the breakup of their apartment. Knowing their home still awaits them serves as a psychological refuge until they establish friendships in the nursing home and adjust to the institutional routines. This delay also postpones the added grief that will occur when their belongings at home have to be stored, distributed to family members, or sold. For families, maintaining the home often means extra yard work and extra bills to pay, but these sacrifices tend to be well worth easing their relative's adjustment to the nursing home. As a symbol of her continued connection to the outside world, a dwelling and the belongings contained within it can make the difference between an older person giving up or staying motivated enough to find a niche in the new environment.

When the hope of leaving the nursing home "in a few months" is vital to the person, family members should feel free to support this hope with positive statements: "Mom, after three or four months, we'll see how much progress you've made with your physical therapy." Using the phrase "when you go home" instead of "if you go home" is encouraging rather than deceptive, as long as it is accompanied by references to the physical improvements necessary before a return home is possible. It may also be helpful to delay implementing signs of permanence, such as changing the address on magazines, until the person has reached a greater degree of acceptance.

Handling Roommate Conflicts

During a hospital stay, most people cope with their roommate's annoying habits by defining them as a temporary plight to be endured. On a short-term basis, violations of privacy can often be tolerated, along with inconsiderate behavior about noise levels, unduly prolonged bathroom usage, and other irritations. When someone enters a nursing home, however, the prospect of putting up with such aggravations indefinitely may evoke rage and very little tolerance. For this reason, complaints about roommates tend to dominate new residents' conversations with their families.

Some older people, having coped with roommates in other contexts, possess good negotiation skills. In contrast, those who have spent a large part of their lives residing alone or in situations where they did not have to make compromises may lack these abilities. Instead of negotiating, they may retreat into silent resentment or assail roommates with unreasonable demands. Family members can try to model respectful negotiation by settling the more trivial issues on their relative's behalf: "We were wondering if you'd be willing to turn off the TV by 8:00 at night if she'd be willing to keep it off until at least 8:00 in the morning." In their zeal as advocates for their relative, however, they should be careful not to "gang up" on a roommate and exact unfair concessions. When conflict between roommates is not resolved after their first few weeks together, family members should request the assistance of the home's social worker or another staff person capable of serving as a mediator.

Sensitivity to the fact that open beds are usually created by the death of a previous roommate is also helpful. Typically, only a few days are allowed to elapse between a resident's death and the introduction of someone to fill the opening: "The bed's not even cold and they've stuck a new person in with me." Anger toward the person taking a beloved friend's place may be at the root of a roommate's initial coldness. Frustration at yet another uncontrollable change and reluctance to bond with someone else who might die are feelings which may underlie withdrawn or gruff behavior. Families may want to ask staff about the nature of the roommate's previous relationships and the circumstances ending them in order to gain insight into the current dynamic.

When negotiation and understanding fail, family members often ask nursing home staff to arrange a room change. They then encounter the reality that until an opening occurs somewhere in the facility, staff cannot move one person without displacing another. Finding someone else willing to change rooms is not easy. In addition, if the roommate in question has an unappealing personality, staff know that they would only make someone else unhappy if they arrange a room change. Staff sometimes manage these dilemmas by placing a resident who does not have the persistent advocacy of family members with less desirable roommates.

Personalizing and Protecting the Room

To help their relative cope with the shrinkage of personal space and feelings of intrusion from roommates, family members should try to personalize the area around the person's bed as soon as possible. Family photographs posted on a cork board, posters and paintings on the wall or closet door, favorite books and magazines on the night table, and a plant to take care of may help the older person to assert her identity. In the pressure of the first few weeks, families may put off extensive decoration unless professionals emphasize its importance.

Fear of theft may interfere with this process of settling in. Even in the best nursing homes, residents' rooms are vulnerable to theft because they cannot be locked. As a result, residents usually exclude from their rooms the objects which hold the most meaning for them. For instance, a retired music professor with a precious collection of concert tapes may confine her listening to one hour per week when her daughter brings in her tape player and some of her tapes. To protect these items from theft, she limits her access to them and thus the frequency of her enjoyment. Another example is a daughter who is unsure whether to allow her confused mother to wear her wedding ring in the nursing home. Her choice is between risking the theft of this valuable family heirloom and depriving her mother of a link with the past which she can touch and look at each day. This protectiveness is a tragic necessity, given the restricted range of experiences and pleasures accessible to people living in nursing homes.

Loss of control over the safety of belongings is one of the most frustrating aspects of nursing home life to residents and their families. If the home permits personal furniture, obtaining a night table with a locked drawer or cabinet can make a difference. Even a small locked space is psychologically significant. Older people lacking enough manual dexterity to handle a key may nevertheless prefer to keep their cabinet locked and to wear the key around their neck as a symbol of control. Some may prefer to have precious items kept at a family member's home or in the nursing home's safety deposit box, despite the resulting loss of contact with these items.

Coping with Loss of Control Over Medications

People who have gone for years managing their own medicines tend to feel outraged and demeaned by nurses taking over this function. Pain medications, sleeping pills, and tranquilizers are examples of medications which most people like to control on their own. Putting on a call light and waiting until someone responds is only the first step in obtaining an extra pain pill during the night. The resident must next wait until the aide finds the nurse in charge of evening medications, and then the nurse must complete the tasks already occupying her attention. When appropriate physician's orders are not listed in the resident's record, the nurse cannot dispense the pill until she reaches the doctor by phone. In the meantime, someone accustomed to reaching into a night table and taking an extra pill to relieve pain must lie there unable to control her suffering.

Loss of control over medications can be just as infuriating for family members, especially when they were previously able to dispense relief at will. A common scene at nursing stations is an angry family member trying to get the staff to hurry up and get their relative needed medications. Staff coping with multiple demands on their time may respond defensively: "Look, I've got thirty other people here to worry about besides your mother." Family members are often overwhelmed to the point of tears by the helplessness entailed in asking staff busy with other priorities to attend to a beloved person's needs. They feel humiliated by having to plead with staff to get them moving on their relative's request, a necessity which also drives home the fact that their relative's care is no longer in their hands. To a large extent, the family's losses mirror those of their relative as they confront the same institutional rigidity.

Adapting to Changes in Hygiene and Clothing

One of the most difficult adaptations for new residents is finding out that they can only bathe once a week. The relief of getting into a hot tub or shower is constrained by the reality of limited bathing facilities and staff to assist with this time-consuming task. Even in the best nursing homes, residents are unable to bathe more often. Assistance with sponge baths is usually available daily, but most homes assign a weekly bath day to each resident to manage this limited resource in a fair and orderly manner. Such scheduling tends to appall lifelong daily bathers when they first enter a nursing home.

Another unwelcome change is garments sent to the centralized laundry which never return, or other people's clothing appearing regularly in place of what had been sent. For instance, a woman whose blouses had not yet come back from the laundry may be offered someone's else's blouse to wear for the day. Some people would not be bothered by these occurrences, while others would feel personally violated. In addition, family members may feel upset when they find their relative dressed in someone else's clothes. Each loss, however trivial, compounds upon the others, with explosions of tears and rage not uncommon among new residents of nursing homes and their families. Often, families cope by taking some of their relative's laundry home with them as a gesture of protective control.

Learning How to Visit

For the first several weeks, the major problem family members face in visiting is their relative's unhappiness. Professionals need to remind families that nursing home placement instigates a grieving process which lessens over time and is not indicative of how their relative will react later on. Listening with empathy to their relative's complaints about the roommate, the food, the nurse's aides, the laundry, the medicines, and the infrequency of bathing is a vital part of helping the person adjust. Trying to act as if these are not personal assaults only adds loneliness to the grief over so much lost control.

Arranging for some form of daily contact from the outside world may hasten the person's adjustment. Phone calls, notes in the mail, flowers, and visits from friends can substitute on the days when family members cannot visit. Such frequency of contact affirms the continuity of relationships when the person most needs this reassurance. Gradually, this contact can be tapered as the person becomes convinced that she will not be abandoned by family and begins to build ties with people in the facility.

A valuable use of time during the family's visits to the nursing home is getting acquainted with staff and helping them get to know the older person. By providing anecdotes to staff about the person's life history and personal habits, family members enhance staff's understanding and interest in the person. Acknowledging extra thoughtfulness is also important: "Thanks so much. My father is really looking good these days." When staff are aware that family members will notice whether someone's hair is neatly combed or their socks match, that person is likely to receive extra attention.

CARE OVER THE LONG RUN

The long run, or the months and years following the adjustment period, offers a different set of challenges for residents and their families. In some ways the situation gets easier, and in other ways it gets harder. The older person gradually abandons the hope of leaving the facility, and family members confront the consequences of this acceptance. Defining what it means to extend their care into the nursing home changes. Their relative's circumstances shift, and the effects of time present new questions.

Becoming Adjusted

As their relative's complaints about being in the nursing home begin to subside, family members may notice that their relative has also stopped asserting herself on certain matters or has ceased altogether to express her preferences. The price of adaptation tends to be some degree of personal surrender. Giving in to the way of life in a nursing home protects residents from frustration. Instead of straining against institutional routines, residents usually shed the aspects of their individuality that do not fit into the environment. The paradox for family members is further grief as they watch their relative become an adjusted nursing home resident.

Alternatively, the people who refuse to adjust become the "difficult" residents. They hang on tenaciously to their idiosyncratic style and their own way of doing things. Their self-assertions are troublesome and inconvenient for staff: "Mrs. Jones, you've got to realize you're not the only person here." It is no accident that those who refuse to accede to the facility's routines retain a spark in their eyes, compared to the dullness in the eyes of those who become fully institutionalized. Family members of a resident who does not capitulate may find that their role becomes that of listening to staff's complaints about their relative and thanking them for their tolerance.

Over the long run, the rebels become a tiny minority. Facing repeated defeats of their preferences, day after day, most nursing home residents gradually shut down their sensitivity. When family members arrive for an hour's visit once or twice a week, they want their relative to rise out of this protective numbness in response to their presence. They especially want their relative to show some signs of gladness upon their arrival in the doorway of the room. Instead, they may be hurt when their relative immediately makes requests without saying "hello" or does not look up from the television. From the older person's standpoint, staying in her shell may be easier than to become stimulated for an hour, only to feel a sense of absence more deeply for having taken in the pleasure of the visit. Nursing home residents often comment, "I want them to visit, but I feel more lonely after they leave."

Another hurt occurs for family members when their relative asks to be taken to the dining room, even though they have just arrived for a visit and it is an hour before mealtime: "Why on earth do you want to go down there when all you'll do is just sit there?" Family members may be astonished to find many residents lined up outside the dining room far in advance of serving time. Unlike visitors, who arrive unpredictably and not nearly so often, meals can be counted on for gratification three times a day, every day. Mealtimes are anchors for getting through the day. The habit of gathering near the dining area to wait for the meal gradually becomes part of the event itself. Asking their relative, "Mom, can't you just get to lunch a little late today?" generally evokes distress. In some instances, an older person may vehemently resist such disruption of her anchoring routine.

Helping Residents Maintain Aliveness

As they become steeped in their new environment, nursing home residents often stop seeing beyond themselves. They may lose interest in others' lives to the point that they change the topic back to themselves when family members try to tell stories about their own situations. One strategy is for families to take relatives home with them for an overnight or all-day visit once a month. Time away from the institutional milieu often jolts people back into awareness of the outside world. It helps them renew their acquaintance with the stresses confronted by their families. For instance, as a mother sits at the kitchen table and hears her daughter tend to a series of phone calls, she gains an immediate view of life circumstances that are unrelated to her needs as a nursing home resident. This view may renew her interest in her daughter's life.

To compensate for the blandness of institutional food, family members can establish a weekly routine of bringing in a home-cooked meal. By allowing their relative to suggest what they bring, family members restore a partial sense of control. Bringing in food is also a powerful way for family members to satisfy their need to nurture their relative, especially when they watch her enjoy special treats. Nursing home residents, confined to eating what is placed before them, often become envious of the family's ability to eat whatever they want. Taking a nursing home resident to a restaurant, even to a drive-in where she need not leave the car, provides a chance to make choices and to consume foods not normally served in nursing homes.

Another helpful practice is for family members to visit once a week on a particular day rather than intermittently or unpredictably. This routine allows their relative to anticipate that day: "Tomorrow is Saturday, the day my daughter comes." Such regularity gives the person a reason to keep track of the days as well as a feeling of security once the schedule is set. The understanding can be established that unless family members phone to cancel, they will appear sometime on that day, eliminating the need to call in advance or to aim toward an exact time.

It can be laborious to make conversation week after week with a relative who has little to say due to the uneventful nature of her life. Reporting on their personal news and asking for advice about their problems is one way family members can stimulate conversation and give the older person a sense of participation in their lives. Generally, nursing home residents benefit from being informed about family conflicts rather than being artificially shielded from life outside the nursing home: "When my daughter tells me about fights with her husband—even though it gets me upset—I feel like I'm still her mother, I'm still somebody."

Even if unable to attend, many people enjoy helping to plan family events, such as a wedding or a trip. Family members may be tempted to hold back from talking about these events, fearful that they will only make their relative feel badly about not being able to go. For nursing home residents, vicarious pleasures are a way of life and should not be limited. The family can enhance their relative's inclusion in these happenings by sending postcards, taking pictures, or bringing in some of the decorations and food to the nursing home.

Forming rituals for visits is also helpful, such as drinking a glass of sherry together after reading a few pages of poetry or jointly working on an oral history. Rituals are especially valuable when families have little to say, providing a structured sequence of things to do during each visit. Assisting with letter-writing, watching a favorite television show, going for a walk outside, and looking through mail-order catalogs for gifts are other ways to make visits more satisfying. Another is to read magazine articles aloud and discuss reactions to the issues presented, thereby spurring their relative's interest in current political and social events. The naturalness of young children can also serve to fill awkward silences during visits. When they are permitted in the facility, pets can be especially evocative of memories and the urge to nurture.

In a further effort to counter the shrinkage of their relative's world, family members can try to encourage activities that involve reaching out to others. A wheelchair-bound resident may be able to read to a visually impaired roommate or to assist another with writing letters or recording audiotapes. A longtime community activist may find her niche on the facility's resident council or in assisting with the nursing home newsletter. Family members can join with their relative in visiting other residents, assisting with special holiday activities, leading sing-alongs, stuffing envelopes for the home's fund-raising effort, or making handicrafts for the home's bazaar. Transporting a resident to vote, to a club, or to church tends to be well worth the family's effort in terms of maintaining the person's sense of connection with a wider community.

Over time, family members may learn to be more comfortable with quiet activities or silences during visits. Simply being present and gently touching their relative can convey their caring. Massaging her back with lotions or manicuring her nails can be a powerful way to express tenderness. When words seem to fail, physical contact can be a meaningful substitution.

People who work in nursing homes witness the phenomenon of adaptation over and over again. The new resident enters, complains vociferously for weeks or months, and gradually incorporates aspects of the institution into herself. As they watch their relative change, family members experience sorrow, but also relief from the lessening of complaints and depictions of unhappiness. It takes time to learn not to be hurt by a relative's unresponsiveness and to accept the loss of personality traits discarded for the sake of adaptation. A year after admission, families often marvel at the pain of the first few months contrasted with the reconciliation of later months.

Much can be done to give a person in a nursing home a feeling of connection to the outside world and a sense of belonging to an involved family. When family members establish a predictable routine for visiting, they allow their relative to count on them and to look forward to the visits. When they maintain regular contact with the nurses and the aides, exchanging information and offering appreciation, they ensure that the staff continue to take a personal interest in their relative. In these ways, placing a loved one in a nursing home can become a relocation of the family's care, rather than its cessation.

SUGGESTED RESOURCES

Articles

Everen, Lisa. "Long-Term Care Ombudsmen: A National Survey of their Views," *Generations*, 11, 4 (1987),43–48.

This article reflects concerns about the inadequacy of community resources by older people who do not want to reside in a nursing home.

Morycz, Richard. "Caregiving Strain and the Desire to Institutionalize Family Members with Alzheimer's Disease," Research on Aging, 7 (1985), 329–361.

Strain was found to increase the desire of caregivers to place their relative in a nursing home, except among male and African-American caregivers. Intensity of strain or stress was related to the availability of social support to the caregiver.

Books

Richards, Marty, Nancy Hooyman, Mary Hansen, Wendy Brandts, Kathy Smith-DiJulio, and Lynn Dahm. *Choosing a Nursing Home* (Seattle, WA: University of Washington Press), 1985.

A concise, easy-to-read guide for families, available directly from the publisher: (800) 441–4115. Discusses selection factors, the transition to nursing home life, and ways for families to work effectively with nursing home staff.

Diamond, Timothy. *Making Gray Gold: Narratives of Nursing Home Care* (Chicago: University of Chicago Press), 1993.

Based upon participant observation, the author paints a moving portrayal of daily life in a nursing home. He concludes with practical recommendations for change, including unions for nursing assistants and resident input into care.

Salamon, Michael J., and Gloria Rosenthal. *Home or Nursing Home: Making the Right Choice* (New York: Springer), 1990.

Discusses the benefits of nursing home life, the process of making the decision, choosing a facility, and easing the transition. Life satisfaction was found to be higher among a sample of nursing home residents compared to those receiving home care.

Sarton, May. *As We Are Now* (Ontario, CA: Penguin Books, 1973.

A beautifully written account of experiencing a nursing home through the eyes of a resident.

Tisdale, Sally. *Harvest Moon: Portrait of a Nursing Home* (New York: Henry Holt), 1987.

A moving, sensitive, and insightful view of life in a nursing home. The author intertwines descriptions of daily life for nursing home residents and staff with discussion of policy and practice issues, including the right to die.

Organizations

American Association of Homes for the Aging (AAHA). 901 E Street, N.W., Suite 500, Washington, DC 20004. 202–783–2243.

Members of this private nonprofit group work with each other and the government in trying to identify and solve problems in nursing homes.

Long-Term Care Ombudsman. (There is no national program. Each state has its own program.)

As mandated by the Older Americans Act, each state has an ombudsman who is charged with protection of the rights and welfare of nursing home residents. Nursing home residents, their relatives and friends, professionals in the community, or nursing home staff may report concerns about deficient care for investigation by the ombudsman. The ombudsman's office can be found through a state's department of aging or social and health services.

National Citizens' Coalition for Nursing Home Reform. 1224 M Street, N.W., Suite 301, Washington, DC 20005. (202) 393–2018.

The coalition is comprised of groups and individuals committed to improving the quality of life and care for nursing home residents. They serve as a voice enabling consumers to be heard. They publish a journal, *Collation*, for advocates working on nursing home issues.

National Council of Senior Citizens. 1331 F Street, N.W., Washington, DC 20004. (202) 347–8800.

The Council's Education and Research Center operates the Nursing Home Information Service, a referral center for consumers of long-term care services. They offer information on how to select a nursing home as well as alternative community and health services.

Index

List of Charts in Sequential Order